Transcatheter Aortic Valve Replacement Program Development

A Guide for the Heart Team

Transcatheter Aortic Valve Replacement Program Development

A Guide for the Heart Team

Clinical Editors

Marian C. Hawkey, RN
Columbia University Medical Center
New York, NY

Sandra B. Lauck, PhD, RN
Centre for Heart Valve Innovation
Vancouver, BC

Elizabeth M. Perpetua, DNP, ACNP-BC, AACC
Empath Health Services
Seattle, WA

Amy E. Simone, PA-C, AACC
Clinical Director, Marcus Heart Valve Center
Atlanta, GA

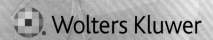
. Wolters Kluwer

Philadelphia • Baltimore • New York • London
Buenos Aires • Hong Kong • Sydney • Tokyo

Acquisitions Editor: Nicole Dernoski
Development Editor: Maria M. McAvey
Editorial Coordinator: Kerry McShane
Production Coordinator: Sadie Buckallew
Design Coordinator: Joan Wendt
Manufacturing Coordinator: Kathleen Brown
Marketing Manager: Linda Wetmore
Prepress Vendor: TNQ Technologies

9 8 7 6 5 4 3

Printed in China

Library of Congress Cataloging-in-Publication Data

Names: Hawkey, Marian C., editor. | Lauck, Sandra B., editor. | Perpetua, Elizabeth M., editor. | Simone, Amy E., editor.
Title: Transcatheter aortic valve replacement program development : a guide for the heart team / clinical editors, Marian C. Hawkey, Sandra B. Lauck, Elizabeth M. Perpetua, Amy E. Simone.
Description: Philadelphia : Wolters Kluwer, [2020] | Includes bibliographical references and index.
Identifiers: LCCN 2018057129 | ISBN 9781975105228 (pbk.)
Subjects: | MESH: Transcatheter Aortic Valve Replacement | Aortic Valve Stenosis–surgery | Patient Care Team–organization & administration | Patient Care Planning–organization & administration
Classification: LCC RD598 | NLM WG 265 | DDC 617.4/12–dc23
LC record available at https://lccn.loc.gov/2018057129

shop.lww.com

CCS0920

Dedicated to our patients, who are the reason for this journey.

Contributors

Leslie Achtem, RN, BSN
St. Paul's Hospital
Vancouver, BC

Russell A. Brandwein, MS, PA-C
New York Presbyterian Hospital/Columbia
University Medical Center
New York, NY

Marjo J.A.G. De Ronde-Tillmans, RN
Erasmus Medical Center
Department of Cardiology
The Netherlands

Kimberly A. Guibone, ACNP
Beth Israel Deaconess Medical Center
Cardiology - Structural Heart Program
Boston, MA

Marian C. Hawkey, RN
Columbia University Medical Center
New York, NY

Patricia A. Keegan, DNP, NP-C, AACC
Emory Healthcare
Atlanta, GA

Amanda Kirby, DNP, APNP, ACNP-BC
Aurora Healthcare
Milwaukee, WI

Bettina Hoejberg Kirk, RN, MSN
Rigshospitalet
The Heart Center
Copenhagen

Sandra B. Lauck, PhD, RN
Centre for Heart Valve Innovation
Vancouver, BC

Joan Michaels, MSN, CPHQ, AAC
American College of Cardiology
Washington, DC

Tone M. Norekvål, PhD, RN
University of Bergen
Department of Clinical Science
Bergen, Norway

Roseanne Palmer, MSN, RN
Dartmouth Hitchcock Medical Center
Structural Heart Program
Lebanon, NH

Elizabeth M. Perpetua, DNP, ACNP-BC, AACC
Empath Health Services
Seattle, WA

Jopie Polderman, BSN, RN
St. Paul's Hospital
Center for Heart Valve Innovation
Vancouver, Canada

Amy E. Simone, PA-C, AACC
Clinical Director, Marcus Heart Valve Center
Atlanta, GA

Martina Kelly Speight, MSN, FNP-BC
Stanford Health Care
Stanford, California

Janet Fredal Wyman, DNP, RN-CS, ACNS-BC
Henry Ford Health System
Detroit, MI

Preface

The modern history of heart valve surgery dates back more than 60 years with the development of simple, primitive, but often effective repair procedures and early versions of implantable valves. From these ground-breaking beginnings, surgical valve therapy has evolved into a family of sophisticated and reproducible therapies for many patients with valvular heart disease.

The modern history of transcatheter valve therapy dates back less than 20 years with the feasibility cases of early pulmonary and aortic valve implantation and mitral valve repair procedures. Similar transcatheter ground-breaking beginnings led to an accelerated second revolution in valve therapy culminating in the current era of safe and efficacious transcatheter aortic valve implantation/replacement (TAVI/TAVR) procedures.

Owing to favorable clinical outcomes, surgical aortic valve replacement has been the accepted gold standard for treating patients with severe symptomatic aortic stenosis (AS). Consequently, TAVR has been held to a higher standard of evidence development, requiring randomized clinical trials that progressed according to patient risk strata (from highest to lowest surgical risk patients). Ironically, the more rigorous evidence requirements for TAVR have resulted in an avalanche of clinical data that have hastened the acceptance of this new less-invasive approach to aortic valve replacement. TAVR is now viewed as the preferred therapy for patients who are not suitable for surgery or have high-risk surgical profiles and an equivalent alternative to surgery in intermediate-risk patients. Moreover, dramatic technology enhancements over a short timeframe have (1) reduced the device profiles permitting transfemoral access in most patients, (2) markedly decreased the incidence of para-valvular regurgitation, and (3) improved the precision of device deployment resulting in predictable, safe, and more user-friendly procedures.

Increasingly, TAVR is becoming the dominant intervention for AS, and several developed countries, including Germany and the United States, now perform more transcatheter than surgical aortic valve replacements. In the past, the conversation had been about who are poor candidates for surgery who might benefit from TAVR. Now, after innumerable rigorous randomized trials, the conversation has become reversed to who are good candidates for TAVR, such that surgery can be avoided under most circumstances. Clearly, there is still more work to be done, as TAVR has not been validated as an acceptable alternative to surgery in low-risk patients and patients with bicuspid aortic valve disease. Nevertheless, TAVR has captured the imagination of practitioners worldwide and has provided a platform for extending transcatheter therapies to patients with other valvular lesions.

An unexpected important by-product of TAVR has been the emergence of the heart valve team as a central force to direct clinical care pathways. The "Heart Team" includes multidisciplinary health care professionals, such as surgeons, interventionalists, imaging experts, cardiologists, anesthesiologists, other physician subspecialists (as indicated), and many nonphysician caregivers who help to evaluate the patients and coordinate the clinical care before, during, and after TAVR procedures. The collective expertise of this aligned group of valve experts surpasses the skills of any individual and helps to provide an environment for respectful optimized clinical decision making.

The astounding growth and dispersion of TAVR has provided an interesting opportunity to refine the efficiencies of patient care by employing this Heart Team approach. The reference text entitled **TAVR Program Development: A Guide for the Heart Team** is a first-of-its-kind guide that helps to articulate the systems of care required to create a modern, efficient, comprehensive TAVR center. Importantly, this book is presented through the lens of nonphysicians, with distinguished international experts from across North America and Europe. This book takes its audience through every stage and step of the TAVR experience, from initial referring physician contacts, to valve clinic visits, to diagnostic workup requirements, to the procedure itself, and finally to the postprocedure management requirements. The expressed goal is to help create strong TAVR programs, increasingly led by nursing professionals who provide seamless care from referral to follow-up. Undoubtedly, a broad audience of physicians, nonphysician valve experts, hospital administrators, and others will greatly benefit from the insights, sensitivity, tips and tricks, spirit, and meaningful content provided by this fresh approach to clinical care of patients undergoing TAVR. As the TAVR revolution continues to inform our notions of modern cardiovascular care, we desperately need "Go-To" references like this, intended for a diverse audience, to lead the path to improved and enlightened care for our patients.

JOHN G. WEBB, MD
MARTIN B. LEON, MD

Acknowledgments

We gratefully acknowledge:

Our contributors for their collaboration, expertise, and commitment.

The dedication and expertise of this international community of leaders who continue to improve the way we care for patients.

Our families for their love and support.

Introduction

Transcatheter Aortic Valve Program Development: The Road So Far

The first ground-breaking transcatheter aortic valve replacement (TAVR) was performed in 2002 by Dr Alain Cribier and his colleagues in Rouen, France. The earliest feasibility study of the first device commenced in the United States in 2006 led by Dr Martin Leon and the Columbia University Hospital team (New York, USA) utilizing the retrograde access approach that was pioneered by Dr John Webb at St. Paul's Hospital (Vancouver, Canada). The patients enrolled in these early clinical trials were almost exclusively elderly and at high, if not extreme, risk for surgical aortic valve replacement. Research nurses, coordinators, and other clinical leaders involved with these pioneering studies initiated the early work of crafting evaluation and procedural pathways that were both protocol-compliant and focused on the needs of the patient population and emerging technology. This leadership was instrumental in recognizing the challenging programmatic moving parts and the critical importance of program development to support changes in the management of heart valve disease. The value of TAVR program development strengthened as clinical trials and other studies led to international regulatory approval of the risk-stratified use of TAVR with various devices and within various subsets of patients.

The complementary skillsets offered by the Heart Team have been fundamental to program development, with the cardiac surgeon and interventional cardiologist as foundational members. The central importance of the valve program clinician gained early visibility and recognition and was soon credited as an integral component of successful programs. As TAVR technology further developed and was made available to increasing numbers of patients, the Heart Team model expanded to include a heterogeneous group of imaging experts, anesthesiologists, geriatric specialists, and clinicians involved along the continuum of patients' journey of care. In the past decade, the role of the valve program clinician has become a standard of care. This group of clinicians have strongly advocated for the need for evidence-based program development and for training and education matched to their responsibilities.

Valve program clinicians are most frequently registered nurses, advanced practice nurses, or physician assistants. This unique role has emerged across multiple regions and developed over the years; it is now embedded in recommendations for best practices and international guidelines. Key responsibilities include program coordination, facilitation of patient-focused processes of care, and fostering of communication pathways, in addition to program-wide clinical leadership from referral to follow-up. An early appreciation of the need for a specialized education and professional development pathway highlighted opportunities to develop a training curriculum that complements the required competencies of this unique role.

The Moving Parts of Successful Programs

The implications of the paradigm shift that TAVR has instigated in the management of heart valve disease reach far beyond the development of successful devices and procedural approaches. Few cardiac or other innovations have been associated with the intensity of changes in the expertise and configurations of teams, processes and delivery of care, and monitoring to adapt to the rapidly evolving clinical and operational needs. These needs have emerged and changed over time and created opportunities for innovative programs to tailor their operations and practices to meet the unique needs of the procedure and patients. In the absence of programmatic planning and careful scrutiny to meet these imperatives, programs can experience significant challenges and barriers that may jeopardize the quality of care and the delivery of services. In contrast, careful attendance to these moving parts can help TAVR programs optimize patient access and outcomes and lay a solid foundation to successfully integrate transcatheter heart valve therapies as one of the pillars of cardiac care. The purpose of this resource is to help address 4 priorities of TAVR program development and strengthen the role and contributions of valve program clinicians.

New Expertise to Lead the Heart Team

The silos of care within cardiac programs, including the distances that have historically separated the cardiology and cardiac surgery services, have been bridged by TAVR program development. The clinical needs and the regulatory requirements have combined to create opportunities for the development of new expertise and to redesign care delivery models across patients' journey from referral to follow-up. The skillset and leadership of valve program clinicians have been instrumental in the significant progress made to date. Across programs, there has been an increasing awareness that limiting the operationalization of the Heart Team to the collaboration of cardiologists and cardiac surgeons is insufficient to promote successful TAVR program development. The contributions of valve program clinicians extend from the essential activities of program coordination to the provision of periprocedure and postprocedure care to ensure that programmatic success is when the patient returns home to enjoy a longer and better life. TAVR programs are increasingly recognizing that achieving this goal consistently requires expert knowledge and unique competencies, as well as championing the role and contributions of valve program clinicians.

Yet, there continues to be a lag in evidence, recommendations, and sharing of resources to help guide this bridging and integration of best practices in TAVR programs. To date, there has not been a resource to support the unique expertise of valve program clinicians, discuss how their role is a pivotal point of connection within the TAVR Heart Team, and strengthen their leadership, knowledge, and impact on patients and health services.

Processes of Care

The slow and sometimes unpredictable disease progression of AS, the clinical complexity of the primarily elderly patient population, and the intense multimodality TAVR assessment require unique processes of care. To date, little has been documented about the components of the multidisciplinary evaluation pathway; valve program clinicians have led initiatives across programs to establish processes and protocols to standardize care. To this end, much attention has focused on operationalizing a comprehensive Heart Team approach and developing innovative approaches to organize the referral, assessment, treatment decision, procedure planning, and postprocedure care.

The essential expertise required spans a strong grasp of foundational knowledge related to the presentation, progression, and treatment of AS; a comprehensive understanding of the core and adjunctive assessments; a working knowledge of diagnostic imaging; and the capacity to organize patient-centered and multidisciplinary care.

Delivery of Patient Care

In TAVR programs, the delivery of care occurs along the continuum from assessment to follow-up. Valve program clinicians gained an early appreciation for the importance of measuring frailty and functional status to inform case selection, risk-stratified procedure planning, postprocedure care, and follow-up. The heterogeneity of the age-related physiological reserves of people with advanced valve disease raises unique challenges to capture patients' health vulnerabilities and plan accordingly. Highlighting the intersections between best cardiac and geriatric practices has been a hallmark of the contributions of valve program clinicians.

Although indications continue to evolve, careful case selection remains essential to TAVR program success. Determining who is the right patient for TAVR demands the consideration of multimodality diagnostics, multidisciplinary expertise, consensus agreement, and patient and family engagement. Thus, strategies for patient-centered care inclusive of patient and family education and shared decision making are particularly important to achieve excellent program outcomes and patient satisfaction. Similarly, procedure planning and postprocedure care must be tailored to patient and procedural needs to reflect patient profiles, devices, and approaches while mitigating the risks of adverse events and deconditioning. Providing the right care in the right place, for both the procedure and the recovery period, requires the expertise of valve program clinicians who can lead the development of specialized competencies, protocols, and clinical pathways to establish best practices.

Monitoring and Adapting Requirements

TAVR programs are resource intensive and continue to have rapidly changing needs. The high cost of devices, the unique multidisciplinary and multimodality requirements, and the complexity of patients call for careful scrutiny of program evaluation, including clinician and patient-reported outcomes, health service utilization, and benchmarking performance across jurisdictions. Valve program clinicians play an important role in monitoring access and quality of care and in the stewardship of health resources. From data collection to the interpretation of quality reports and the championing of continuous quality improvement, valve program clinicians act as the catalyst for this essential surveillance.

The transformation of TAVR is under way. Following the first decade of intense development in technology and procedural approaches, there is growing interest in improving outcomes by optimizing anatomical and functional screening, streamlining the procedure to match patient needs, promoting rapid mobilization and reconditioning, and reducing length of stay. Remaining at the forefront of program development, valve program clinicians continue to exhibit early leadership to promote best practices in this rapidly evolving clinical context.

A Resource for Valve Program Clinicians

The primary objective in delivering this resource is to formalize the sharing of our collective experience with the intention of supporting the clinical practice of valve program clinicians. The content aims to fill the existing gap in knowledge and provide a practice-ready source of comprehensive information. The project builds on the early collaboration of the contributors who have provided individual and collective leadership to inform clinical practice and accelerate research and knowledge dissemination to improve the care of patients undergoing TAVR. The impetus arose from course curriculum developed to meet the following objectives:

- Create a network of nonphysician clinicians involved in the development of successful TAVR programs
- Share resources, experiences, and learning to promote evidence-based practice and implementation of successful patient-centered programs
- Focus on the processes of care, including the challenges and opportunities, to support TAVR program development and sustained success
- Offer a forum for questions and interactive discussion

The selection of topics discussed in this resource aimed to formalize the content explored in these early professional development courses. The project was also motivated by a call to arms to recognize the unique expertise and contributions of valve program clinicians as integral leaders of the TAVR Heart Team. We sought the collaboration of international nursing and allied health professionals whose clinical, educational, and research contributions have been instrumental in moving the role, expertise, and scientific impact of valve program clinicians forward. We are acutely aware of the challenges of advancing recommendations for best practice for TAVR program development given the limited evidence available at this time. We are equally cognizant of the heterogeneity of health service delivery models, local contexts of care, and variation in access to treatment and quality of care. This resource is the first attempt to propose consensus recommendations and evidence-informed strategies to support best practices across regions and programs. We hope that this resource will be perceived as validating the leadership of valve program clinicians and will provide the Heart Team with valuable information to improve the way we care for patients undergoing TAVR.

MARIAN HAWKEY, RN
SANDRA B. LAUCK, PhD, RN

Contents

CHAPTER 1

Foundational Knowledge: Transcatheter Aortic Valve Replacement

Marjo J.A.G. De Ronde-Tillmans, RN | *Martina Kelly Speight, MSN, FNP-BC*

OBJECTIVES

▶ Describe patients' experience of aortic stenosis
▶ Outline basic understanding of TAVR
▶ Highlight how TAVR fits in the continuum of care

Aortic Stenosis

Historical Perspective

The evolution of transcatheter aortic valve replacement (TAVR) follows a long history of pursuit of management of heart valve disease and innovation. The first pathological descriptions of aortic valve stenosis date back as early as the 17th century. In 1663, a French physician, Lazare Rivière (1589-1655), described a man with symptoms of an "occluded artery" that included palpitations, diminished pulses, and an irregular heartbeat. At necropsy, Rivière described the man's left ventricle (LV) as enlarged and having "round masses occluding the mouth of the aorta." What Rivière described was likely more representative of vegetations associated with infective endocarditis; nonetheless, it was one of the first descriptions of an aortic valve lesion.[1] Théophile Bonet (1620-1689) described osseous fusions of the aortic valve leaflets at necropsy[2] and Jean-Nicolas Corvisart (1755-1821) described a diseased aortic valve as "ossified and united so closely that the end of the little finger could scarcely be introduced."[1] Corvisart is also credited for his detailed descriptions of the physical findings and clinical presentations associated with aortic stenosis (AS). Nineteenth-century physicians could identify the murmur of AS with the use of early stethoscopes, but hemodynamic assessment of AS was limited owing to the belief that retrograde catheterization of these patients was contraindicated. In 1951, the Gorlin formula was adapted to measure aortic valve area, and in 1981, noninvasive Doppler was developed to measure valve gradients and areas.[3]

Theodore Tuffier is credited with carrying out the first cardiac valve surgery by manually dilating the stenotic aortic valve of a 26-year-old patient in 1912 with immediate operative success and recovery but, of course, very little long-term success.[4] In 1953, Charles Hufnagel implanted a self-designed floating ball-valve prosthesis into the descending aorta of a patient with severe aortic valve insufficiency.[5] Cardiopulmonary bypass was developed in 1953, and Harken et al. reported the first successful aortic valve replacement with a mechanical prosthesis in the subcoronary position in 1960.[6] Donald Ross completed the first aortic valve replacement with a homograft in 1962 and, in 1967, also pioneered the Ross procedure in which the pulmonary valve is transferred into the aortic position (pulmonary autograft).[7]

Anatomy

The aortic root is located between the left ventricular outflow tract and the ascending aorta and comprises the aortic valve annulus (ring), cusps, sinuses of Valsalva, coronary ostia, and sinotubular junction (Figure 1.1). The normal aortic valve contains 3 cusps, or leaflets, of similar size and shape. The cusps extend from the sinuses of Valsalva and are named relative to their association with the coronary ostia. The left coronary cusp, right coronary cusp, and noncoronary cusp each have semilunar hinge points attached to the aortic root that open to form an equilateral triangle during systole and coaptation surfaces that close and seal completely during diastole.[8]

Etiology

There are 3 known causes of valvular AS: rheumatic disease, calcific disease, and congenital valve disease. The frequency of these causes varies across continents, with rheumatic valve disease being the most prevalent worldwide.[9] Rheumatic AS, due to rheumatic fever, remains a major burden in lesser developed countries.[10] Rheumatic AS is typically associated with

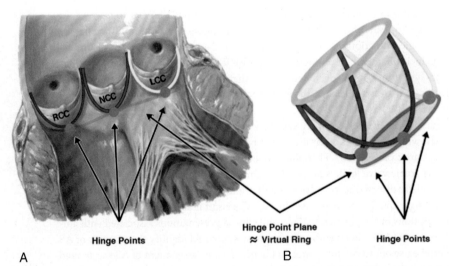

FIGURE 1.1. Components of the aortic root anatomy and representation of the cusps relative to the coronary artery anatomy. LCC, left coronary cusp; NCC, noncoronary cusp; RCC, right coronary cusp.

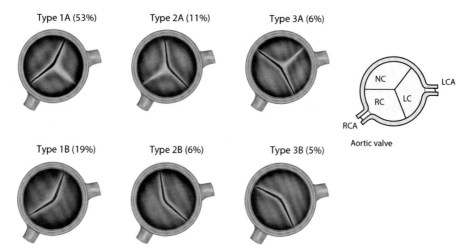

FIGURE 1.2. Distribution of bicuspid aortic valve phenotypes according to Sievers' balloon aortic valvuloplasty nomenclature system. RCA, right coronary artery; LCA, left coronary artery; RC, right coronary cusp; LC, left coronary cusp; NC, non-coronary cusp. (Reproduced from Koenraadt WMC, Bartelings MM, Bökenkamp R, et al. Coronary anatomy in children with bicuspid aortic valves and associated congenital heart disease. *Heart.* 2018;104:385-393, copyright 2018 with permission from BMJ Publishing Group Ltd.)

concurrent mitral valve disease and is characterized by fusion of the commissures between the leaflets, leaving just a small orifice in the center of the valve.[9] This pathology may lead to both AS and aortic regurgitation.

In North America and Europe, calcific disease of a native trileaflet valve or a congenitally bicuspid valve remains the most common cause of valvular AS. The mechanism of calcification is due to an inflammatory process caused by mechanical stress, lipid deposition, and some characteristics similar, but not entirely, to arterial atherosclerosis.[11] These changes are known to occur earlier in bicuspid valves than in tricuspid valves[8] presumably attributed to increased mechanical stress and earlier initiation of the inflammatory process in the asymmetrical bicuspid valve (Figure 1.2).

Prevalence

The prevalence of AS is known to increase with age and is expected to continue to grow in the forthcoming years owing to the aging population.[10] According to Eveborn et al.'s population-based study in Norway that spanned over 14 years, AS was prevalent in 0.2% of people in the 50 to 59-year-old cohort, 1.3% in the 60 to 69-year-old cohort, 3.9% on the 70 to 79-year-old cohort, and 9.8% in the 80 to 89-year-old cohort.[12] The progression of the disease was noted to be accelerated in its more advanced stages of the disease, and mortality was not significantly greater in the asymptomatic group when compared with the "normal" non-AS population.[12]

Bicuspid aortic valve is the most commonly occurring congenital cardiac anomaly affecting 0.5% to 1.4% of the population, with a male predominance.[13] Significant stenosis of a bicuspid aortic valve most commonly occurs in the fifth or sixth decade of life.[8]

Progression of Disease

Progression of AS produces a reduction in the aortic valve area and an increased pressure gradient across the valve. As the aortic leaflets thicken and calcify, antegrade velocity remains normal with minimal change to the valve gradient until the orifice area reaches less than half of normal; normal valve area is about 3 to 4 cm^2 in adults.[9] As AS becomes increasingly hemodynamically significant, there is pressure overload in the LV. This increased wall stress leads to LV hypertrophy (LVH)[14] with increased wall thickness. At this stage, a normal chamber size is maintained. The increased LV wall mass allows the ventricle to generate increased pressure to compensate for the overload, and contractile function is maintained. However, over time, this increased mass of muscle cells and the development of interstitial fibrosis lead to stiffness and diastolic dysfunction that may or may not improve with treatment of the stenosis.[15]

Clinical Presentation

The natural history of AS is known to have a prolonged latent period, and symptoms rarely develop until the stenosis is severe in the setting of normal LV systolic function. Often, patients will develop symptoms of their AS before the onset of left ventricular dysfunction.[16] The onset of symptoms is an important demarcation point in the prognosis of AS, as survival is historically known to be just 2 to 5 years, depending on symptoms, if left untreated.[16] More recent studies confirm this dim prognosis and revealed survival to be 1 to 3 years after the onset of symptoms.[17,18] If there is a reduction in myocardial function and decreased ability of the LV, its failure will result in reduced stroke volume and cardiac output and eventually lead to symptoms of heart failure. AS can be suspected with the finding of a systolic murmur on examination and then confirmed by echocardiogram. Patients with a known and timely diagnosis of AS who are followed routinely and prospectively with serial echocardiogram are likely to present with a decrease in exercise or activity tolerance, fatigue, and/or dyspnea on exertion.[15] In the later stages of the disease, especially when undiagnosed, patients may present with dizziness, syncope, angina, and/or heart failure.[8] LV diastolic dysfunction gives rise to increased end-diastolic pressures and leads to pulmonary congestion. Exertional symptoms are caused by a decreased ability to increase cardiac output with exercise. Both systolic and diastolic dysfunction can occur with AS.

Approximately two-thirds of patients with severe AS will experience angina, and approximately 50% of those will have significant coronary artery disease.[19] Angina in AS is commonly exertional and relieved by rest. Angina that occurs in AS in the absence of significant coronary disease is a result of increased oxygen demand of the hypertrophied myocardium and decreased oxygen delivery to the coronaries due to compression and diastolic dysfunction.[15]

The pathogenesis of syncope in AS can be attributed to various hypotheses.[20] Syncope in AS is usually precipitated by exertion and may be due to the inability to increase cardiac output for cerebral perfusion with exertion, coupled with a decrease in peripheral vascular resistance.[8] Syncope may also be attributed to poor baroreceptor function in the setting of severe AS as well as a vasodepressor response due to increased intraventricular pressure during exercise.[15] Furthermore, syncope may be precipitated by supraventricular or ventricular arrhythmias. Atrial fibrillation associated with AS is typically a late finding as are pulmonary hypertension and systemic venous hypertension.[15] The risk of sudden death related to AS is approximately 1% in the absence of symptoms but as high as 8% to 34% after the onset of symptoms.[21]

Assessment and Diagnosis
Physical Examination

A physical examination will often give an indication to the presence of AS.

The most useful physical examination findings for diagnosing AS include a slow rate of increase in the carotid pulse, a mid to late peaking intensity of the systolic murmur, and a reduced intensity of the second heart sound.[22] Physical examination findings can help correlate the severity of disease; however, echocardiography remains necessary to assess severity reliably.[23] It is important that the physical examination also include an assessment of the signs and symptoms of heart failure.

Echocardiogram

Transthoracic echocardiogram is an important diagnostic modality for assessing the presence and severity of AS. Two-dimensional echocardiography reveals images of calcified aortic valve leaflets and their mobility, valve structure, and anatomy. The extent of LVH can be measured by calculating LV mass; LV ejection fraction can also be measured. Doppler studies are used to accurately quantify the transvalvular pressure gradient and aortic valve area by using standardized equations[24] (Table 1.1). Aortic valve sclerosis is defined as thickening and calcification of the aortic valve leaflets without a significant gradient across the valve (typically defined as an aortic jet velocity ≤ 2 m/s). A diagnosis of AS is made when antegrade velocity across the diseased leaflets is equal to or exceeds 2 m/s. AS is defined as severe once the transvalvular velocity is >4 m/s in the setting of a valve area <1 cm^2. In patients with impaired left ventricular function and low cardiac output, a dobutamine infusion, to increase contractility, may be required to assess the full severity of disease.[15]

Diagnostic Testing

Other useful diagnostic modalities to support the diagnosis of AS include electrocardiography that may demonstrate LVH and chest radiography to assess signs of heart failure, including cardiomegaly, a prominent ascending aorta, and/or pulmonary venous congestion. Cardiac catheterization and angiography can provide important hemodynamic information and are also recommended when noninvasive testing is inconclusive or if there are discrepancies in clinical findings. Measurements of plasma concentrations of B-type natriuretic peptide (BNP) and N-terminal pro-BNP in patients with severe AS may be useful. In patients with severe AS, concentrations are typically higher in symptomatic patients than in asymptomatic patients

TABLE 1.1. Echocardiographic Classification of Aortic Stenosis Severity

	Aortic Jet Velocity (m/s)	Mean Gradient (mm Hg)	Valve Area (cm^2)
Normal	≤ 2.0	<5	3.0-4.0
Mild	<3.0	<25	>1.5
Moderate	3.0-4.0	25-40	1.0-1.5
Severe	>4.0	>40	<1.0

and also typically reduce after aortic valve replacement.[25] Higher baseline concentrations of BNP values are predictive of reduced symptom-free survival[26] and overall survival,[27] so care is required to appropriately interpret the clinical significance of these values.

It is important to differentiate other causes of systolic ejection murmur and left ventricular outflow tract from AS. Other considerations include subvalvular AS and supravalvular AS.[28]

Transcatheter Aortic Valve Replacement: A Game-Changing Treatment of Aortic Stenosis

The First Years

In recent decades, TAVR has become a viable alternative treatment of severe AS in select patients and is now a mainstay treatment option worldwide. The first successful reported use of stented heart valves in an animal heart was in 1992. Henning Anderson et al. mounted porcine aortic valve leaflets onto expandable stents and compressed them over balloon catheters. Catheters were advanced in a retrograde fashion. The team deployed 9 valves into various subcoronary and supracoronary positions along the aortic root of anesthetized pigs.[29] Andersen et al. reported good hemodynamic results in all nine deployments and described a complication of restricted coronary blood flow in 3 of the animals. Despite their relative success, Andersen's animal studies did not immediately lead to human implantations. The first human implantation of a stented valve is credited to Bonhoeffer et al. for implanting a percutaneous valve in the diseased pulmonary artery prosthetic conduit of a 12-year-old boy in 2000.[30]

Between 1993 and 1994, Alain Cribier and colleagues, of Rouen, France, implanted 23-mm Palmaz stents into the diseased aortic roots of cadaver specimens and validated the concept of aortic valvular stenting in human calcific AS.[31] Cribier's team was the first to develop and use catheter-based treatments for AS by successfully performing balloon aortic valvuloplasty (BAV) in humans beginning in 1985.[32] BAV requires a balloon on the distal end of a catheter that, once inflated, stretches the narrowed and calcified aortic valve leaflets, thereby reducing symptoms of obstruction. BAV was (and is) limited by its high rate of restenosis, approximately 80% in 1 year, despite the immediate clinical improvement it often provides.[32,33] As a result, BAV fell out of favor and Cribier's team pressed on with their vision for a better, more permanent solution.

In 1999, Cribier formed Percutaneous Valve Technologies (New Jersey, USA) and developed a balloon-expandable transcatheter heart valve and delivery system to be deployed in the calcific valve of a beating heart.[31] In Rouen, France, in April 2002, Cribier deployed the first human implantation of a transcatheter heart valve in a 57-year-old man with severe AS who had presented with cardiogenic shock and severe left ventricular dysfunction.[34] After the procedure, there was immediate hemodynamic improvement and the procedure was without complication to coronary flow, the mitral valve, or atrioventricular conduction; there was only mild paravalvular regurgitation.[34] This first clinical use was a breakthrough in the world of interventional cardiology and garnered much international attention.[31] Cribier and his colleagues continued their series of human cases and initiated early feasibility studies via compassionate use at their institution.[35] In late 2003, Percutaneous Valve Technologies was acquired by Edwards Lifesciences (Irvine, California, USA),[36] thus enabling rapid improvements and advancements of the technology. Feasibility studies with the updated Edwards balloon-expandable valve (BEV) technology, now called the SAPIEN valve, began in Europe and the United States in 2004. Concurrently, Medtronic, Inc. (Minneapolis, Minnesota, USA) was developing its transcatheter heart valve technology with the self-expanding CoreValve. Feasibility studies of both the SAPIEN and CoreValve led to CE (Conformité Européenne) mark for both valve systems in 2007.[31]

The Era of Early Clinical Trials

Thanks to high-quality, well-designed, randomized clinical trials (RCTs), we have been able to determine the safety and effectiveness of TAVR in various cohorts over the past decade. The pivotal Placement of Aortic Transcatheter Valves (PARTNER) trial began in 2007 at 22 US clinical sites, 3 Canadian sites, and 1 German site. The study was a prospective, multicenter, RCT designed to determine the safety and effectiveness of the SAPIEN transcatheter heart valve and its delivery system in 2 separate cohorts of patients, cohort A and cohort B.[18] Cohort A, the surgical arm of the trial, revealed noninferiority of balloon-expandable TAVR versus surgical aortic valve replacement (SAVR) with respect to all-cause mortality and repeat hospitalization at 1-year and in subsequent follow-up years.[37] Cohort B, the nonsurgical arm of the trial, revealed significant superiority of balloon-expandable TAVR over medical management in inoperable, prohibitive risk patients, with a 20% increase of survival in the treatment (TAVR) group.[18] The trial created a paradigm shift in the treatment of valvular heart disease. It also highlighted the need to improve complications associated with TAVR, namely, stroke and paravalvular leak.[38]

A head-to-head comparison of TAVR with SAVR with a self-expanding transcatheter heart valve (CoreValve, Medtronic) in patients with increased surgical risk was completed in a multicenter, RCT performed at 45 US clinical sites. Risk was defined as a 15% or more estimated risk of mortality within 30 days of surgery or 50% risk of irreversible complications in the same period. Results of this trial showed superior 1-year survival in TAVR compared with SAVR without significantly different rates of neurological events.[39] The incidence of a new permanent pacemaker requirement after TAVR with self-expandable valve (SEV) was 22.3% at 1 year,[38] comparatively higher than reported with the use of BEV.[40]

Given the results of the PARTNER Cohort B study, a randomized trial comparing the self-expanding TAVR system with medical management in extreme-risk patients (estimated 50% or greater risk for mortality or irreversible morbidity at 30 days with SAVR) was abandoned. Instead, a prospective nonrandomized investigation of the self-expanding system was completed and revealed TAVR with a self-expanding system to be a viable alternative to medical management in extreme-risk patients despite limitations related to stroke, paravalvular leak, and new permanent pacemaker requirements.[41]

These powerful data brought a rapid change to the care of cardiac patients as the Edwards SAPIEN balloon-expandable system received US Food and Drug Administration (FDA) approval in October 2012 followed by the approval of the Medtronic CoreValve in January 2014. Both platforms were initially approved for use in patients considered unsuitable for open heart surgery or who were considered high risk for surgery.[31]

Meanwhile, technological refinements were ongoing, with large efforts made to reduce procedural complications and improve valve hemodynamics. In addition to addressing complications associated with TAVR, clinical trials sought expansion of TAVR indications to include intermediate-risk patients. Data from the PARTNER II and Surgical Replacement and Transcatheter Aortic Valve Implantation trials drove FDA approval for TAVR in intermediate-risk patients for the Edwards BEV and Medtronic SEV systems in 2016 and 2017, respectively. To date, these 2 valve systems remain the only TAVR devices with FDA approval and commercial availability in the United States.[42] Other regions have access to different devices. Ongoing RCTs and registries continue to seek approval for new valve system technologies as well as expansion for TAVR use in low-risk and asymptomatic patients with severe AS. In addition, clinical trials are also addressing the treatment of moderate AS with TAVR in the setting of patients with advanced heart failure.[43]

The Role of Transcatheter Aortic Valve Replacement in the Treatment of Aortic Stenosis

Owing to the above-mentioned RCTs, TAVR has become a viable and validated alternative to SAVR in select patients and continues to evolve in other subsets of patients. TAVR is providing a treatment option to many who may have otherwise gone without treatment of their severe AS. The choice of TAVR as a therapy for individual patients involves many steps and careful evaluation by the multidisciplinary heart team. Appropriate criteria are used to determine eligibility, and diagnostic testing helps to determine procedural feasibility and device selection.

Procedural Approaches

The procedural approach to TAVR is largely driven by vascular and cardiac anatomy considerations. Assessment of the iliofemoral system, aorta, and aortic root by multidetector computed tomography is essential for procedural planning. As TAVR has evolved, nearly 95% of cases are performed via transfemoral (TF) access.[42] When TF access for TAVR is not feasible, alternative access approaches may be considered. Alternative access approaches are predominantly transsubclavian, transaortic, transapical, and transcarotid. A TF approach to TAVR remains preferred, as the benefits of TAVR versus SAVR are greatest in TF cohorts.[37]

Transcatheter Aortic Valve Replacement Devices

The evolution of TAVR has driven rapid and impressive technology enhancements that have simplified, standardized, and streamlined the procedure. Fortunately, with these advancements, there has also been a precipitous reduction in complications.[44] Devices now incorporate features that facilitate desired positioning, easier deployment, and optimal hemodynamics. TAVR devices are categorized according to their deployment technique and include BEVs and SEVs.

Balloon-Expandable Valves

BEVs are delivered via catheter by way of the arterial system or LV. A BAV will often be performed to open the narrowed valve and prepare for TAVR. The valve is compressed over another balloon catheter to make it small enough to be delivered via the delivery sheath and is advanced across the aortic valve leaflets and into the aortic root. When positioning is desirable, the balloon is inflated with fluid to expand the transcatheter valve in place within the diseased valve. Rapid ventricular pacing during balloon inflation reduces stroke volume and blood pressure to minimize the risk of ejection or rupture of the balloon. Once fully expanded, the balloon is deflated, the delivery system is removed, and the access site is closed.[45]

The Edwards SAPIEN 3 is the current-generation BEV system with design improvements based on its predecessor transcatheter heart valves, the SAPIEN and SAPIEN XT.[40] The SAPIEN 3 uses bovine pericardial leaflets sutured to a low-height cobalt chromium frame (Figure 1.3). The design includes an outer sealing skirt made of polyethylene terephthalate

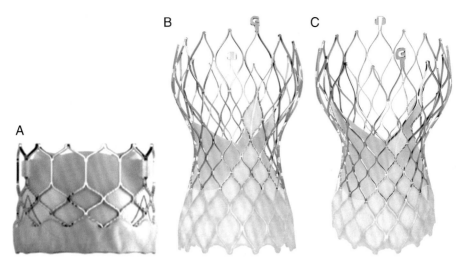

FIGURE 1.3. A, The Edwards SAPIEN 3 transcatheter heart valve. B, Medtronic Evolut R. C, Medtronic Evolut PRO. (Reprinted with permission from Kern MJ. *SCAI Interventional Cardiology Review.* 2nd ed. Philadelphia: Wolters Kluwer Health/Lippincott Williams & Wilkins; 2013.)

that covers the lower portion of the frame to specifically reduce paravalvular leak by sealing the area between the outside frame and native annulus.[45] The SAPIEN 3 is available in 20-, 23-, 26-, and 29-mm sizes and can be accommodated by a minimum vessel size of 5.5 to 6.0 mm. The valve is delivered through a 14F expandable sheath with the exception of the 29-mm valve, which requires a 16F expandable sheath.[40,45] The SAPIEN 3 device can be delivered via TF, direct transaortic, or transapical routes[45] according to the manufacturers; however, additional alternative accesses are technically feasible and are conventionally restricted to operators and institutions with the appropriate skillset.[46]

Self-Expandable Valves

Similar to BEV, SEVs are delivered via catheter by way of the arterial system. A BAV may be performed to open the narrowed valve and prepare for TAVR. The SEV is compression loaded onto a catheter and advanced across the aortic valve leaflets and into the aortic root. When positioning is desirable, the valve is unsheathed and begins to flower until fully deployed and functional. If not fully deployed, the valve can be resheathed and repositioned until placement is desirable. Once disengaged, the delivery system is removed and the access site is closed.[47]

Currently available SEV systems in the United States are part of the Medtronic CoreValve family. The CoreValve Evolut R and Evolut PRO were designed to mitigate the challenges of their predecessor, the CoreValve Classic. The Evolut R and PRO use supra-annular porcine pericardial tissue leaflets in a nitinol frame. The Evolut R is a resheathable valve that allows it to be recaptured and repositioned during deployment.[47] The Evolut R is available in 4 sizes, 23, 26, 29, and 34 mm, and can accommodate a minimal vessel diameter between 5.0 and 5.5 mm. The Evolut PRO is also recapturable and repositionable and indicated for vessels down to 5.5 mm. It was designed with an external pericardial wrap to help mitigate paravalvular leak by increasing surface contact with the native annulus to reduce gaps.[47] The Evolut PRO is available in 23-, 26-, and 29-mm sizes.[48] The Evolut R and PRO can be delivered via the TF route or by alternative access approaches that can be done safely by an individual operator and hospital institution.

Transesophageal and/or transthoracic echocardiogram may be used intraprocedurally or postprocedurally during TAVR to assist with placement/deployment and to assess the hemodynamics of the valve. Fluoroscopy is the mainstay intraprocedural imaging method during TAVR. TAVR with either a BEV or an SEV can be safely performed under general anesthesia, monitored anesthesia, or conscious sedation, and the mode of anesthesia should be determined at the site level by the multidisciplinary heart valve team. Careful consideration should be made to factors that may present higher procedural risk (e.g., alternative access) or instability when customizing the individual anesthesia plan.[46]

Other Devices

Multiple other TAVR devices are in existence both in and out of the United States for either commercial and/or investigational use. Other self-expanding valve systems include the Portico valve (Abbott, Abbott Park, IL), Accurate Neo valve (Boston Scientific, Marlborough, MA), Allegra (NVT, Hechingen, Germany), and Centera (Edwards Lifesciences, Irvine, CA). The Lotus valve (Boston Scientific, Marlborough, MA) is a mechanically expandable valve system. These next-generation devices serve to offer features that can address various anatomical and clinical scenarios.

Comparison of Balloon-Expandable Valve and Self-Expandable Valve

Several observational studies and meta-analyses have been conducted by doing head-to-head comparisons of the early-generation BEVs and SEVs. These comparative studies are limited by their lack of large patient groups and lack of long-term follow-up and should, therefore, be interpreted with caution. The multicenter randomized trial, CHOICE (Randomized Comparison of Transcatheter Heart Valves in High Risk Patients With Severe Aortic Stenosis: Medtronic CoreValve Versus Edwards SAPIEN XT Trial), revealed greater device success and decreased permanent pacemaker requirements at 30 days with balloon-expandable systems. At 1 year, there was no significant difference in mortality between the 2 groups.[49] Recently, comparison between the newer Edwards SAPIEN 3 and Medtronic CoreValve Evolut R was undertaken by Rogers et al.[50] Their single-center experience revealed substantially higher rates of new complete heart block and subsequent permanent pacemaker implantation at 30 days with SEVs (12.7% vs 4.7%, $P = .049$). There was no significant difference in mortality between the 2 cohorts. As discussed, the Edwards SAPIEN and self-expandable Evolut PRO were both designed to include an outer skirt or pericardial wrap design to mitigate paravalvular leak; however, there are no data detailing a comparison between the two. In the PARTNER II SAPIEN 3 trial, moderate paravalvular leak was seen in 3.4% of patients with a 13.3% rate of permanent pacemaker implantation.[51]

In the US Evolut PRO Study, completed on 60 patients in 8 US centers, no patients experienced moderate paravalvular leak at 30 days and the rate of permanent pacemaker implantation was 10%.[52]

Indications

Appropriateness of TAVR in select patients is determined by a comprehensive assessment of technical and clinical suitability as determined by the patient and heart valve team. Indications are rapidly evolving and differ by regions.

United States Guidelines and National Coverage Determination Criteria

The 2014 American Heart Association (AHA)/American College of Cardiology (ACC) Guideline for the Management of Patients with Valvular Heart Disease[28] and the 2017 ACC Expert Consensus Decision Pathway for Transcatheter Aortic Valve Replacement in the Management of Adults with Aortic Stenosis provide useful guidance for clinicians and heart valve teams when approaching patients with severe AS with varying degrees of surgical risk. These guidelines provide recommendations and considerations related to the risks of valvular intervention (either SAVR or TAVR) and medical therapy. The AHA/ACC guidelines provide a framework of evidenced-based statements developed by clinical leaders. These statements are assembled in a peer-reviewed approval process and identified by both level of evidence and classes of recommendations. Guidelines are intended to assist practitioners in clinical decision making for diagnosing and offering treatment options for specific disease processes. Expert Consensus Decision Pathways, in particular, provide clinical decision-making guidance in areas where evidence may be lacking or evolving.[46] In addition, the multisociety 2017 Appropriate Use Criteria for the Treatment of Patients With Severe Aortic Stenosis were also set forth to provide guidance to clinicians based on various and specific clinical presentations and scenarios.[29]

The Centers for Medicare and Medicaid (CMS) is a US agency that administers and provides federal and state health coverage for people of a certain age (65 y or older) and/or certain disabilities. CMS establish their own criteria and requirements to determine Medicare coverage for treatments of diagnoses. These criteria are based on evidence and allow for public participation in the determination.[53] CMS has determined coverage for TAVR in the United States with multiple conditions. These conditions include accordance with FDA approval indications, 2 independent surgical evaluations, care by a multidisciplinary heart team as well as joint procedure participation by an interventional cardiologist and a cardiac surgeon, appropriate hospital infrastructure and procedure volumes, and participation in a prospective, national, audited registry.[53] Currently, FDA approval indications for TAVR include treatment of patients with severe, symptomatic calcific AS who are deemed by a heart team to be at intermediate or greater risk for SAVR. TAVR is also indicated for patients with symptomatic heart disease due to failure of a surgical bioprosthetic aortic or mitral valve who have been determined by a heart team to be at high or greater risk of redo surgery.[45]

European Guidelines

European guidelines for the management of valvular heart disease are supported by the European Society of Cardiology (ESC) and European Association of CardioThoracic Surgery (EACTS) and were most recently updated in 2017. The 2017 update was expansive to include accumulated TAVR data and the technological advancements, including the valve-in-valve technique for failing bioprosthetic valves. Much like the AHA/ACC guidelines, the ESC/EACTS guidelines provide evidenced-based data to guide heart team decision making in the treatment of valvular heart disease, including the decision-making process of SAVR versus TAVR, which is largely based on risk assessment. ESC/EACTS-stated recommendations identify both level of evidence and classes of recommendations. Important aspects include patient evaluation, inclusive of functional and cognitive status, and the severity of the aortic valve disease. Risk stratification is required for weighing related risks and potential benefits of treatment, including the patients' self-reported quality of life and preference for treatment. Most European countries maintain national guidelines based on the ESC/EACTS guidelines and participate in national and European data registries.

Contraindications

Careful consideration of the contraindications for treatment of AS should be made by the heart valve team during the evaluation process. Site and operator experience should also be considered relative to the following recommendations.

SAVR is not recommended in patients with AS with extreme surgical risk owing to major cardiovascular comorbidities (eg, ≥50% predicted risk of death or serious irreversible mortality by Society of Thoracic Surgery [STS] score).[42] Other absolute contraindications for SAVR not captured by the STS score include technical infeasibilities such as circumferential or heavy calcification of the ascending aorta ("porcelain aorta") that make aortic cross-clamping prohibitive. A "hostile chest" due to severe radiation damage or complications from a previous chest surgery is also an absolute contraindication for SAVR.[54] Relative contraindications not captured by the STS score include advanced liver disease, severe pulmonary hypertension, severe right ventricular function, and/or frailty.[42]

TAVR is not recommended in patients with an estimated life expectancy of less than 12 months owing to noncardiac comorbidities, unlikelihood to improve quality of life, or concomitant valve disease that is a major contributor and treatable by surgery. Other anatomic issues and clinical presentations that may prohibit TAVR include active endocarditis, recent untreated thrombus, risk of coronary ostial occlusion, and/or native annulus size that is outside the range of available devices.[55,56] There are a number of other relative contraindications that should be carefully assessed before proceeding with or denying treatment with TAVR. TAVR in bicuspid valves was excluded from the early TAVR pivotal trials owing to concerns related to elliptical deployment. To date, TAVR in congenital bicuspid valves has been successfully performed, although it is recognized that device implantation in this population requires careful assessment and procedure planning to avoid complications.[57]

Conclusion

SAVR and TAVR are both sustaining treatments of severe, symptomatic AS with outcomes that prolong survival and improve quality of life.[42] TAVR has matured to prove efficacy and feasibility in select patients and has truly modernized the management of AS. Heart team evaluation and collaboration remain focused on identifying those patients most likely to benefit from TAVR and optimizing outcomes. Risk-benefit assessments and treatment planning should be individualized with special attention paid to a patient's preference, age, anatomy, life expectancy, and comorbid burdens. Planning for future and lower-risk generations of patients will need to address the issue of durability and limitations associated with quality of life limiting complications, such as cognitive deficits and conduction system interference. As with all developing therapies, future directions will focus on ongoing trials and high-quality, robust data. TAVR remains poised for ongoing success, and its contributions to the cardiovascular community have already served to broaden treatments for many other types of heart disease.

KEY TAKEAWAYS AND BEST PRACTICES

▶ Knowledge of natural history, clinical presentation, and diagnostic confirmation of AS is essential when caring for patients undergoing evaluation for TAVR.

▶ Familiarity with approved treatment indications for severe, symptomatic AS, as well as contraindications, is fundamental to the clinical practice of the valve program clinician.

▶ Clinical practice guidelines provide a framework to assist practitioners with evidence-based decision making.

References

1. Vaslef SN, Roberts WC. Early descriptions of aortic valve stenosis. *Am Heart J*. 1993;125(5):1465-1474. doi:10.1016/0002-8703(93)91036-e.
2. McGinn S, White PD. Clinical observations on aortic stenosis. *Am Heart J*. 1934;10(2):273-274. doi:10.1016/s0002-8703(34)90385-9.
3. Wood FO, Abbas AE. General considerations and etiologies of aortic stenosis. *Aortic Stenosis*. 2015:1-20. doi:10.1007/978-1-4471-5242-2_1.
4. Shumacker HB. *The Evolution of Cardiac Surgery*. Bloomington: Indiana University Press; 1992.
5. Hufnagel CA. Surgical correction of aortic insufficiency. *Mod Concepts Cardiovasc Dis*. 1955;24(8):287-289.
6. Harken DE, Soroff HS, Taylor WJ, Lefemine AA, Gupta SK, Lunzer S. Partial and complete prostheses in aortic insufficiency. *J Thorac Cardiovasc Surg*. 1960;40:744-762.
7. Ross D. Homograft replacement of the aortic valve. *Transplantation*. 1968;6(4):627-631. doi:10.1097/00007890-196807000-00036.
8. Topol EJ, Califf RM. *Textbook of Cardiovascular Medicine*. Philadelphia: Lippincott Williams & Wilkins; 2007.
9. Gaasch WH. *Natural History, Epidemiology, and Prognosis of Aortic Stenosis*. UpToDate; May 10, 2016. http://www.uptodate.com/. Accessed 5 January 2018.
10. Nkomo VT, Gardin JM, Skelton TN, Gottdiener JS, Scott CG, Enriquez-Sarano M. Burden of valvular heart diseases: a population-based study. *Lancet*. 2006;368(9540):1005-1011. doi:10.1016/s0140-6736(06)69208-8.
11. Otto CM, Kuusisto J, Reichenbach DD, Gown AM, Obrien KD. Characterization of the early lesion of degenerative valvular aortic stenosis. Histological and immunohistochemical studies. *Circulation*. 1994;90(2):844-853. doi:10.1161/01.cir.90.2.844.
12. Eveborn GW, Schirmer H, Heggelund G, Lunde P, Rasmussen K. The evolving epidemiology of valvular aortic stenosis: the Tromsø study. *Heart*. 2012;99(6):396-400. doi:10.1136/heartjnl-2012-302265.
13. Wang L, Ming Wang L, Chen W, Chen X. Bicuspid aortic valve: a review of its genetics and clinical significance. *J Heart Valve Dis*. 2016;25(5):568-573.
14. Grossman W, Jones D, Mclaurin LP. Wall stress and patterns of hypertrophy in the human left ventricle. *J Clin Invest*. 1975;56(1):56-64. doi:10.1172/jci108079.
15. Otto CM, Bonow RO. *63 valvular heart disease*. In: *Braunwald's Heart Disease: A Textbook of Cardiovascular Medicine*. 10th ed. Elsevier; 2015:1446-1523.
16. Ross J, Braunwald E. Aortic stenosis. *Circulation*. 1968;38(1S5). doi:10.1161/01.cir.38.1s5.v-61.

17. Bach DS, Siao D, Girard SE, Duvernoy C, Mccallister BD, Gualano SK. Evaluation of patients with severe symptomatic aortic stenosis who do not undergo aortic valve replacement: the potential role of subjectively overestimated operative risk. *Circ Cardiovasc Qual Outcomes.* 2009;2(6):533-539. doi:10.1161/circoutcomes.109.848259.

18. Leon MB, Smith CR, Mack M, et al. Transcatheter aortic-valve implantation for aortic stenosis in patients who cannot undergo surgery. *N Engl J Med.* 2010;363(17):1597-1607. doi:10.1056/nejmoa1008232.

19. Green SJ, Pizzarello RA, Padmanabhan VT, Ong LY, Hall MH. Relation of angina pectoris to coronary artery disease in aortic valve stenosis. *Am J Cardiol.* 1985;55(8):1063-1065.

20. Lombard JT, Selzer A. Valvular aortic stenosis. *Ann Intern Med.* 1987;106(2):292. doi:10.7326/0003-4819-106-2-292.

21. Sorgato A, Faggiano P, Aurigemma GP, et al. Ventricular arrhythmias in adult aortic stenosis: prevalence, mechanisms, and clinical relevance. *Chest.* 1888;113(2):482-491.

22. Etchells E, Bell C, Robb K. Does this patient have an abnormal systolic murmur? *JAMA.* 1997;277(7):564-571. doi:10.1001/jama.277.7.564.

23. Munt B, Legget ME, Kraft CD, Miyake-Hull CY, Fujioka M, Otto CM. Physical examination in valvular aortic stenosis: correlation with stenosis severity and prediction of clinical outcome. *Am Heart J.* 1999;137(2):298-306. doi:10.1053/hj.1999.v137.95496.

24. Foster E. Echocardiographic Evaluation of the Aortic Valve. Login. https://www.uptodate.com/login. Accessed 11 January 2018.

25. Weber M, Arnold R, Rau M. Relation of N-terminal pro-B-type natriuretic peptide to progression of aortic valve disease. *ACC Curr J Rev.* 2005;14(9):34. doi:10.1016/j.accreview.2005.08.219.

26. Bergler-Klein J. Natriuretic peptides predict symptom-free survival and postoperative outcome in severe aortic stenosis. *Circulation.* 2004;109(19):2302-2308. doi:10.1161/01.cir.0000126825.50903.18.

27. Clavel MA, Malouf J, Michelena H, Enriquez-Sarano M. Impact of type-B natriuretic peptide on survival in aortic stenosis. *Eur Heart J.* 2013;34(suppl 1):1816. doi:10.1093/eurheartj/eht308.1816.

28. Nishimura RA, Otto CM, Bonow RO, et al. 2014 AHA/ACC guideline for the management of patients with valvular heart disease: a report of the American College of Cardiology/American Heart Association Task Force on Practice Guidelines. *Circulation.* 2014;129(23). doi:10.1161/cir.0000000000000031.

29. Bonow RO, Brown AS, Gillam LD, et al. ACC/AATS/AHA/ASE/EACTS/HVS/SCA/SCAI/SCCT/SCMR/STS 2017 appropriate use criteria for the treatment of patients with severe aortic stenosis. *J Am Coll Cardiol.* 2017;70(20):2566-2598. doi:10.1016/j.jacc.2017.09.018.

30. Bonhoeffer P, Boudjemline Y, Saliba Z, et al. Percutaneous replacement of pulmonary valve in a right-ventricle to pulmonary-artery prosthetic conduit with valve dysfunction. *Lancet.* 2000;356(9239):1403-1405. doi:10.1016/s0140-6736(00)02844-0.

31. Cribier AG. The Odyssey of TAVR from concept to clinical reality. *Tex Heart Inst J.* 2014;41(2):125-130. doi:10.14503/thij-14-4137.

32. Letac B, Cribier A, Koning R, Bellefleur JP. Results of percutaneous transluminal valvuloplasty in 218 adults with valvular aortic stenosis. *Am J Cardiol.* 1988;62(9):598-605. doi:10.1016/0002-9149(88)90663-7.

33. Percutaneous balloon aortic valvuloplasty. Acute and 30-day follow-up results in 674 patients from the NHLBI balloon valvuloplasty registry. *Circulation.* 1991;84(6):2383-2397. doi:10.1161/01.cir.84.6.2383.

34. Cribier A, Eltchaninoff H, Tron C, et al. Early experience with percutaneous transcatheter implantation of heart valve prosthesis for the treatment of end-stage inoperable patients with calcific aortic stenosis. *J Am Coll Cardiol.* 2004;43(4):698-703. doi:10.1016/j.jacc.2003.11.026.

35. Cribier A, Eltchaninoff H, Tron C, et al. Treatment of calcific aortic stenosis with the percutaneous heart valve. *J Am Coll Cardiol.* 2006;47(6):1214-1223. doi:10.1016/j.jacc.2006.01.049.

36. Edwards Lifesciences Completes Acquisition of Percutaneous Valve Technologies for $125 Million. 2004. www.edwards.com.
37. Kodali SK, Williams MR, Smith CR, et al. Two-year outcomes after transcatheter or surgical aortic-valve replacement. *N Engl J Med.* 2012;366(18):1686-1695. doi:10.1056/nejmoa1200384.
38. Svensson LG, Tuzcu M, Kapadia S, et al. A comprehensive review of the PARTNER trial. *J Thorac Cardiovasc Surg.* 2013;145(3). doi:10.1016/j.jtcvs.2012.11.051.
39. Adams DH, Popma JJ, Reardon MJ, et al. Transcatheter aortic-valve replacement with a self-expanding prosthesis. *N Engl J Med.* 2014;370(19):1790-1798. doi:10.1056/nejmoa1400590.
40. Wiegerinck EM, Van Kesteren F, Van Mourik MS, Vis MM, Baan J. An up-to-date overview of the most recent transcatheter implantable aortic valve prostheses. *Expert Rev Med Devices.* 2016;13(1):31-45. doi:10.1586/17434440.2016.1120665.
41. Popma JJ, Adams DH, Reardon MJ, et al. Transcatheter aortic valve replacement using a self-expanding bioprosthesis in patients with severe aortic stenosis at extreme risk for surgery. *J Am Coll Cardiol.* 2014;63(19):1972-1981. doi:10.1016/j.jacc.2014.02.556.
42. Brecker SJ, Aldea GS. *Choice of Therapy for Symptomatic Aortic Stenosis.* UpToDate; June 2, 2017. http://www.uptodate.com/. Accessed 1 December 2017.
43. Transcatheter Aortic Valve Replacement to UNload the Left Ventricle in Patients With Advanced Heart Failure (TAVR UNLOAD) – Full Text View. ClinicalTrials.gov. 2016. https://clinicaltrials.gov/ct2/show/study/NCT02661451. Accessed 18 January 2018.
44. Harold JG. Harold on history: the evolution of transcatheter aortic valve replacement. *Cardiology.* 2017;46(7):38.
45. Edwards Lifesciences – the Leader in Heart Valves & Hemodynamic Monitoring | Edwards Lifesciences. Devices: SAPIEN 3. http://www.edwards.com/. Accessed 1 January 2018.
46. Otto CM, Kumbhani DJ, Alexander KP, et al. 2017 ACC expert consensus decision pathway for transcatheter aortic valve replacement in the management of adults with aortic stenosis. *J Am Coll Cardiol.* 2017;69(10):1313-1346. doi:10.1016/j.jacc.2016.12.006.
47. Transcatheter Aortic Valve Replacement. www.medtronic.com.
48. Mahtta D, Elgendy IY, Bavry AA. From CoreValve to Evolut PRO: reviewing the journey of self-expanding transcatheter aortic valves. *Cardiol Ther.* 2017;6(2):183-192. doi:10.1007/s40119-017-0100-z.
49. Abdel-Wahab M, Mehilli J, Frerker C, et al. Comparison of balloon-expandable vs self-expandable valves in patients undergoing transcatheter aortic valve replacement. *JAMA.* 2014;311(15):1503. doi:10.1001/jama.2014.3316.
50. Rogers T, Steinvil A, Buchanan K, et al. Contemporary transcatheter aortic valve replacement with third-generation balloon-expandable versus self-expanding devices. *J Interv Cardiol.* 2017;30(4):356-361. doi:10.1111/joic.12389.
51. Kodali S, Thourani VH, White J, et al. Early clinical and echocardiographic outcomes after SAPIEN 3 transcatheter aortic valve replacement in inoperable, high-risk and intermediate-risk patients with aortic stenosis. *Eur Heart J.* 2016;37(28):2252-2262. doi:10.1093/eurheartj/ehw112.
52. Forrest JK, Mangi AA, Popma JJ, et al. Early outcomes with the Evolut PRO repositionable self-expanding transcatheter aortic valve with pericardial wrap. *JACC Cardiovasc Interv.* 2018;11(2):160-168. doi:10.1016/j.jcin.2017.10.014.
53. Decision Memo for Transcatheter Aortic Valve Replacement (TAVR) (CAG-00430N). *Home – Centers for Medicare & Medicaid Services*; 14 December 2017. http://www.cms.gov. Accessed 15 January 2018.
54. Kappetein AP, Head SJ, Généreux P, et al. Updated standardized endpoint definitions for transcatheter aortic valve implantation: the valve academic research consortium-2 consensus document. *J Thorac Cardiovasc Surg.* 2013;145(1):6-23. doi:10.1016/j.jtcvs.2012.09.002.
55. Holmes DR, Mack MJ, Kaul S, et al. 2012 ACCF/AATS/SCAI/STS expert consensus document on transcatheter aortic valve replacement. *J Am Coll Cardiol.* 2012;59(13):1200-1254. doi:10.1016/j.jacc.2012.01.001.

56. Vahanian A, Alfieri O, Andreotti F, et al. Guidelines on the management of valvular heart disease (version 2012): the joint task force on the management of valvular heart disease of the European Society of Cardiology (ESC) and the European Association for Cardio-Thoracic Surgery (EACTS). *Eur J Cardiothoracic Surg*. 2012;42(4). doi:10.1093/ejcts/ezs455.
57. Bauer T, Linke A, Sievert H, et al. Comparison of the effectiveness of transcatheter aortic valve implantation in patients with stenotic bicuspid versus tricuspid aortic valves (from the German TAVI Registry). *Am J Cardiol*. 2014;113(3):518-521. doi:10.1016/j.amjcard.2013.10.023.

CHAPTER 2

The Heart Team Approach

Amy E. Simone, PA-C, AACC

OBJECTIVES

▶ Present a multidisciplinary perspective of the Heart Team that highlights the contributions of nursing and allied health professionals

▶ Highlight the rationale for a Heart Team approach

Introduction to the Heart Team

Background

The concept of a multidisciplinary Heart Team for the provision of comprehensive, collaborative care to patients with valvular heart disease (VHD) was formalized with the inception of transcatheter valve therapy. The Heart Team model is a class I recommendation from both American and European professional societies and is required in the United States for reimbursement following transcatheter aortic valve replacement (TAVR).[1,2] This team-based approach aims to leverage the strengths and skills of its members to optimize safety and quality of patient care.

The Heart Team navigates the patient in a personalized manner through each stage of the journey from time of diagnosis to referral, initial consultation, screening, shared decision making, procedure, recovery, and follow-up. This patient-centric model of individualized care is made possible through standardized processes implemented by the members of the team. The Heart Team construct will not be identical between institutions, and this embodies the beauty and uniqueness of the concept. There is, however, the undeniable overarching role of the Heart Team that includes providing high-quality care across the continuum spanning a variety of medical specialties through reliable, forthright, and clear lines of communication. This is facilitated via empowerment of each member to contribute their unique insights, ideas, and opinions openly to the group for the provision of safe, comprehensive care.

Construct

The construct of the Heart Team differs slightly from program to program; however, the fundamental elements remain constant. "The management of patients with complex severe VHD is best achieved by a Heart Valve Team composed primarily of a cardiologist and a surgeon…there may be a multidisciplinary, collaborative group of caregivers, including cardiologists, structural valve interventionalists, cardiovascular imaging specialists, cardiovascular surgeons, anesthesiologists, and nurses."[2] In the past, Cardiology and Cardiothoracic Surgery existed in mutually exclusive silos.[3] The development of a multidisciplinary Heart Team is seen as a blending of these silos to ultimately enhance patient selection, procedural performance, and outcomes.[3]

The Heart Team comprises core and extended members who collectively provide care across the continuum (Figure 2.1). Although the foundation of the team may be the cardiothoracic surgeon (CTS) and interventional cardiologist (IC), each additional member provides value. There are multiple layers of investment across a myriad of specialties, roles, and training. The formal responsibilities in patient selection and procedural planning are site specific, but all play pivotal roles in shepherding patients on the pathways of diagnosis, treatment, and follow-up. Ideally, the nonphysician members of the team are equal participants and partners in complex decision making. Notably, in the United States and Canada, the role of the valve program clinician (VPC) has emerged as instrumental to the cohesive nature of the Heart Team and aims to facilitate procedural success, positive clinical outcomes, and an optimal postprocedure recovery.

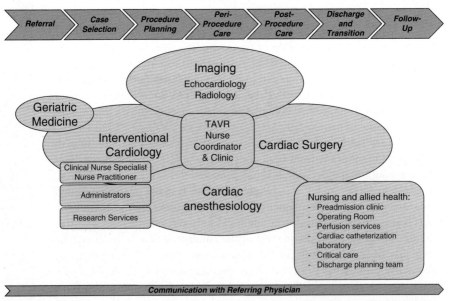

FIGURE 2.1. The expanded heart team model along the transcatheter aortic valve replacement (TAVR) continuum of care. (Reprinted with permission from Lauck SB, Wood DA, Baumbusch J, et al. Vancouver transcatheter aortic valve replacement clinical pathway minimalist approach, standardized care, and discharge criteria to reduce length of stay. *Circ Cardiovasc Qual Outcomes.* 2016;9(3):312-321. *Wolters Kluwer Health, Inc.*)

Rationale and Purpose

The rationale supporting the value and necessity of the Heart Team is clearly described in the 2014 American Heart Association/American College of Cardiology (ACC) Valvular Heart Disease Guidelines, and the responsibilities are clearly delineated. The Heart Valve Team (1) reviews the patient's medical condition and valve abnormality; (2) determines the possible interventions that are indicated, technically feasible, and reasonable; and (3) discusses the risks and outcomes of these interventions with the patient and family.[2] The duties described included patient selection, optimal care plans, shared decision making, and an avoidance of poor outcomes, with focus on anticipated improvement in quality of life. Concise, clear criteria are embedded in the guidelines to determine which interventions are *indicated* and to quantify the severity of VHD. The issue of *technical feasibility* is one that is best addressed utilizing the clinical acumen and expertise of the CTS, IC, cardiovascular imaging specialist, and anesthesiologist. Procedural viability requires extensive preprocedure screening and testing, including advanced imaging techniques, to ensure no anatomical barriers exist that may preclude a successful procedure.

The question of which intervention is considered *reasonable* is a far more nuanced discussion between the members of the Heart Team, which includes the contributions of patient-facing, nonphysician members, including advanced practice providers (APPs, ie, physician assistants and nurse practitioners), nurses, and the VPC. The Heart Team is responsible for educating patients and families regarding disease progression, prognosis, and treatment options, while taking patient preferences and values into account. This is applied via a shared decision making (SDM) method.[1] Patient selection is one of the crucial roles of the team "through a comprehensive understanding of the risk-benefit ratio of different treatment strategies."[2] There are psychosocial aspects that may negatively affect recovery after the procedure and must be incorporated into the decision making. Also, understanding patient motivation requires Heart Team members to ask the right questions in the right situation within the SDM process, with a focus on anticipated improvement in patient-defined quality of life.[4,5]

Potential Benefits

Although the distinct benefits associated with the Heart Team approach have yet to be evaluated, the aim is to provide high-quality, patient-centered care. Continuity is established and maintained from the time of initial consultation, procedure, and follow-up, which, in similar specialties, has been found to affect the overall patient experience. The concept of multidisciplinary teams providing care for complex patient populations has history in transplant, oncology, and heart failure management. For example, in a study of heart failure management utilizing multidisciplinary, team-based care, both hospital readmission and length of stay were reduced.[6,7]

The transcatheter valve therapy arena is rapidly evolving, and the Heart Team approach may facilitate establishment and implementation of best practices. These best practices are established nationally through the formation of guidelines and implemented at the level of the institution.

Challenges and Barriers

Changing culture and practice may present challenges for the Heart Team. Among the most common challenges is the establishment and maintenance of effective communication and scheduling processes. Given the very nature of procedural-oriented specialists and a complex and often high-acuity patient population, "rallying the troops" may be required for the most fundamental team functions, ranging from clinic consultations to meeting attendance.

Engaging the core members of the Heart Team and inspiring a shared vision while cultivating this change in culture and shift in care paradigm can feel like a full-time endeavor. Posing yet another challenge, these efforts are difficult to track by conventional metrics of productivity. In countries using a designated coordination role (eg, United States and Canada), change management responsibilities may be embraced by the VPC. To traverse these changes in culture and practice, the VPC frequently embodies the implicit role requirements of resilience and meticulousness.

Barriers to implementation of an effective Heart Team may include culture of institution and clinicians, physical location of providers, challenging schedules, physical meeting space, presence of support staff, funding, and leadership.[1] The Heart Team must function as a cohesive unit to identify and reconcile any barriers to create a highly functional and resilient team (Table 2.1).

TABLE 2.1. Potential Benefits of and Barriers to Heart Teams

Benefits of Heart Teams	Barriers to Heart Teams
Incorporating broader input by different physician and clinical experts into a complex decision-making process	Engaging different physicians from a broad range of specialties into a complex decision-making process
Minimizing fragmented decision making and improving coordination of care	Ensuring a streamlined process for integrating and summarizing input from multiple viewpoints in a Heart Team in a systematic manner
Facilitating shared decision making with patients and families	Including active participation by patients and families into the decision-making process by Heart Teams while maintaining efficiencies
Improving timeliness and consistency of decisions when multiple providers are likely to be involved, increasing satisfaction for both patients and physicians	Ensuring accurate communication of discussions held by Heart Teams to patients and their families
Minimizing concerns related to physician self-referral	Improving mechanisms for fair and equitable remuneration of services provided by physicians and health systems, particularly across specialists and between cognitive and procedural services
Allowing more intricate and patient-centered treatment plans to be developed (eg, "hybrid" revascularization)	
Enhancing patient enrollment in research protocols	

Reprinted with permission from Nallamothu BK, Cohen DJ. No "I" in heart team: incentivizing multidisciplinary care in cardiovascular medicine. *Circ Cardiovasc Qual Outcomes.* 2012;5(3):410-413.

Roles and Responsibilities of Heart Team Members

Caring for patients with the diagnosis of complex VHD requires "a village." The road on which a prospective patient with TAVR embarks is long, winding, and tedious at times. Although the pillars of the Heart Team include the CTS and the IC, each care team member plays a role in the patient journey.

Each team member serves to navigate the harrowing process of screening, decision making, treatment, recovery, and follow-up. Broad responsibilities of the Heart Team are outlined in Table 2.2. There is need for a systematic approach and coordination (eg, via the VPC in the United States and Canada), as managing patients with VHD and multiple confounding comorbidities is challenging. There is a multitude of data points collected through the screening process for each patient. It is easy to become "fogged over" by the amount and minutia of data—point after point, measurement after measurement. The Heart Team serves as a beacon through this fog of data, ensures that key information is not lost along the way, and positions the patient at the center of the discussion. It is the responsibility of the Heart Team to ask all of the pertinent questions, including those regarding psychosocial aspects (eg, lives alone with limited resources), which may negatively affect recovery potential.

The Heart Team may be classified into the Core Heart Team (ie, primary responsibility for patient care and coordination across the continuum) and Extended Heart Team (ie, episodic or transitional responsibility for patient care and coordination on the continuum).

TABLE 2.2. Broad Responsibilities of the Heart Team

- Navigate the patient through the entire process and provide individualized treatment plans
- Establish baseline health, cognitive, and functional statuses
- Use preprocedure shared decision making
- Define social support structure
- Manage expectations of patients, families, and referring providers
- Proper patient selection
- Technical planning for procedural success
- Streamline the procedure
- Emphasize patient safety
- Strive for early and safe discharge planning
- Educate regarding disease process and heart failure diagnosis
- Outline postprocedure care and anticipated recovery
- Discuss follow-up recommendations
- Apply effective communication techniques for all involved

Core Heart Team
Cardiothoracic Surgeon

The CTS provides an expert opinion regarding surgical risk/operability and options for invasive therapy. The surgeon may perform TAVR or surgical aortic valve replacement and documents surgical risk using multiple measures such as the Society of Thoracic Surgeons' (STS) risk model score and functional assessments. In the United States, it is required at this point for 2 CTSs to formally assess patients via a face-to-face encounter and weigh available clinical data to form, document, and share opinions designating surgical risk stratification. Subsequently, in the Unites States, the CTS participates in the procedure alongside the IC. The CTS may be assigned as the attending service for postprocedure care; however, this model varies per institution. These individuals are certified and licensed per their region and hospital requirements. There are a growing number of physicians who are double board certified as Cardiothoracic Surgeons and Interventional Cardiologists; this is a remarkable endeavor that clearly requires years of dedicated training and expertise. It is this type of dual certification that illustrates the "marriage" of the 2 specialties and the hybrid approach necessary for screening and treating patients with VHD via transcatheter valve therapies.

Interventional Cardiologist

The IC embodies proficiency using catheter-based technologies and brings a high level of technical skill to the Heart Team. As alluded to earlier in this chapter, procedural eligibility and technical feasibility must be thoroughly investigated before offering a treatment plan and scheduling a procedure. To keep patient safety and optimal clinical outcomes at the forefront, all screening data must be meticulously compiled and reviewed. Once the Heart Team agrees that the degree of VHD indicates treatment, the CTS and IC work collaboratively and draw upon their individual technical skill and clinical acumen to discuss procedural success. Issues affecting the plan and sequence for treatment (eg, concomitant coronary artery disease and VHD) must be explored diligently and options discussed. Maintaining open communication with the members of the Heart Team as well as the referring provider is critical at this juncture. This is commonly the "jumping-off point" for candid conversations involving key members of the team to discuss *reasonable* in conjunction with *feasible*. This dialogue includes conjecture based on concrete data abstracted through screening tests, including functional and cognitive assessments. This is the very crux of proper patient selection. With careful attention, Heart Team members candidly discuss the patient's risk to benefit ratio, recovery potential, and likelihood for improved quality of life.

Cardiovascular Imaging Specialist

The cardiovascular imaging specialist is essential in procedural planning through interpretation of high-quality studies obtained via dedicated protocols. The role of the cardiovascular imaging specialist has evolved on pace with the technology. The technique for appropriately and thoroughly sizing aortic annuli as part of procedural planning has shifted a great deal in recent years. Initial sizing during the early days of TAVR technology as seen within the PARTNER (Placement of Aortic Transcatheter Valve) randomized clinical trial included sizing parameters based on measurements obtained from 2-dimensional echocardiography. In contrast,

3-dimensional (3-D) multidetector computed tomography with angiography (CTA) has been shown to provide comprehensive and superior anatomical information further supporting proper patient selection and prosthesis sizing.[9] As transcatheter technology and operator experience matured, the paradigm for annular sizing shifted from 2-dimensional echocardiogram to gated CTA as the modality of choice in this arena.[8] The cardiovascular imaging specialist in the past may have referred only to the physician performing intraprocedural transesophageal echocardiography. With the advent of electrocardiography-gated 3-D multidetector CTA for transcatheter valve sizing, the radiologist or cardiologist interpreting the CTA may serve as the cardiovascular imaging specialist.

Currently, advanced imaging is an essential part of the preoperative assessment for TAVR, as well as a crucial topic for discussion and investigation by the Heart Team. Multimodality 3-D imaging, which has emerged as a critical component of every facet of evaluation and treatment, is discussed in detail in chapter 5. To determine technical feasibility of TAVR, the Heart Team must ensure that there are no limiting factors to performing TAVR or surgical aortic valve replacement, including unfavorable or dangerous calcium distribution in the annulus or left ventricular outflow tract, short distance between the aortic annulus and coronary artery ostia, aortopathy or porcelain aorta, congenital leaflet malformation, unusually large or small annuli, hostile chest, critical structures in close proximity to the sternal table (eg, right ventricle, coronary artery bypass graft), or adverse vascular access.

Given the likelihood for incidental findings on a near full-body scan, the radiologist or cardiologist reviewing CTAs plays an important role in elucidating the significance of such findings and recommending the appropriate evaluation or follow-up. It is not uncommon in this patient population to encounter incidental findings such as suspicious pulmonary nodules, a variety of potential malignancies, occluded vasculature, or thrombus in the left atrial appendage or other portions of the heart. Incidental findings with the potential to affect life expectancy or quality of life need to be thoroughly evaluated by the appropriate specialty before TAVR. If further investigation of a suspicious finding is warranted and treatment is delayed, a patient under evaluation for severe aortic stenosis may undergo balloon aortic valvuloplasty (if anatomically and technically feasible) as a bridge to treatment or may be referred to palliative care.[8] Thus, the interpretation of the CTA and subsequent recommendations by the cardiovascular imaging specialist may influence the patient's options and timeline to treatment.

Cardiac Anesthesia

The level of involvement for cardiac anesthesia in TAVR cases varies greatly between programs and institutions. The use of monitored anesthesia care or moderate/conscious sedation for appropriate transfemoral TAVR cases is growing across the globe, but practice variations remain.[8] Engagement is based on a number of factors including historical relationships, procedural availability, and buy-in to the Heart Team and the specific anesthetic approaches used in this patient population. The Heart Team and institution may define patient and procedure-level criteria for the appropriate anesthesia approach (moderate or conscious sedation, general anesthesia), airway, and associated invasive lines. It is best practice to discuss the type and level of sedation, as well as who will administer medications, on a case-by-case basis, ideally during the Heart Team meeting. This decision is multifaceted and nuanced; for further reference please see chapter 9.

Valve Program Clinician

The VPC contributes to Heart Team discussions on patient selection, with emphasis on the anticipated improvement in quality of life and recovery potential. As the member of the team likely to spend the greatest quantity of time interacting directly with the patient and the family, the VPC is well positioned to develop a trustworthy rapport and maintain this across the continuum of care. Frequently, it is through this relationship that details emerge regarding psychosocial aspects of the patient's case, which are not readily accessible through routine testing but may negatively affect recovery. For instance, defining the patient's social structure is critical; identification of the patient's caregivers, confidants, friends, and family gives insight into the patient's postprocedure support. The procedure is only the first step to recovery. The subsequent steps require diligence and dedication to regain strength and stamina via physical activity and cardiac rehabilitation.

The VPC investigates logistics important to define before the procedure: on discharge, what support measures are in place to check on the patient, ensure prescriptions and groceries are available, help with necessary activities of daily living, and provide companionship during the initial stages of recovery? This assessment aims to facilitate early and safe discharge planning as well as reduced readmission rates.

The VPC acts as a constant along the care continuum and may serve as a source of comfort to the patient and family. The unique insight supplied by the VPC (ie, the "voice of reason") may embody the old adage "Just because we can doesn't mean that we should." Often the difficult and nuanced responsibility of managing expectations belongs to the VPC. This includes expectations of patients, family members, caregivers, and referring providers. Please see chapter 4 for further discussion and role delineation.

Nursing/Nurse Navigator/Patient Navigator

Education for patients, family members, and caregivers is essential at every stage of the journey when considering, preparing for, and recovering from TAVR. Although all members of the Heart Team may educate patients and families, the central responsibility of teaching "what to expect when expecting" and recovering from TAVR typically lies with the nonphysician members of the Heart Team: the VPC, allied health professionals, APPs, and nurses.

Some centers have adopted a designated navigator role, typically staffed by nurses. This role has emerged from professional society cardiovascular quality initiatives (eg, ACC FOCUS MI to support hospital discharge and reduce readmissions), with an emphasis on education and care coordination and evidence-based practice to improve patient experience and outcomes.[10] In contrast to the VPC who may have overarching coordination responsibilities for the program as a whole, the navigator position frequently has specific, patient-facing duties and objectives. On a Heart Team with a VPC and a navigator, it may be the navigator who serves as a central point of contact for patients and their families. Common items addressed by the navigator include addressing expectations before and after the procedure, questions regarding medications, education, instructions regarding preoperative testing, logistics of where and when to report on procedure day, and questions during recovery.

As patient care plans and best practices evolve, Core and Extended Heart Team members require the most current information. Typically, education, empowerment, and engagement of the Heart Team membership is provided by nurses, navigators, VPCs, and APPs. Role delineation may vary from team to team; for example, the nurse navigator may conduct functional and cognitive assessments. The nurse on the Heart Team serves as a source of information for preprocedure planning, such as medication adjustments or anticoagulation protocols before TAVR. Communication and patient education are among the notable strengths of the nurses on the Heart Team.

With understood variation between programs that utilize these positions, the nurse navigator, VPC, and APP may have distinct but complementary responsibilities. For example, the workup of incidental findings necessitates vigilant and timely coordination so that a prognosis may be adjudicated and appropriate tests or treatment may be expedited. For patients who meet criteria for extreme frailty, these 3 valuable members of the team may be responsible for arranging prehabilitation and/or a bridging balloon aortic valvuloplasty to aid in symptom alleviation and strength training before re-evaluation with the Heart Team. The dynamic care and coordination provided by any permutation of nurse navigator, VPC, and APP is particularly highlighted in complicated cases or scenarios requiring additional evaluation or treatment before TAVR.

Advanced Practice Providers

In countries that utilize these roles, APPs have emerged as vital members of the Heart Team. Although scope of practice and licensure vary, APPs may serve as the front line of provider-level care along the entire continuum. For example, physician assistants and nurse practitioners commonly participate in initial patient consultations with the CTS and IC, as well as contribute to the preliminary treatment plan based on risk stratification (STS risk scores, functional and cognitive assessments) and imaging studies (echocardiography, CTA). In accordance with licensure and scope, the APP may perform a preprocedure history and physical, obtain informed consent for procedures, and review preadmission testing (eg, chest x-ray, electrocardiogram, and laboratory studies). The APP may also prescribe or adjust medications in advance of diagnostic tests and procedures (eg, medication protocols for contrast allergy, diabetes, or anticoagulation/antiplatelet).

APPs may also manage the postoperative course of patients with TAVR, serve as stewards of evidence-based practice as standards evolve, and ensure that patient safety remains paramount at all times. For example, assuring early mobilization for patients who do not require a higher level of intensive care unit care is essential to timely recovery and decreased delirium.[11,12] Fast-track, minimalist recovery care pathways and protocols exist for safe yet swift transition to cardiac units bypassing intensive care when appropriate.[12] The benefits of these care pathways include safety with decreased morbidity and mortality, decreased length of stay, and decreased resource utilization, which significantly lowers hospital costs.[12] Next-day discharge after minimalist transfemoral TAVR has been shown to be safe while achieving similar 30-day and superior 1-year clinical outcomes.[13] Physician members of the team, frequently in the operating room or cardiac catheterization laboratory performing procedures, may collaborate with APPs to assess and intervene as appropriate to optimize the patient's course of hospitalization. If there is an unexpected deviation from the postprocedure trajectory, the APP may expeditiously assess and relay findings to the members of the Heart Team, as well as recommend or provide subsequent interventions.

In some institutions, there are inpatient as well as outpatient provider-level duties assigned to APPs (eg, preprocedure history and physical, hospital admission after the procedure, daily rounds, hospital discharge, and follow-up visits). The APPs, VPC, and nursing staff partner diligently to ensure patient safety and optimal clinical outcomes. For example, the efforts of the VPC to explore the patient's social support structure and psychosocial needs during the evaluation process in turn give the APP the tools to facilitate early and safe discharge planning with the inpatient team. This continuity of care serves the patient and the family and can be incredibly gratifying for the APP.

APPs may perform follow-up visits and based on program need may have dedicated follow-up clinics to improve throughput in busy clinics with limited patient access. At these visits, there is careful attention paid to data points required for research trials as well as the national registries such as the STS/ACC TVT Registry. In this visit, the APP also documents adverse events and provides reassurance and encouragement, as well as education on cardiac rehabilitation and endocarditis prophylaxis. Follow-up echocardiograms may also be ordered and reviewed by APPs to ensure that there is no evidence of premature valve degeneration, leaflet thrombosis, or increasing central or paravalvular aortic insufficiency.

Administrative Staff

A patient diagnosed with severe VHD is referred to a Valve Center to discuss disease state and severity, progression, and potential treatment options. The first point of contact between the patient and the Valve Center, and often the referring provider, is the administrative support team (eg, administrative assistants, schedulers, telephone receptionists, front desk personnel, and billing specialists). This initial communication (via telephone call, voice mail, or e-mail) is critical, as this "first impression" sets the tone for the initial visit to the institution and for the overall patient and referring provider experience.

Establishing initial contact and scheduling a consultation is a daunting first step in the process for patients and families. It is important to engage administrative support staff to provide a seamless and pleasant experience throughout all interactions with the Valve Center, Heart Team, and institution. Equally important are frequent reminders of the impact that the work of the administrative staff, both behind the scenes and patient facing, has on overall experience. This concept also applies to providers who are referring patients for Heart Team evaluation. Effective communication is the cornerstone of best practice with an emphasis on empathetic patient and family interactions.

Extended Heart Team
Referring Provider

The referring provider is an important extended member of the Heart Team. This is a relationship enriched by a foundation of timely and concise communication. Like any relationship, this needs to be cultivated and encouraged to flourish. The Heart Team should investigate ideal methods of communication for referring providers. These methods not only vary owing to personal preference but also are evolving in the digital age in which we live. Perhaps old fashioned, but the ideal may be a personal phone call from a member of the Heart Team to the referring provider with updates on procedural plan, clinical course, complications, medication changes, and follow-up expectations. These telephone calls are likely supplemented with written or digital documentation of the hospital course and pertinent details. Institutions may choose to include the referring provider in the Heart Team meeting in which his or her patient will be reviewed. There may also be opportunities for joint education including procedural observation if schedules allow.

Consultative Specialties

As alluded to throughout this text, patients with severe VHD and a myriad of comorbidities have a complex condition and may require multiple specialists to address their specific needs. With "more cooks in the kitchen," accuracy and timeliness of information become even more critical to a patient's journey. Consultative specialties may include gerontology, palliative care, oncology, hepatology, hematology, neurology, psychiatry, nephrology, vascular surgery, pulmonary, heart failure, and intensivists. These specialists are extended members of the Heart Team and, when needed, prove integral to a patient's clinical course and outcome. The addition of specialists and subspecialties increases the complexity of care coordination. Nurses, the VPC, or APPs on the Heart Team serve as patient advocates and may provide a central voice to succinctly explain and clarify recommendations into terminology more easily digestible for the patient. With the addition of consultative specialties, effective communication transparent to the entire care team is increasingly critical and must be followed closely to ensure clarity and safety of the treatment plan.

Administrative Leadership

The engagement of an institution's administrative leadership (eg, managers, directors, executives) is key to a program achieving its full potential. This potential may be influenced by infrastructure and resources to support expedited patient screening processes, optimal procedural capacity and throughput, staffing models to accommodate evolution in postprocedure care, and financial sustainability.

A physician champion may be the central voice of the Heart Team representing goals, vision, and programmatic strategy to the hospital administrators. A high level of commitment to the program by administration facilitates the implementation of planned change when the Heart Team aims to adjust staffing models, shift culture, modify current processes, engage nursing, increase procedural throughput, and evolve patient care pathways. Buy-in from the institution's administrative leadership, which has financial, strategic, and operational oversight, is essential to the success of the program.

Hospital Staff

The hospital staff may comprise various departments and units in an institution. Broadly, these members of the Extended Heart Team include the clinical staff (physicians, nursing, and allied health) caring for patients during their TAVR hospitalization. These staff implement pathways through admission (eg, nurses), procedure (eg, operating room technicians and nurses, cardiac catheterization laboratory technicians and nurses, anesthesia technicians and nurses), postprocedure (eg, APPs, physicians, nurses, physical therapists, respiratory therapists, social workers, consultative specialties), and discharge (nurses, coordinators). Also critical to this continuum are the echocardiography sonographers/technicians and, if applicable, research coordinators and quality registry/data managers.

As each of the roles of the members of the Heart Team have been described in this section, please note that these members may not be standard across all programs. Each member of the team is encouraged to draw on their experience and strengths to work within the scope of their license and competency to ensure that all aspects of care coordination are addressed.

How to Build a Functional Heart Team

Mechanisms to Increase Effectiveness of the Heart Team

To build an effective, productive, efficient Heart Team, a certain fundamental element needs to be understood: each member must recognize and embrace the importance of his/her work and how it affects patients' lives (Table 2.3). The work being done by the Heart Team can be the difference between life and death. Maintaining this perspective is of the utmost importance for every member of the Heart Team to keep top of mind. The next section reviews key ingredients for a "recipe for success" in forming, maintaining, and cultivating a Heart Team. As stated previously, the model and best practices described here may differ between institutions and there is credence given to each unique construct.

Meeting Structure

Regularly scheduled meetings are the essential forums to discuss care of the patients who have entrusted their health to the Heart Team. These meetings are platforms to discuss patients under evaluation for VHD and considered for potential treatment. Attendance

TABLE 2.3. Tips for Improving Effectiveness of the Heart Team

- Foster engagement and buy-in of all team members
- Decide, as a group, on common goals and how to define success of the Heart Team
- Emphasize repeatedly this shared vision and make this your mantra
- Define the purpose of the Heart Team and discuss what rewards or incentives may exist
- Delineate roles utilizing individual's strengths and expertise
- Embrace camaraderie and solidarity as a group
- Treat each team member in a respectful manner
- Stress that the success of the team is about the members as a whole and not centered on a particular individual
- Hold each member accountable, strive to honor agreements, and meet agreed-upon expectations
- Keep morale as high as possible. Team-building events are a good way to reconnect and relax with your teammates
- Celebrate successes of the Heart Team and congratulate members for a job well done
- Discuss openly all cases, particularly those with unexpected or undesirable outcomes to identify lessons learned and practice changes to apply in the future

TABLE 2.4. Example of Best Practices for Assembling Effective Heart Team Meetings

- Determine the Heart Team member roles for the meeting (eg, coordinated and led by the valve program clinician [VPC])

- Determine whose attendance is required (ie, typical Heart Team members who must be in attendance include cardiothoracic surgeon(s), interventional cardiologist, cardiac imaging specialist, anesthesiologist, VPC, and, if applicable, nurse navigator and research coordinator)

- Set the agenda beforehand, including a list of patients to discuss and making readily available all pertinent information

- Establish a routinely scheduled day and time that works for key stakeholders/Core Heart Team members to attend

- Foster mutual agreements among team members for meeting attendance (eg, the meeting is essential and they will be present unless circumstances beyond their control arise)

- Dedicate a physical meeting space with capability to review the electronic medical record (EMR) and diagnostic images (eg, echocardiograms, CT scans, cardiac catheterizations)

- Set ground rules to facilitate respect and support of team members and allow for all opinions and voices to be heard. By these rules, the multidisciplinary team members should each be given the chance to contribute to the discussion and final consensus will be reached as a group

- Document Heart Team decisions (eg, clinical dispositions, procedural plans) in the EMR for all members to access and reference

CT, computed tomography.

is often mandatory for core members. Meetings comprise a strict agenda, which may be organized and steered by the VPC, and includes reviewing screening tests, frailty and cognitive assessments, patient preferences and shared decision making, social support, and procedural planning (ie, procedure, valve type and size, vascular access, sedation preference, location of procedure, and procedural date). It is advisable that meetings use best practices (Table 2.4).

Communication Within the Heart Team

Interpersonal communication differs between each Heart Team, as they are unique entities in and of themselves. Identification of the most effective means of communication within the group frequently becomes a responsibility of the VPC. In this digital age, there are various modalities to remind team members of meetings, such as e-mails, text messages, and calendar invitation reminders. For time-sensitive matters or complex issues, direct communication (eg, phone call) is often preferable. When electronic communication methods are used, specific patient-related questions and discussions occur via encrypted, secure environments. A patient's privacy and sensitive medical information need only be addressed by immediate members of the care team, and privacy laws (ie, in the United States, Health Insurance Portability and Accountability Act or HIPAA) are to be respected at all times.

Ongoing effort of all Heart Team members to ensure that effective communication remains intact and the methods evolve as necessary is essential. At times, teams may face an element of "communication fatigue." Should this occur, it is recommended that the group be reinvigorated by readdressing the shared vision and common goals. What is it we are doing? Why does it matter? What does success look like? It is human nature to lose focus on objectives if inundated by the minutia of the day-to-day routine. Communication between the Heart Team members is crucial to success, and solidifying effective channels to connect will benefit everyone, especially the patient.

How to Manage Differing Opinions of Heart Team Members

Not uncommonly there will be differing opinions between Heart Team members regarding patient care. These can be difficult conversations to navigate, and at times a moderator may be required. This role can be held by any member of the team, including the VPC. These nuanced discussions must be handled in a thoughtful, respectful, and nonjudgmental manner. Ideally, the opinions of all members of the team are heard and decisions made after consideration of all viewpoints. The formerly agreed upon shared vision and goals for the program and patient care can serve as a framework to house these difficult discussions. Avoidance of abrasive language, dismissive behavior, or poor conduct is advised and should not be tolerated by the members of the team. The 2012 expert consensus document on TAVR highlights a Heart Team "demonstrating mutual trust and commitment."[1,14] It is unreasonable to think that the Heart Team will unanimously and harmoniously agree on all aspects of every patient's care plan. However, the methods by which these discussions are conducted are critical to the ultimate sustainability of the team. Respect for all team members should be observed and reflected in behavior at all times and may be facilitated by the use of a moderator, reference to shared goals, and application of guidelines and expert recommendations.

Heart Team Responsibilities

Setting Expectations

Challenges relayed by patients, families, referring providers, and extended members of the care team may involve this central theme: the desire for clear expectations and concise communication. The Heart Team must implement methods to communicate with patients and families while clearly outlining team members and roles as well as what to expect during the processes of screening, treatment, recovery, and follow-up.

Expectations are set via education, which is essential in both written and verbal forms. Programs that use a standard packet of information with team photographs, names, and roles find this piece instrumental in outlining central members of the care team. In the era of modern technology, educational videos can be used as adjuncts to written and verbal teachings and instructions. Whatever the modalities used, a standardized approach using materials that can be easily understood by a variety of reading and education levels should be developed.

Constant reinforcement of expectations is preferred, and no one will complain about overcommunication! Setting expectations and in turn building confidence and trust in the members of the Heart Team start at first impression and are commonly solidified at time of the initial consultation. In an ideal world, a patient leaves the consultation appointment with the impressions listed in Table 2.5.

TABLE 2.5. Ideal Patient Impressions After Initial Consultation With the Heart Team

- "I met all of the members of the team and know what their roles are in my care."

- "I had plenty of time with the doctor(s) on my first visit and he/she answered all of my questions."

- "I am clear about the treatment options."

- "The team asked what I wanted and I really feel that my wishes were heard and honored."

- "By the end of the visit my family and I knew what the plan was and had a very good idea of when it would happen."

- "By the end of the visit I had a clear understanding of my disease and my prognosis with and without a procedure."

- "My local doctor had good communication with the Heart Team and was kept in the loop."

Setting realistic expectations for referring providers is critical in regard to treatment options, timeline of procedure, recovery, and follow-up. As an extended member of the Heart Team, the referring provider may be asked to participate at various stages of a patient's journey. He/she may be asked to attend in person or via telephone the team meeting in which results and final disposition for the patient will occur. Providers may wish to attend the procedure if possible and kept apprised of postprocedure clinical course. Time of discharge, changes to medication regimen, anticoagulation, adverse events or complications, and detailed description of the procedure should be made readily available and communicated to the provider.

Some programs use personal phone calls as well as the medical record to convey important pieces of information. Discharge packets can be sent to the referring provider with pertinent items such as the hospital discharge summary, procedure or operative report, most recent echocardiogram, laboratory values, discharge medication list, and follow-up plans. A personalized letter accompanying these documents is a nice touch, which may aid in cultivating and maintaining the strength of this relationship. It is important to emphasize to the patient that the referring provider is involved in each decision the Heart Team makes and that after the procedure, he/she will continue to direct and manage cardiac care.

Shared Decision Making

"The goal of TAVR is to prolong life and either improve poor quality or maintain high quality of life."[15] The Heart Team is responsible for initiating complex conversations with the patient during the screening portion of the process to explore potential factors that may predispose the patient to a poor outcome. First, how do we define a poor outcome? Arnold and colleagues define poor outcome 6 months following TAVR as "death or KCCQ <45 or KCCQ decrease of ≥10 points."[16] Of note, as an end point, quality of life is as important as mortality.[5] The Heart Team must address the reasonable anticipated improvement in quality of life the patient can expect. In elderly patient populations, goals of treatment may favor quality of life over survival.[5]

Professional guidelines recommend using a SDM process to lead to decisions and treatment care plans that are aligned with patient-defined goals of care.[5] In attempts to personalize the procedure and explore potential benefit for each patient, comprehensive screening must include comorbidities, overall baseline health status, functional capacity, cognitive impairment,

TABLE 2.6. Examples of Questions to Elicit Candid Patient Responses in Shared Decision Making

- In your own words, how would you describe your current quality of life?
- What are you not able to do at this point that you would like to resume?
- Do you think TAVR might offer improvement in your overall quality of life?
- What matters most to you?
- What confuses you the most in talking about the treatment options?
- What is your most feared outcome?
- Do you believe the benefit of TAVR will outweigh the risks?

TAVR, transcatheter aortic valve replacement.

social support, and motivation. SDM is a unique process in which pointed conversations and decision aids are used to illustrate a patient's prognosis and available treatment options. For example, an effective inquiry at the time of consultation might include the question "What do you hope to accomplish by having your valve replaced?"[5] Additional examples of questions used to elicit a patient's preferences and goals of care can be seen in Table 2.6.

The ability to perform a specific activity and spend time with loved ones are the most common patient-defined goals, and these outweigh the goal of simply staying alive.[5] By focusing on patient-centered goals for therapy, treatment options can be chosen while incorporating the patient's specific goals of therapy. Identifying patient preferences is a pivotal step in SDM, and members of the Heart Team can be successful in obtaining preferences and goals.[5] The SDM process (Figure 2.2) is one that must be embraced and perpetuated by the Heart Team for every patient and applied in standardized and methodical ways (Figures 2.3–2.5).

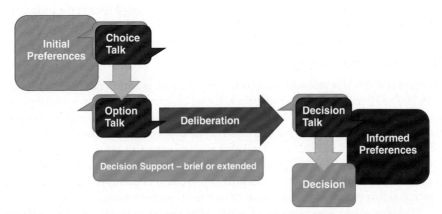

FIGURE 2.2. Overview of the shared decision making conversation. (Courtesy of Megan Coylewright. The Call for Shared Decision Making in Severe Aortic Stenosis. From Policy to Implementation. Dartmouth-Hitchcock Medical Center, The Dartmouth Institute for Clinical Practice and Health Policy. Adapted from Joseph-Williams N, Lloyd A, Edwards A, et al. Implementing shared decision making in the NHS: lessons from the MAGIC programme. *BMJ.* 2017;357:j1744.)

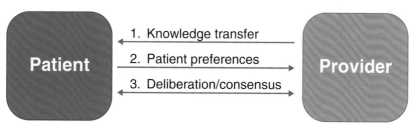

FIGURE 2.3. Broad overview of the shared decision making process and transfer of information. (Courtesy of Megan Coylewright. The Call for Shared Decision Making in Severe Aortic Stenosis. From Policy to Implementation. Dartmouth-Hitchcock Medical Center, The Dartmouth Institute for Clinical Practice and Health Policy. Data from Charles C, Gafni A, Whelan T. Decision-making in the physician-patient encounter: revisiting the shared treatment decision-making model. *Soc Sci Med.* 1999;49(5):651-661 and Spatz ES, Spertus JA. Shared decision making: a path toward improved patient-centered outcomes. *Circ Cardiovasc Qual Outcomes.* 2012;5(6):e75-e77.)

Patient Selection

At times, it is necessary for the group to participate in candid, sometimes uncomfortable, conversations regarding patient selection. These scenarios may include futility or lack of procedural options from an anatomic standpoint. Other times, the team may believe a patient is a good candidate for the procedure, but the patient wishes to have medical management without invasive interventions and those wishes need to be honored. There are chapters

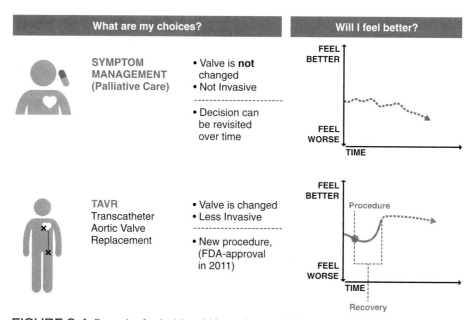

FIGURE 2.4. Example of a decision aid in aortic stenosis (used in discussing the disease and its progression, pros and cons of treatment options, and procedural risk). FDA, US Food and Drug Administration; TAVR, transcatheter aortic valve replacement. (Courtesy of Megan Coylewright. The Call for Shared Decision Making in Severe Aortic Stenosis. From Policy to Implementation. Dartmouth-Hitchcock Medical Center, The Dartmouth Institute for Clinical Practice and Health Policy.)

1. **Name** the choices
2. **Explain** shared decision making
3. **Describe** the choices using the decision aid
4. **Listen** to what matters most to the patient
5. **Make a decision together** using patient preferences

FIGURE 2.5. Key components in implementation of shared decision making. (Courtesy of Megan Coylewright. The Call for Shared Decision Making in Severe Aortic Stenosis. From Policy to Implementation. Dartmouth-Hitchcock Medical Center, The Dartmouth Institute for Clinical Practice and Health Policy.)

in this text dedicated to the nuances of patient selection. However, here it is reiterated that Heart Team consensus is essential in all circumstances but even more critical for complex cases. Even when there are no anatomic barriers to proceeding with a procedure, it is the responsibility and duty of the Heart Team to consider all aspects of the patient's baseline health and functional and cognitive status before moving forward with intervention. For example, in the aforementioned instance in which a patient's anatomy is desirable but he/she demonstrates extreme frailty, what reasonable anticipated improvement in quality of life can be expected? In cases such as these it is not uncommon for the Heart Team to consider bridging balloon aortic valvuloplasty or prehabilitation with close monitoring on clinical improvement before scheduling intervention. At the heart of each patient disposition are these questions for the Heart Team: "Does the benefit outweigh the risk? Just because we can do this procedure, should we?"

Procedural Planning

Members of the Heart Team decide on crucial aspects of procedural planning, including the type of intervention, sedation, location of procedure and subsequent recovery, type of imaging required preprocedure and periprocedure, required personnel, equipment, and bail-out or contingency planning. Procedural planning is discussed in detail in chapter 10.

Conclusions

Just as the paradigm and role of the Heart Team has evolved in the brief history of transcatheter valve therapy, it will continue to change over time. The Heart Team will need to demonstrate flexibility in accommodating future iterations as the technology and the care pathways for patients continue to mature. There is also speculation that the model of the team meeting may advance to include increasing patient involvement as well.[1] Furthermore, the number of institutions that offer additional transcatheter therapies for structural heart disease will continue to grow. TAVR has prompted a revision of the care model for patients suffering from aortic stenosis, and this shift will likely affect other specialties in the future. Multidisciplinary, team-based, patient-centric, high-quality, cost-effective care will continue to permeate all aspects of modern medical practice.

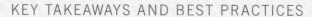

KEY TAKEAWAYS AND BEST PRACTICES

▶ The overarching purpose of the Heart Team is to provide team-based, patient-centric, high-quality, cost-effective care for patients with aortic stenosis.

▶ The construct of the Heart Team will vary slightly between programs; however, it fundamentally comprises core and extended members who collectively provide care across the continuum.

▶ Building an effective Heart Team demands engagement of its members, and the success of the team as a whole depends on each member embracing designated roles and responsibilities.

▶ Consistent, high-level communication within the team is mandatory to provide optimized patient care as well as member satisfaction. This includes ongoing efforts to avoid communication fatigue by regular reiteration of the team's shared vision and common goals.

▶ The Heart Team will function as a cohesive unit and strive to set reasonable expectations, emphasize SDM, ensure proper patient selection, detail procedural planning, and implement optimized clinical care pathways.

References

1. Coylewright M, Mack MJ, Holmes DR, O'Gara PT. A call for evidence-based approach to the heart team for patients with severe aortic stenosis. *J Am Coll Cardiol*. 2015;65(14):1472-1480.

2. Nishimura RA, Otto CM, Bonow RO, et al. 2014 AHA/ACC guideline for the management of patients with valvular heart disease: a report of the American College of Cardiology/American heart association task force on practice guidelines. *J Am Coll Cardiol*. 2014;63(22):e69-e70.

3. Holmes DR, Mohr F, Hamm CW, Mack MJ. Venn diagrams in cardiovascular disease: the heart team concept. *Ann Thorac Surg*. 2013;95(2):389-391.

4. Nallamothu BK, Cohen DJ. No "I" in heart team: incentivizing multidisciplinary care in cardiovascular medicine. *Circ Cardiovasc Qual Outcomes*. 2012;5(3):410-413.

5. Coylewright M, Palmer R, O'Neill ES, Robb JF, Fried TR. Patient-defined goals for the treatment of severe aortic stenosis: a qualitative analysis. *Health Expect*. 2016;19(5):1036-1043.

6. Del Sindaco D, Pulignano G, Minardi G, Apostoli A, et al. Two-year outcome of a prospective, controlled study of a disease management programme for elderly patients with heart failure. *J Cardiovasc Med (Hagerstown)*. 2007;8(5):324-329.

7. Ducharme A, Doyon O, White M, Rouleau JL, Brophy JM. Impact of care at a multidisciplinary congestive heart failure clinic: a randomized trial. *CMAJ*. 2005;173(1):40-45.

8. O'Gara PT, Grayburn PA, Badhwar V, et al. 2017 ACC expert consensus decision pathway on the management of mitral regurgitation. A report of the American College of Cardiology task force on expert consensus decision pathways. *J Am Coll Cardiol*. 2017;70(19):2421-2449.

9. Apfaltrer P, Henzler T, Blanke P, Krazinski AW, Silverman JR, Schoepf UJ. Computed tomography for planning transcatheter aortic valve replacement. *J Thorac Cardiovasc Surg*. 2012;144(3):e29-e84.

10. American College of Cardiology. *Patient Navigator Program Completes Hospital Selection: Team Approach Will Smooth Transition Home for Patients, Reduce Readmissions* [Press release]. Available at: http://www.acc.org/about-acc/press-releases/2014/10/28/13/06/patient-navigator-program-national-release-2; October 28, 2014.

11. Lauck SB, Wood DA, Baumbusch J, et al. Vancouver transcatheter aortic valve replacement clinical pathway minimalist approach, standardized care, and discharge criteria to reduce length of stay. *Circ Cardiovasc Qual Outcomes*. 2016;9(3):312-321.

12. Babaliaros V, Devireddy C, Lerakis S, et al. Comparison of transfemoral transcatheter aortic valve replacement performed in the catheterization laboratory (minimalist approach) versus hybrid operating room (standard approach): outcomes and cost analysis. *JACC Cardiovasc Interv*. 2014;7(8):898-904.

13. Kamioka N, Wells J, Keegan P, et al. Predictors and clinical outcomes of next-day discharge after minimalist transfemoral transcatheter aortic valve replacement. *JACC Cardiovasc Interv*. 2018;11(2):107-115.

14. Holmes DR, Mack MJ, Kaul S, et al. 2012 ACCF/AATS/SCAI/STS expert consensus document on transcatheter aortic valve replacement. *J Am Coll Cardiol*. 2012;59:1200-1254.

15. Green P, Arnold SV, Cohen DJ, et al. Relation of frailty to outcomes after transcathter aortic valve replacement (from the PARTNER trial). *Am J Cardiol*. 2015;116(2):264-269.

16. Arnold SV, Reynolds MR, Lei Y, et al. Predictors of poor outcomes after transcatheter aortic valve replacement: results from the PARTNER (Placement of Aortic Transcatheter Valve) trial. *Circulation*. 2014;129(25):2682-2690.

CHAPTER 3

The Valve Program Clinician

Marian C. Hawkey, RN | *Bettina Hoejberg Kirk, RN, MSN*

OBJECTIVES

▶ Highlight the importance and unique role of the valve program clinician
▶ Describe required competencies and specialized knowledge for the valve program clinician

The Central Importance of the Valve Program Clinician

As discussed in the previous chapter, international guidelines recommend a multi-disciplinary Heart Team approach across the continuum of care for patients undergoing transcatheter aortic valve replacement (TAVR). A successful program with favorable patient outcomes relies on ongoing efforts to optimize practice and care pathways. Central to the multidisciplinary Heart Team is the clinician who leads the coordination of the program, facilitates patient-focused processes of care, and fosters communication pathways. The role of these clinicians is the central focus of this chapter. As we proceed, it is important to remember that there is variability and diversity across programs; the role we discuss may not perfectly describe the role or perspective of the individual reader. We are drawing from our collective experience and expertise to provide as comprehensive a representation as possible, inclusive of the experiences of our US, Canadian, and European colleagues.

As transcatheter valve programs have evolved over the past decade or so, this role has historically been identified as the "Valve Clinic Coordinator" or "TAVR Program Coordinator." Neither label perfectly defines the role and its associated competencies and by no means intends to minimize the magnitude of expertise and responsibility. During the development of this text, we recognized the need to reconsider the nomenclature for the role to better capture the associated clinical responsibilities. We are acutely aware of the challenges of identifying a universally acceptable and appropriate title but feel compelled to propose a more inclusive professional designation. To this end, we use valve program clinician (VPC) to describe this essential role on the Heart Team. Our intention is to acknowledge the diverse clinical backgrounds of the health care professionals who function in this position and the wide scope of responsibilities that are primarily grounded in clinical practice.

It should be noted that much of our knowledge base and understanding of this role is anecdotal and a product of our collective experience. Thus far, there has been a dearth of relevant evidence to support delineating the responsibilities and measuring the impact of VPCs. There are, however, references supporting the benefits of nurses' central, coordinating role in other clinical subspecialties, such as the management of patients with heart failure.[1] The first foundation for the VPC role was established by research nurses and coordinators during the early feasibility and pivotal TAVR clinical trials. These members of the research teams were essential in the coordination and development of clinical pathways and processes of care for the patients at every point of their journey from referral to long-term follow-up. Indeed, many of these practices remain part of our current standards with iterations that have occurred over time in response to the evolution of TAVR technology, patients' needs, and program growth.

Valve Program Clinician Role Description

The central importance of the VPC cannot be emphasized strongly enough and has been established as the standard of care to meet the needs of patients and sustain the success of TAVR program development.[2] The VPC is often integral to the fostering of collaborative and mutually supportive interdepartmental relationships and maintaining essential processes of communication. Frequently, the VPC has a nursing background as a registered nurse or nurse practitioner, and physician assistants also function as VPCs in many settings. The scope of practice is subject to professional regulations, and responsibilities depend on the level of education and training. The role can be well adapted across the continuum of allied health care professionals. Although this diversity enriches the position, it also highlights the challenges of guiding practice to manage the complexity of TAVR program coordination. The VPC role is multifunctional by necessity to adequately attend to TAVR patient and program needs (Figure 3.1).

The challenges of the VPC role are in large part related to the complexity of the patient population diagnosed with valvular heart disease and living with multiple health vulnerabilities. Our patients are primarily geriatric with varying degrees of comorbid burden as well as cognitive and/or functional decline in many cases. Patient needs vary along the trajectory of care. The coordination of the evaluation pathway is essential to support careful case selection. Best practice is to facilitate the completion of diagnostic tests, consultations with cardiologists and surgeons, and assessment of functional status and frailty in a comprehensive clinic visit that minimizes patient burden.[3] Facilitation and delivery of patient-centered processes of care rely heavily on the skillset of the VPC. The VPC is instrumental in attending to patient and family education and expectations, case managing preprocedure optimization protocols, and coordinating early planning for postprocedure and discharge care needs. In collaboration with the postprocedure team, the VPC facilitates discharge and safe transition home and the coordination of follow-up to prevent gaps in care. As patients recover and reintegrate with their primary health care provider, the VPC may continue to act as an expert clinician and ongoing contact for patients and their family.

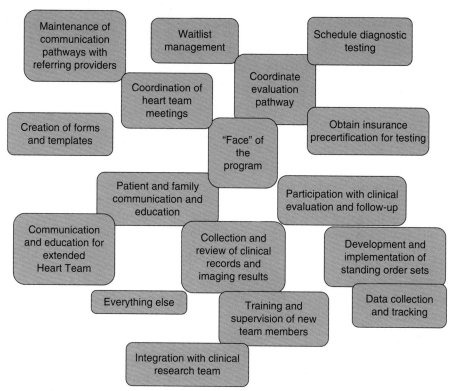

FIGURE 3.1. The many moving parts of the valve program clinician role.

The VPC can influence the quality and method of local or registry-required data collection as well as implement initiatives to strengthen utilization of these metrics to improve outcomes, processes, and program structure. For example, the regular reporting of quality and outcome data to the Heart Team supplies essential information to improve practice. Transparency and ease of accessibility to these quality indicators raise the awareness and engagement of senior administrative and medical leadership; this in turn accelerates quality and program improvement strategies.

A single and potentially isolated VPC may be in place when a program is in its early stages of growth and development. However, as programs expand and volume increases in response to new indications and the growing availability of catheter-based structural heart procedures, there may be multiple personnel required to adequately manage the full array of VPC-designated activities. For example, once the essential clinical operations are in place, an important addition to the team may be in a clerical/administrative role to handle time-consuming, day-to-day tasks, such as scheduling, obtaining and distributing records, and managing health insurance–related requirements. The amount of time diverted from clinical to administrative tasks can be a significant source of dissatisfaction and suboptimal use of VPC qualifications and competencies. This must be considered when choosing a course of action to expand the staff.

Valve Program Clinician Responsibilities

The VPC role is not identical from one institution to another but broadly encompasses the following areas of responsibility (Table 3.1):

- Program leadership and coordination
- Facilitation of patient-focused processes of care
- Fostering of Heart Team communication pathways

Program Leadership and Coordination

The VPC is a foundational Heart Team member and is often perceived by patients, clinicians, and administrators as the "face of the program" with the primary responsibility of developing programmatic processes, including throughput of referrals, efficient evaluation and postprocedure pathway logistics, fostering relationships with ancillary departments, and organization of clinical data. VPCs are instrumental in program growth and optimization in collaboration with the Heart Team. Inherent in these responsibilities is the capability to sustain engagement of the extended Heart Team by the implementation of durable communication pathways and educational initiatives that ensure consistency and quality across the continuum of care. These responsibilities may require management by more than one person, especially as a program grows and patient volume increases.

Facilitation of Patient-Focused Processes of Care

Navigation through the diagnostic testing required for evaluation can be arduous as our patients are frequently elderly with varying degrees of symptoms and mobility challenges. Most are accompanied by at least one, if not many, family members, whereas some may lack social support. It is commonly within the scope of the VPC to develop an evaluation pathway model that is efficient while simultaneously tailored to the limitations of our patients. This requires consideration of diagnostic testing schedules and locations and is often a balance of the benefit of consolidating appointments in a single versus multiple visits. Patients and their families often have a preference as to what may work best for them; the VPC takes these preferences into account whenever possible. The best laid plans are, however, not a guarantee that we will not find some tired, hungry, and possibly grumpy clients in our waiting rooms at the end of a long clinic day. The VPC can play a pivotal role in anticipating seemingly minor needs that can cause significant patient and family stress. For example, provision of information about the expected duration and itinerary for the day and the suggestion to bring a snack in case a meal break is not feasible can have a significant impact on patient and family satisfaction.

The VPC contributes to the development and maintenance of efficient and comprehensive periprocedural and postprocedural pathways; this activity involves extensive engagement with the extended Heart Team. Procedural planning requires careful integration of not only the procedural operators and imaging experts but also anesthesiology, cardiac catheterization laboratory and/or operating room clinical staff, cardiac perfusion, and the clinical research team where applicable. Optimization of the postprocedure recovery pathway necessitates clear communication and adherence to the established processes of care, as well as engagement with the nursing staff in the areas where patients recover after the procedure.

TABLE 3.1. Valve Program Clinician Role Description

Program Leadership and Coordination

- Serves as foundational Heart Team member

- Supports program development in collaboration with the Heart Team

- Participates in program evaluation and supports the implementation of interventions to optimize patient outcomes and length of stay

- Assists with outreach initiatives

Facilitation of Patient-Focused Processes of Care

- Supports program development, including standardization of processes and clinical pathways

- Develops and coordinates processes for evaluation pathway, including diagnostic testing and functional assessments, and clinical triage

- Coordinates scheduling of diagnostic testing

- Assists with conduct of comprehensive history and physical examinations and cognitive/functional assessments

- Facilitates referrals to subspecialty consultants

- Assists with collection/review of clinical records and imaging data

- Contributes to treatment decision-making process

- Contributes to procedural planning and scheduling

- Coordinates early planning for postprocedure and discharge needs

- Develops processes for data collection and tracking, including for required registry

- Provides information and education to patient/family regarding disease management, evaluation pathway, treatment decision process, postprocedure care, and so on

- Assists patients and families with navigation of the evaluation process

- Assesses and manages patient/family expectations

Fosters Communication Pathways

- Serves as the primary point of contact across the continuum of care

- Participates in organization and leadership of team meetings

- Provides in-services and program updates for the extended Heart Team

- Supports ongoing communication with referring providers

- Identifies communication gaps and develops remedial processes

A common thread through all phases of the care continuum is the need for patient and family education as well as the management of expectations. Our patients may come to their initial clinic evaluation with preconceived ideas of their treatment options, the timing for delivery of care, and expectations about recovery. Our aim is to foster conversations, provide easily accessible information, and facilitate the process for shared decision making.[4] The VPC frequently develops a rapport based on extensive, ongoing communication with patients and families and thus plays a key role in the delivery of information and education. The evaluation pathway and decisions about treatment options are quite complex and require that information be provided in a clear and comprehensive manner. Information may be introduced at the time of the initial clinical evaluation by discussion as well as with written materials. Additional opportunities for ongoing teaching are often required. This is a particular area where family support can be especially valuable as some of our patients may have limited capacity to fully understand or recall all information that is provided. These discussions also facilitate the management of expectations. Patients may present with limited or erroneous understanding of the evaluation process, available treatment options, and anticipated benefits. The VPC is instrumental in assisting patients and families to align their expectations with Heart Team recommendations and a realistic appraisal of what may constitute a successful outcome. We commonly carry the "small" details about each individual patient that enable us to serve as knowledgeable advocates as they proceed on this journey.

Fostering Heart Team Communication Pathways

Some of the most critical and challenging processes are associated with the development and maintenance of communication pathways. Our first consideration is to develop foundational communication practices for our Heart Team. This will typically include the initiation of weekly team meetings for patient review and discussion of clinical and operational issues. Most programs find this to be an essential forum for making team-based treatment decisions and having a regular opportunity for group consideration of topics that affect programmatic growth and success. There may also be a periodic agenda for morbidity and mortality review and discussion to focus on quality improvement and critical examination of established practices.

The VPC may be responsible for engaging the extended Heart Team, which is inclusive of referring providers, cardiac catheterization laboratory and operating room staff, anesthesiologists, subspecialty consultants, critical care and cardiac unit staff, and ancillary departments. There is a need to coordinate communication with anyone who may be involved with our patients as they proceed through their evaluation and treatment pathways. Some extended Heart Team members may be included at team meetings. Other forms of communication such as wide-distribution e-mails are useful to circulate information regarding upcoming procedures. They can frequently be useful to organize meetings with the staff of treatment and clinical areas to share information on processes and goals of care. This is also an opportunity to proactively address questions and concerns and avert potential barriers to appropriate provision of care to our patients undergoing TAVR.

Communication with referring providers is essential throughout the continuum of care. Strategies may involve physician-to-physician communication and formal meetings. Nevertheless, the VPC remains the key point person to keep providers engaged and informed as patient evaluation proceeds and treatment decisions are made. This consistent sharing of information helps to maintain a strong relationship with referring providers and enables them to maintain a seamless delivery of care to our mutual patients.

Competencies and Specialized Knowledge

Most of us came to the VPC role from another position at our institutions with little or no training processes in place other than "trial by fire." As described by Benner's nursing novice to expert model, we may have started out as "advanced beginners" in the VPC role[5] with a solid clinical background to support us as we found our way through this new territory with the goal of becoming program experts. Our practice demands that we stay current on the latest evidence and guidelines in the rapidly developing field of TAVR. Although there are existing core curricula for cardiovascular allied health professionals,[6] there is, thus far, no established training curriculum across institutions for VPCs, a gap that we hope this text will bridge at least in part.

The VPC requires competency in cardiovascular and geriatric care, clinical leadership, and clinical program development. The specialized knowledge of clinical presentation, pathophysiology, and disease progression of aortic stenosis is foundational to the expertise of the VPC. An in-depth understanding of the trajectory of illness, including symptoms and disease progression, diagnostic testing and imaging modalities, and the array of available treatment options are particularly relevant to patient assessment, decision support, and clinical triage (Table 3.2).

TAVR programs are unique in their intensive reliance on imaging diagnostics, including echocardiography, computerized tomography, and cardiac catheterization, although perhaps outside of the scope of practice of the VPC, a degree of imaging literacy is a significant asset to specialized TAVR practice. Training focused on the basic principles of diagnostic imaging, and a road map to the landmarks of standard images, can help develop the appropriate alerts during the eligibility assessment and increase the professional development of the VPC.

Multidisciplinary case selection and consensus treatment decision informed by the expertise of cardiology, cardiac surgery, imaging specialists, and other members of the Heart Team are core functions of TAVR programs. The coordination of eligibility decision, risk stratification, and procedure planning is a key function of the VPC role. Team agreements, standardized processes, and ongoing coordination are vital to overcome logistical challenges, ensure the availability of clinical documentation, and facilitate multidisciplinary communication. Following treatment decision, the VPC may be responsible for coordinating the scheduling of the procedure and liaising with vendors to ensure the availability of required specialized devices and personnel. Lastly, TAVR programs require the implementation of a standardized postprocedure clinical pathway and the coordination of follow-up to optimize outcomes and monitor quality of care.

The health vulnerabilities of the elderly patient population and the programmatic costs associated with resource utilization continue to place TAVR programs under significant institutional and health policy scrutiny. In the United States, the VPC holds significant responsibility for coordinating the completion of the mandatory data requirements of the STS/ACC TVT Registry[7] that reports on case selection and quality of care. VPCs in other regions and jurisdictions may have similar responsibilities. A detailed understanding of TAVR health economics and reimbursement policies is essential to sustain the success of the program.

The past several years have seen the development of industry-sponsored educational forums for VPCs that address foundational learning needs as well as more advanced concepts for the experienced VPC. These programs are aimed at supporting the competencies and

TABLE 3.2. Valve Program Clinician Key Competencies

Area of Competency	Core Curriculum
Cardiovascular care	• General anatomy and physiology • Cardiovascular anatomy and function • Anatomy, pathophysiology, and clinical manifestation of aortic stenosis • TAVR-specific knowledge, including indications, case selection, device options, access methods, and potential procedural complications
Knowledge of patient population	• Basics of geriatric care, including assessment of cognitive capacity and mobility • Understanding of the concepts of frailty and disability and application of assessment tools • Quantitative and qualitative metrics for evaluating likelihood to benefit from therapy (including palliative care)
Clinical assessment	• Essential components of the clinical evaluation pathway • Required imaging modalities and at least basic literacy regarding how the acquired data are used • Risk stratification models
Patient and family education	• Assessment of learning needs and potential barriers • Engagement of patient and family throughout the continuum of care • Facilitation of shared decision-making process
Coordination of complex processes of care	• Collaborative engagement as essential member of multidisciplinary Heart Team • Development of functional relationships with essential ancillary departments • Surveillance of valve clinic processes and recommendations for change as needed • Implementation and optimization of periprocedural and postprocedural care pathways • Participation in collection and reporting of required data both to internal and to external agencies • Fundamental understanding of health care economic policies related to TAVR
Program leadership	• Engagement of the extended Heart Team • Establishment of functional and durable communication pathways • Incorporation of processes for education and training of the extended Heart Team • Participation in quality and outreach initiatives

TAVR, transcatheter aortic valve replacement.

accelerating the expertise of the allied health professionals who are engaged with TAVR programs as well as promoting the growth of networking opportunities within this professional community. In the first published recommendations for best practices for TAVR program development, the expertise, competencies, and responsibilities of the VPC were highlighted.[2] The necessity for articulating learning needs and enabling nurses and allied health professionals to gain expertise and develop a network of community of practice was apparent.

In 2012, a formal training curriculum for VPCs in the United States was independently developed by a team of TAVR nurse leaders with extensive experience in the clinical practice and operational aspects of TAVR programs. The objectives included the development of curricula for foundational as well as advanced programmatic concepts inclusive of the patient's journey from referral to follow-up, the promotion of evidence-based best practices, and the fostering of a national network of VPCs with an emphasis on shared experiences. Similarly, a formal program to foster the network of Canadian VPCs was implemented in 2014, and nursing symposia focusing on transcatheter valve therapy have been presented in Europe as well. The unique learning needs of VPCs center on clinical knowledge of the TAVR population, conduct of TAVR program coordination, leadership of a multidisciplinary team, and program evaluation. The components of the core curriculum are included in Table 3.2.

Of interest, in the years that have elapsed since the inception of these educational efforts, we have seen a shift in the attendees from sole and/or "founding" VPCs to the inclusion of new replacements in mature programs as well as VPCs who are supplemental to an existing team. Although these nuances may seem subtle, there is an impact on learning needs as well as urgency to achieve competency, especially for an inexperienced VPC who is assuming a role with an established program.

The Role of the Valve Program Clinician in Developing a Successful Valve Clinic

The VPC has a key role in the organization of the valve clinic. Although the components of the evaluation pathway are standardized as described in chapter 4 there can be a variety to the valve clinic underpinnings. This is largely dictated by the practice environment and physical resources, as there is no clinic model that is "one size fits all" (Table 3.3).

It is commonly agreed that it is most ideal to have a set clinic day (or days) usually on a weekly basis but at a minimum with a frequency that accommodates the current patient volume. A regular clinic day allows for practitioners to organize their schedules accordingly. Although we describe the valve clinic as existing in a single, brick-and-mortar location, it may be structured to occur in more than one location, especially if there are multiple provider practices represented on the Heart Team.

The VPC or a designee may be responsible for clinic scheduling, collection of intake information, and obtaining clinical records. Ideally, clerical staff are available to perform these administrative functions, thus allowing the VPC to focus on clinical practice. It is most efficient for the evaluation process if an interventional cardiologist and cardiac surgeon are both available on clinic days if the program has a requirement for mandatory in-person review by both specialists. The number of necessary personnel is largely dependent on clinic volume, and it is not uncommon for patient volume growth to precede an attendant increase in staffing.

TABLE 3.3. Essential Tasks for a Successful Valve Clinic

Receipt of referral	Obtain basic intake information
	Collect clinical records and available imaging
Preparation for valve clinic appointment	Review available records and imaging
	Schedule appointment(s)
	Schedule necessary testing (obtain insurance authorization as needed)
	Inform patient and family of plan, send preliminary information and patient education resources and any special instructions regarding medications, fasting status, and how to prepare for assessment visit(s)
	Keep referring provider informed
Valve clinic evaluation	Conduct comprehensive history and physical examination
	Ascertain patient and family understanding and expectations of the evaluation process and potential treatment options
	Provide patient and family education
	Integration of shared decision-making process
	Conduct cognitive and functional assessments according to site protocol
	Collection of data required by mandatory and/or clinical registries
	In-person evaluation by required Heart Team members
	Plan for second surgeon evaluation if required
	Acquisition of necessary diagnostic imaging
	Plan for subsequent diagnostic tests, ie, cardiac catheterization
	Engage clinical research team as indicated
	Keep referring provider informed
Postclinic evaluation	Review and team discussion of clinical data and imaging results
	Consider need for further testing or subspecialist evaluation(s)
	Multidisciplinary team decision of individualized treatment plan
	Incorporate elements of shared decision making with patient and family

TABLE 3.3. Essential Tasks for a Successful Valve Clinic   (Continued)

Procedural planning	Schedule date, location of procedure, team required (insurance authorization as needed)
	Arrangements to obtain preoperative bloodwork, consent, and so on
	Communicate plan and logistics to patient and family
	Keep referring provider informed

In addition to oversight of clinic operations, the VPC is often involved with obtaining patient history and physical examinations as well as completing cognitive and functional assessments. There may be time and facilities available for real-time review of imaging during clinic, but this may also occur during team meetings. The VPC is likely involved in compiling the necessary information and imaging data for patient review and discussion of treatment options. The VPC is uniquely positioned to assess valve clinic operations on an ongoing basis and make recommendations for course corrections and adjustments as needed. The flexibility to allow for growth and change is inherent to the role of the VPC.

Also essential is an understanding of the full array of treatment options and the patient-specific factors associated with the selection of a particular therapy. There will be patients who, because of frailty, adverse anatomy, or significant comorbidities, are not appropriate candidates for TAVR, and introduction to a palliative care pathway may be necessary. There will also be patients who will need to be referred for a surgical treatment option or perhaps enrollment in a clinical trial. The VPC is frequently involved in these conversations and can facilitate the alignment of the patient's understanding and expectations with the Heart Team decision for treatment allocation.

Looking to the Future

Most of our accumulated knowledge regarding the VPC role is based on our collective experience and is contingent on further study, networking opportunities, and consideration of the evolving clinical evidence base in transcatheter valve therapy. We are a small but growing group of professionals, and it is in our best interest to establish shared goals, competencies, and professional development pathways.

There has been some excellent work initiated by the American College of Cardiology to establish policy regarding cardiovascular team-based care, in particular the clinical, technical, and programmatic contributions of advanced practice providers.[8] We are also aware that there is work yet to be done to improve on the evidence for the delivery of cardiovascular care to the elderly.[9] Although there is no professional organization or certification designed specifically for the VPC, many of us are members of organizations that support our professional aspirations and advocacy as cardiovascular experts. Our area of practice remains novel and can be well served by the ongoing development of standardized training and education pathways with a focus on current guidelines and evidence-based care. This should be inclusive of educational opportunities that include attendees from a geographical array of centers as well as the development of site-based training curricula.

We would be remiss in closing this chapter without mentioning the importance of VPC self-advocacy. We commonly refer to ourselves as advocates for our patients and their families, and also for our Heart Teams and programs. We must also advocate for ourselves. This may be by approaching senior administration with data relevant to increasing resources or reporting on quality of care and services or by attending professional meetings or other forums where there are opportunities to network with others who work in this specialized area.

Transcatheter valve therapy is ever growing and changing; the role of the VPC can be expected to evolve in tandem. One of the most beneficial features that has emerged from the existing educational forums is the creation of a VPC network that facilitates the sharing of ideas, challenges, and insights and provides the support of knowing that one is not alone on this journey.

KEY TAKEAWAYS AND BEST PRACTICES

▶ The VPC is of central importance for the provision of patient-focused processes of care.

▶ Essential components of the VPC role include the fostering of collaborative and mutually supportive interdepartmental relationships and maintenance of functional communication pathways.

▶ Competency in cardiovascular and geriatric care and knowledge of clinical presentation with an in-depth understanding of the trajectory of illness are foundational to the expertise of the VPC.

References

1. Ensign CM, Hawkins SY. Improving patient self-care and reducing readmissions through an outpatient heart failure case management program. *Prof Case Manag.* 2017;22(4):190-196.
2. Hawkey MC, Lauck SB, Perpetua EM, et al. Transcatheter aortic valve replacement program development: recommendations for best practice. *Catheter Cardiovasc Interv.* 2014;84:859-867.
3. Otto CM, Kumbhani DJ, Alexander KP, et al. 2017 ACC expert consensus decision pathway for transcatheter aortic valve replacement in the management of adults with aortic stenosis: a report of the American College of Cardiology Task Force on Clinical Expert Consensus Documents. *J Am Coll Cardiol.* 2017;69:1313-1346.
4. Coylewright M, Palmer R, O'Neill ES, et al. Patient-defined goals for the treatment of severe aortic stenosis: a qualitative analysis. *Health Expect.* 2016;19(5):1036-1043.
5. Benner P. From novice to expert. *AJN.* 1982;82(3):402-407.
6. Astin F, Carroll D, De Geest S, et al. A core curriculum for the continuing professional development of nurses working in cardiovascular settings: developed by the Education Committee of the Council on Cardiovascular Nursing and Allied Professions on behalf of the European Society of Cardiology. *Eur J Cardiovasc Nurs.* 2015;14(S2):S1-S17.
7. Grover FL, Vemulpalli S, Carroll JD, et al. 2016 annual report of The Society of Thoracic Surgeons/American College of Cardiology Transcatheter Valve Therapy Registry. *J Am Coll Cardiol.* 2017;69(10):1215-1230.

8. Brush JE, Handberg EM, Biga C, et al. 2015 ACC health policy statement on cardiovascular team-based care and the role of advanced practice providers. *J Am Coll Cardiol.* 2015;65:2118-2136.

9. Rich MW, Chyun DA, Skolnick AH, et al. On behalf of the American Heart Association Older Populations Committee of the Council on Clinical Cardiology, Council on Cardiovascular and Stroke Nursing, Council on Cardiovascular Surgery and Anesthesia, and Stroke Council; American College of Cardiology; and American Geriatrics Society. Knowledge gaps in cardiovascular care of the older adult population: a scientific statement from the American Heart Association, American College of Cardiology, and American Geriatrics Society. *Circulation.* 2016;133:2103-2122.

CHAPTER 4

From Referral to Procedure: Clinic Evaluation Pathway

Patricia A. Keegan, DNP, NP-C, AACC | *Leslie Achtem, RN, BSN*

OBJECTIVES

▶ Describe key assessments required to determine eligibility and guide procedure planning

▶ Highlight importance of case selection

▶ Present models of clinic flow

Introduction

The field of transcatheter aortic valve replacement (TAVR) has grown substantially since the first human implant performed in Rouen, France, in 2002. Patient selection has become key to the success and evolution of the field. As part of the workup and screening process, the patient will undergo full evaluation of anatomy, physiology, and psychosocial issues. This information can be used to guide patient procedural planning and predict those who may at be at risk for complications or extended length of stay. Patient evaluation not only determines technical feasibility of TAVR but also analyzes if the potential benefits outweigh the potential risks.

TAVR is indicated for the treatment of severe, symptomatic aortic stenosis (AS). The presence of severe AS is approximately 3% to 4% in persons aged 75 years and older.[1,2] The worldwide population of persons older than 65 years is expected to double by the year 2050.[3] With the increasing prevalence of patients with valvular heart disease, an individualized approach is needed to determine a patient's optimal plan of care. A personalized approach can help to determine the testing required, valve procedure timing, and transcatheter heart valve selection to optimize the risk-benefit ratio for the procedure.[1] Patient testing should be completed and interpreted by qualified individuals at a valve center that meets national standards to perform the indicated testing.[4]

The evaluation to determine the appropriate treatment of symptomatic severe AS is a resource-intensive process requiring an individualized plan of care. Given the economic climate, an emphasis on patient selection and effective resource utilization is essential to the viability of structural heart programs.[5] Care should be given to ensure that the patient is engaged in the process of evaluation with clear expectations and instructions regarding the visit and testing. A standardized pathway may help improve patient outcomes, in addition to decreasing procedural risk.[6]

Also presenting for evaluation are patients with aortic bioprosthetic valve failure (eg, stenosis and/or regurgitation). Bioprosthetic valves are associated with a higher long-term risk of reoperation and endocarditis but a lower risk of stroke and hemorrhage.[7] Biological surgical valves include porcine or bovine pericardial tissue, homografts, and pulmonary autografts (Ross procedure). Structural valve disease can be secondary to stenosis, regurgitation, or a combination of both problems.[8] Evaluation for valve degeneration is similar to that for TAVR and typically starts with a transthoracic echocardiogram (TTE).[9] Guidelines suggest that TTE be performed when there are clinical signs or symptoms. Surveillance TTE is recommended 5 years after surgery.[10] Rarely, structural valve disease presents before 5 years post surgery, but incidence is increased after 7 to 8 years post surgery.[8] Transcatheter aortic valve-in-valve replacement is indicated for use in patients who are at least at high surgical risk for open aortic valve replacement (AVR).

For patients with previous bioprosthetic valves, attention and caution should be paid to those with prosthesis-patient mismatch (PPM). PPM occurs when the valve area is too small in relation to patient body size.[11] Severe PPM occurs when the effective orifice area index is <0.65 cm^2/m^2.[12] Patients with small valves in relation to body surface area (BSA) need to be carefully examined before committing to a valve-in-valve procedure. Factors influencing PPM post-TAVR include increased body mass index (BMI), younger age, small aortic valve area (AVA) index, and increased BSA in the setting of small left ventricular outflow tract (LVOT).[12] Patients with PPM are typically not suitable candidates for valve-in-valve TAVR as the cause of the problem is not addressed in this scenario. Studies to evaluate hemodynamics and the effect of PPM are ongoing.

Guidelines for Evaluation and Treatment of Aortic Stenosis

The content in these guidelines is specific to the United States only. A number of position papers have been released to share best practices gleaned from research and expert opinion regarding the treatment of AS. In 2017, 4 multisociety papers were published to highlight guidelines related to the evaluation and treatment of AS. Papers published included *American College of Cardiology (ACC) Expert Consensus Decision Pathway for Transcatheter Aortic Valve Replacement in the Management of Adults With Aortic Stenosis, European Society of Cardiology (ESC)/European Association for Cardio-Thoracic Surgery (EACTS) Guidelines For the Management of Valvular Heart Disease, Appropriate Use Criteria (AUC) for Treatment of Patients With Severe Aortic Stenosis,* and *A Focused Update to the ACC 2014 Guidelines For Management of Patients With Valvular Heart Disease.* The purpose of these documents is to guide clinical decisions and criteria regarding the diagnosis, management, and treatment of AS.

The AUC specify the appropriateness of interventions to diagnose and treat AS. The AUC integrate existing guidelines, clinical trial data, and expert opinion to provide recommendations for the evaluation of severe AS and treatment options.[4] Interventions are classified as "Rarely Appropriate," "May be appropriate," or "Appropriate" based on various clinical scenarios.[4] The AUC also help to serve as a quality improvement tool by allowing for the adoption of best practices and elimination of testing that is not indicated.[4]

The *American College of Cardiology (ACC) Expert Consensus Decision Pathway for Transcatheter Aortic Valve Replacement in the Management of Adults With Aortic Stenosis* was designed with the intent to provide information and guidance regarding TAVR pathways[6]

(Figure 4.1). The document is separated into 4 sections: Preprocedure Evaluation, Imaging, TAVR Procedural Issues, and Recommended Follow-up.[6] The Expert Consensus Decision Pathway assumes that the patient will be under the care of the Heart Team throughout the evaluation and treatment process.[6]

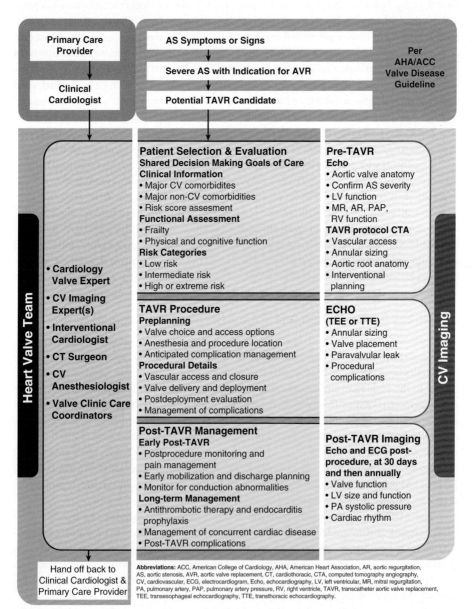

FIGURE 4.1. TAVR decision pathway outline. (Reprinted with permission from Otto CM, Kumbhani DJ, Alexander KP, et al. 2017 ACC expert consensus decision pathway for transcatheter aortic valve replacement in the management of adults with aortic stenosis. *J Am Coll Cardiol.* 2017;69(10):1313-1346. doi:10.1016/j.jacc.2016.12.006.)

In 2014, the *AHA/ACC Guidelines for the Management of Patients With Valvular Heart Disease* was released. This executive summary is a collaborative work between the American Association for Thoracic Surgery, American Society of Echocardiography, Society for Cardiovascular Angiography and Interventions, Society of Cardiovascular Anesthesiologists, and Society of Thoracic Surgeons (STS).[13] The guidelines address the diagnosis and management of adult patients with valvular heart disease. The goal of the document is to provide the clinician with evidence-based, clear, current recommendations for the evaluation, diagnosis, and treatment of valvular disease.[13] Classification of recommendations and levels of evidence are provided allowing the clinician to access the supporting documentation. The field of valvular heart disease is rapidly evolving. There has been new knowledge gleaned in the areas of patient selection, diagnosis, and therapies. Improvements have been made to both catheter and surgical interventions. With this in mind, the AHA/ACC released a focused update to the 2014 guidelines in 2017.[14]

Medical devices require manufacturer-defined indications for use (IFU) and approval by regulatory agencies. The IFU describe the condition(s) the device will treat. The IFU also describe the target patient population. Manufacturers of TAVR valves must list the IFU for their products. At present, there are two transcatheter aortic valves approved by the Food and Drug Administration in the Unites States. The manufacturers of both valves indicate that their IFU is "to treat native AS in symptomatic disease in patients felt to be at intermediate or greater risk for open surgical therapy or in symptomatic heart disease due to failure of surgical bioprosthetic aortic valve in patients found to be at high or greater risk for open heart surgery." In Europe, transcatheter valves go through a process to receive the *Conformité Européenne* (CE) mark, which indicates that the products have been assessed to meet safety, environmental, and health requirements.

Patient Evaluation

The purpose of the Heart Team is to use a patient-centered approach to determining treatment of severe AS.[15] It is a class I indication (recommended) for patients with severe valvular heart disease to be evaluated by a multidisciplinary Heart Valve Team if intervention is being considered.[13] It is a class IIa recommendation (reasonable) for patients who are asymptomatic with severe disease or have multiple comorbidities to be referred to a Heart Valve Center of Excellence (Figure 4.2).[13]

Treatment options for severe AS include surgical aortic valve replacement (SAVR), TAVR, or medical management. So far, no medical therapy has convincingly shown a reduction in AS progression or improvement in prognosis. The definitive treatments for treating AS are SAVR and TAVR. Assessment of treatment options comprises psychosocial and physiological components. It is imperative for the Heart Team to determine if symptomology is secondary to valvular disease or due to comorbid conditions.[15] If symptoms are secondary to causes other than AS, valve replacement is not indicated in these patients.

As symptomatic, severe AS carries a poor prognosis, it is paramount to elucidate the presence or absence of symptoms.[16] Patients with AS can present with various symptoms or potentially be asymptomatic. Patients with AS may present with a murmur or symptoms, or AS may be discovered as an incidental finding during routine imaging. For a patient with known valvular disease, a thorough history and physical examination should be performed, as well as a chest x-ray and echocardiogram.[13] Depending on the severity of AS, the patient may undergo ancillary

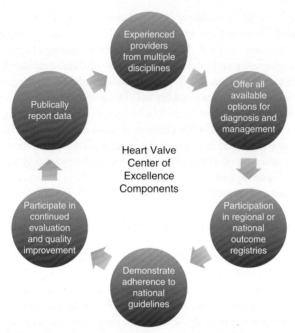

FIGURE 4.2. Heart valve center of excellence components.

testing, which may include multidetector computed tomography (MDCT), cardiac magnetic resonance (CMR) imaging, and/or hemodynamic heart catheterization to determine the optimal treatment of the patient.[13] The patient should also have a full surgical risk assessment to determine candidacy for therapy to include medical management, TAVR, and SAVR. The classification for determining severity of AS has been defined in previous chapters of this text.

The patient experience during the evaluation process can be overwhelming. For example, the consultation and testing appointments are typically lengthy in duration and may require multiple trips to the center. Efforts should be made to streamline the process to keep the patient discomfort at a minimum. Streamlining efforts include triaging patients to ensure that proper testing ordered, blocking time in Echocardiography and Radiology departments to ensure that testing can be completed on the day of visit, as well as ensuring that the proper staff is present for patient visit. The day of evaluation may include a clinic visit with an interventional cardiologist, a cardiothoracic surgeon, echocardiogram, computed tomography angiography (CTA), as well as a meeting with the valve program clinician (VPC) (see chapter 3 for more detailed information on the VPC role). Additional testing may include pulmonary function testing (PFT), carotid ultrasound imaging, coronary angiogram, and dental evaluation. At this point in the United States, 2 face-to-face surgical consultations are required by the Centers for Medicare Services for a patient to undergo TAVR.

Shared decision making including discussing goals of care should be occurring throughout the patient evaluation (Table 4.1).[6] The dialogue between the patient, Heart Team, and family should be transparent. The patient should be in agreement with the process for evaluation and encouraged to have open, honest conversations with the Heart Team as well as their family and loved ones. Shared decision making is expanded on elsewhere in this text.

TABLE 4.1. Checklist for Pre-TAVR Patient Selection and Evaluation

Key Steps	Essential Elements	Additional Details
1. Approach to Care		
Shared decision making	☐ Heart Valve Team	☐ Cardiology: general
		☐ Cardiology: interventional
		☐ Cardiology/radiology: imaging
		☐ CT surgeon
		☐ CV anesthesiologist
		☐ Valve clinic care coordinators
	☐ Referring physician	
	☐ Patient input	
	☐ Family input	
2. Goals of Care		
Live longer, feel better	☐ Life expectancy	☐ Life table estimates
	☐ Patient preferences and values	☐ Symptoms and/or survival
	☐ Goals and expectations	
	☐ End of life construct	☐ What complications to avoid?
		☐ Ideas about end of life?
3. Initial Assessment		
AS symptoms and severity	☐ Symptoms	☐ Intensity, acuity
	☐ AS severity	☐ Echocardiography and other imaging (see Imaging Checklist)
Baseline clinical data	☐ Cardiac history	☐ Prior cardiac interventions
	☐ Physical examination and labs	☐ Routine blood tests, PFTs
	☐ Chest irradiation	☐ Access issues, other cardiac effects
	☐ Dental evaluation	☐ Treat dental issues before TAVR
	☐ Allergies	☐ Contrast, latex, medications
	☐ Social support	☐ Recovery, transportation, postdischarge planning

(Continued)

TABLE 4.1. Checklist for Pre-TAVR Patient Selection and Evaluation   (Continued)

Key Steps	Essential Elements	Additional Details
Major CV comorbidity	☐ Coronary artery disease	☐ Coronary angiography
	☐ LV systolic dysfunction	☐ LV ejection fraction
	☐ Concurrent valve disease	☐ Severe MR or MS
	☐ Pulmonary hypertension	☐ Assess pulmonary pressures
	☐ Aortic disease	☐ Porcelain aorta (CT scan)
	☐ Peripheral vascular disease	☐ Prohibitive re-entry after previous open heart surgery (CT scan)
		☐ Hostile chest
		☐ See imaging for PVD
Major non-CV comorbidity	☐ Malignancy	☐ Remote or active, life expectancy
	☐ Gastrointestinal and liver disease, bleeding	☐ IBD, cirrhosis, varices, GIB—ability to take antiplatelets/anticoagulation
	☐ Kidney disease	☐ eGFR <30 cc/min/1.73 m^2 or dialysis
	☐ Pulmonary disease	☐ Oxygen requirement, FEV1 <50% predicted or DLCO <50% predicted
	☐ Neurological disorders	☐ Movement disorders, dementia
4. Functional Assessment		
Frailty and disability	☐ Frailty assessment	☐ Gait speed (<0.5 or <0.83 m/s with disability/cognitive impairment)
		☐ Frailty (Not frail or frail by assessments)
	☐ Nutritional risk/status	☐ Nutritional risk status (BMI <21 kg/m^2, albumin <3.5 mg/dL, >10-lb weight loss in past year, or ≤11 on MNA)
Physical Function	☐ Physical function and endurance	☐ 6-min walk <50 m or unable to walk
	☐ Independent living	☐ Dependent in ≥1 activities
Cognitive Function	☐ Cognitive impairment	☐ MMSE <24 or dementia
	☐ Depression	☐ Depression history or positive screen
	☐ Prior disabling stroke	
Futility	☐ Life expectancy	☐ <1 y life expectancy
	☐ Lag-time to benefit	☐ Survival with benefit of <25% at 2 y

TABLE 4.1. Checklist for Pre-TAVR Patient Selection and Evaluation (Continued)

Key Steps	Essential Elements	Additional Details
5. Overall Procedural Risk		
Risk categories	☐ Low risk	☐ STS-PROM <4% and
		☐ No frailty and
		☐ No comorbidity and
		☐ No procedure specific impediments
	☐ Intermediate risk	☐ STS-PROM 4%-8% or
		☐ Mild frailty or
		☐ 1 major organ system compromise not to be improved postoperatively or
		☐ A possible procedure-specific impediment
	☐ High risk	☐ STS-PROM >8% or
		☐ Moderate-severe frailty or
		☐ >2 major organ system compromises not to be improved postoperatively or
		☐ A possible procedure-specific impediment
	☐ Prohibitive risk	☐ PROMM >50% at 1 y or
		☐ ≥3 major organ system compromises not to be improved postoperatively or
		☐ Severe frailty
		☐ Severe procedure-specific impediments
6. Integrated Benefit-Risk of TAVR and Shared Decision-Making		
No current indication for AVR	☐ AS not severe or	☐ Periodic monitoring of AS severity and symptoms
	☐ No AS symptoms or other indication for AVR	☐ Re-evaluate when AS severe or symptoms occur
AVR indicated but SAVR preferred over TAVR	☐ Lower risk for surgical AVR	☐ SAVR recommended in lower-risk patients
	☐ Mechanical valve preferred	☐ Valve durability considerations in younger patients
	☐ Other surgical considerations	☐ Concurrent surgical procedure needed (eg, aortic root replacement)

(Continued)

TABLE 4.1. Checklist for Pre-TAVR Patient Selection and Evaluation   (Continued)

Key Steps	Essential Elements	Additional Details
TAVR candidate with expected benefit > risk	☐ Symptom relief or improved survival	☐ Discussion with patient and family
	☐ Possible complications and expected recovery	☐ Proceed with TAVR imaging evaluation and procedure
	☐ Review of goals and expectations	
Severe symptomatic AS but benefit < risk (futility)	☐ Life expectancy <1 y	☐ Discussion with patient and family
	☐ Chance of survival with benefit at 2 y <25%	☐ Palliative care inputs
		☐ Palliative balloon aortic valvuloplasty in selected patients

AS, aortic stenosis; AVR, aortic valve replacement; BMI, body mass index; CT, computed tomography; CV, cardiovascular; DLCO, diffusing capacity of the lung for carbon monoxide; eGFR, estimated glomerular filtration rate; FEV1, forced expiratory volume in 1 s; GIB, gastrointestinal bleeding; IBD, inflammatory bowel disease; LV, left ventricular; MMSE, mini mental state examination; MNA, mini nutritional assessment; MR, mitral regurgitation; MS, mitral stenosis; PFT, pulmonary function test; PROMM, predicted risk of mortality or major morbidity; PVD, peripheral vascular disease; SAVR, surgical aortic valve replacement; STS-PROM, predicted risk of mortality; TAVR, transcatheter aortic valve replacement.
Reprinted with permission from Otto CM, Kumbhani DJ, Alexander KP, et al. 2017 ACC expert consensus decision pathway for transcatheter aortic valve replacement in the management of adults with aortic stenosis. *J Am Coll Cardiol.* 2017;69(10):1313-1346. doi:10.1016/j.jacc.2016.12.006.

History

Careful assessment of the past medical history and current state is imperative to avoid patient mismanagement.[16] Calcific AS is typically a disease of the elderly and is commonly associated with atherosclerosis.[16] Common symptoms seen in patients with severe AS include dyspnea, angina, and/or syncope. The patient should be questioned if they have or are currently experiencing chest pain or discomfort. Angina pectoris in patients with aortic valve disease is usually precipitated by exertion and relieved with rest. The incidence of angina with severe AS has been reported to be between 30% and 40%.[19] When the clinician is taking the patient history, it is important to note the Canadian Cardiovascular Society grading of angina pectoris. This score notes angina on a scale from I to IV, describing angina occurrence with levels of activity. Clinical skills, including adequate history taking and physical assessment, are an important part of the patient evaluation.[18] The evaluation for AS is multifaceted and includes subjective and objective data. Utilization of this information will help to develop the patient's individualized plan of care.

The appearance of symptoms signifies a sharp decline in survival. Ross and Braunwald (1968) described that nearly all symptomatic patients with severe AS die within 5 years.[17] Depending on the symptoms, the survival can be varied. The mean survival after presenting with angina is 5 years. For those presenting with syncope, the average survival is 3 years. Heart failure symptoms carry the worst prognosis, with an average mortality of 2 years after appearance of symptoms in the setting of severe AS.[16] Syncope in patients with severe AS is frequently described as occurring with exertion. The exact mechanism of syncope in AS is unknown.[19]

There is systemic vasodilation with a fixed forward stroke volume (SV). It is hypothesized that the change causes the arterial systolic blood pressure to drop.[20] Other potential causes are related to arrhythmia and sudden failure of an overloaded left ventricle during exercise. Syncope may additionally occur at rest. Potential causes are transient ventricular tachycardia, atrial fibrillation, and (if calcification of the valve extends into the conduction system) atrio-ventricular block.

Heart failure symptoms have the worst prognosis for patients with severe AS.[19] Heart failure symptoms include orthopnea, paroxysmal nocturnal dyspnea, dyspnea with exertion, edema, early satiety, or shortness of breath. Dyspnea is likely caused by altered left ventricular function with increased filling pressure.[20] An important part of the assessment is to note the New York Heart Association classification, which is derived from symptom severity and the degree of exertion needed to elicit symptoms (Table 4.2).

Assessment of symptoms can be difficult in this patient population. Patients may deny symptoms owing to lifestyle adaptation, or they may believe symptoms are related to other comorbid conditions or to their perception of the aging process.[16,21] Patients with severe AS who seem to be asymptomatic based on consultation and by their own report should be further evaluated. Exercise treadmill testing (ETT) or cardiopulmonary exercise testing to confirm or deny symptoms is a recommendation per guidelines.[13,21] The prognosis for patients with severe AS with positive ETT is the same as for those who present with symptoms.[16]

Patients should be carefully assessed for the presence of comorbid conditions. Comorbidities associated with a life expectancy of less than 1 year are typically considered to be a contraindication to TAVR.[6,10,13] Comorbid conditions such as chronic obstructive pulmonary disease, pulmonary hypertension, cirrhosis, history of stroke, cognitive deficit, and chronic kidney disease (CKD) should be noted for inclusion in the calculation of surgical risk as well as for Heart Team discussion regarding treatment allocation. Prior gastrointestinal bleeding, liver disease, and blood dyscrasias are noted as potential contributory factors to increased risk of bleeding secondary to use of antiplatelet and anticoagulation agents. A history of chest irradiation and deformities should also be assessed. Owing to improvement in cancer survival, structural heart programs may see

TABLE 4.2. New York Heart Association Classification of Symptoms of Heart Failure

Class	Patient Symptoms
I	No limitation in physical activity. Ordinary physical activity does not cause excess fatigue, rapid/irregular heartbeat, or dyspnea
II	Slight limitation in physical activity. Comfortable at rest, but normal activity results in fatigue, rapid/irregular heartbeat, or dyspnea
III	Marked limitation in physical activity. Comfortable at rest, but less than ordinary activity causes fatigue, rapid/irregular heartbeat, or dyspnea
IV	Unable to carry out any activity without symptoms of fatigue, rapid/irregular heartbeat, or dyspnea. If any activity is undertaken, symptoms increase

Data from Yancy CW, Jessup M, Bozkurt B, et al. 2013 ACCF/AHA guideline for the management of heart failure: a report of the American College of Cardiology Foundation/American Heart Association Task Force on Practice Guidelines. *Circulation*. 2013;128(16):e240-e327.

more patients affected by radiation-induced heart disease. For patients who have a history of radiation-acquired heart disease, SAVR is connected with increased long-term mortality.[26] Patients should also be assessed for a history of conditions that are procedural-specific impediments for TAVR. Examples of impediments include tracheostomy, calcified ascending aorta, chest malformation, arterial coronary grafts posterior to the sternum, as well as radiation damage. Any of these conditions may increase the risk or decrease the feasibility of performing SAVR.

Evaluation of patients' social support structure is a crucial component of the evaluation process. This includes defining their social support structure and identifying any barriers to their ongoing participation in the evaluation and care pathways (eg, access to transportation). A comprehensive evaluation process that takes into account both physiologic and social factors can contribute to individualized treatment plans and optimization of postprocedure outcomes (Figure 4.3).

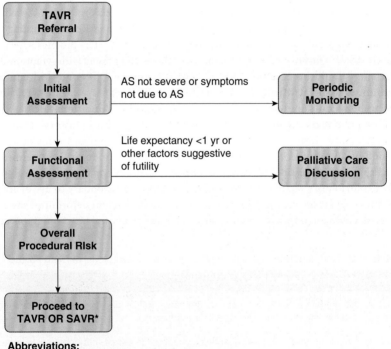

Abbreviations:
AS, aortic stenosis, AVR, aortic valve replacement,
TAVR, transcatheter aortic valve replacement

*per current AHA/ACC Guideline for the Management
of Patients with Valvular Heart Disease

FIGURE 4.3. Pre–transcatheter aortic valve replacement considerations by the heart valve team. (Reprinted with permission from Otto CM, Kumbhani DJ, Alexander KP, et al. 2017 ACC expert consensus decision pathway for transcatheter aortic valve replacement in the management of adults with aortic stenosis. *J Am Coll Cardiol.* 2017;69(10):1313-1346. doi:10.1016/j.jacc.2016.12.006.)

Physical Examination

The physical examination is an integral part of the provider-patient relationship and provides the opportunity to garner otherwise unattainable information.[18] The information gleaned from the physical examination can help delineate the need for further testing.[18]

Vital sign assessment is an integral part of the patient evaluation. Height and weight measurements are used to calculate BMI and BSA. The BMI is used to calculate some measures of frailty, whereas the BSA is a portion of the formula for indexed valve area. The height and weight are also collected as part of the STS score, which is used as a determinant of surgical risk. Other vital signs to be obtained and documented include oxygen saturation, blood pressure, heart rate and rhythm, as well as pain assessment.

The patient typically presents with a systolic murmur. A murmur of AS is typically a mid-systolic ejection murmur, heard best over the right second intercostal space, with radiation into the right neck. The murmur is typically described as harsh in quality. The patient may have a soft or absent S2 depending on the quality of the murmur. Another finding characteristic of AS is tardus et parvus, which is on palpation the pulse is weak (parvus) and late (tardus).

The patient visit allows the clinician to determine the acuity of a patient's disease process.[6] Addressing acute comorbid conditions and allergy assessment should occur during the visit to help guide the remaining evaluation. Careful attention to addressing contrast or latex allergies should occur at this stage of the patient evaluation. Patients with documented intravenous dye allergies will need to be pretreated before contrast administration, which will be necessary during CTA (should renal function allow) as well as heart catheterization.

Pertinent Testing
Exercise Treadmill Testing

Exercise testing is an appropriate test to risk stratify patients with asymptomatic AS who are able to exercise. Contraindications to performing an ETT are (1) an established reason to have AVR, (2) uncontrolled hypertension, (3) uncontrolled or symptomatic arrhythmia (eg, rapid atrial fibrillation and supraventricular tachycardia), or an (4) inability to perform the test.[22] It is essential to ensure that the patient is not symptomatic before performing the ETT. The goal is for the patient to reach 80% to 85% age-predicted maximum heart rate.[22] Abnormal results include development of AS-related symptoms, drop in blood pressure, ventricular arrhythmia, or ST depression. Cardiopulmonary exercise test can also be used to identify if patients are truly asymptomatic.[23]

Echocardiogram

There are 3 types of echocardiogram used in the assessment of AS. The 3 types are (1) TTE, (2) transesophageal echocardiogram (TEE), and (3) dobutamine stress echocardiogram (DSE).

Transthoracic Echocardiogram

According to the guidelines, TTE is indicated to establish a diagnosis of AS and valvular heart disease.[10,13] The TTE provides information about the severity of valve disease, the anatomy of the valve, concomitant valvular lesions, as well as ejection fraction and wall motion abnormalities. TTE also provides information regarding the presence of atrial or ventricular septal defects, pericardial effusion, or LVOT obstruction. TTE is performed to assess the cause of aortic valve stenosis, size of valve, extent of calcification, leaflet motion, and shape of valve.

TTE works by placing the transducer on the chest and creating high-frequency sound waves to create pictures of the heart. The images can be used to confirm the diagnosis of AS and provide specific information on left ventricular function. Three findings on TTE are indicative of severe AS: limited cusp motion, decrease in the maximal cusp separation, and the presence of left ventricular hypertrophy.[28] Echocardiogram can determine the anatomy of the aortic valve and delineate if the valve is tricuspid, bicuspid, unicuspid, or quadricuspid. The common view indicated to assess the aortic valve is the parasternal long view.[27] Patients with bicuspid aortic valves should be evaluated for aortopathy, as aortic root dilation is present in up to 50% of these patients.[29] TAVR is indicated in patients with trileaflet, symptomatic, severe AS.[4,6,13]

The mean gradient, maximum velocity, SV, and AVA are the most powerful predictors of the need for AVR.[6,30] Determinations for severity of AS are made by obtaining the AVA, maximum velocity (Vmax), and the mean and peak aortic gradient. Using this information, the severity of valvular disease can be determined. The AVA is a measurement that determines the opening orifice area of the aortic valve. The 4 hemodynamic variants of severe AS include asymptomatic severe AS, severe AS with preserved EF, low-flow (LF) low-gradient (LG) AS with left ventricular dysfunction, and LF/LG AS with preserved EF also known as paradoxical LF, LG severe AS (Table 4.3).[31]

There are a number of ways of determining the AVA. Planimetry is tracing the opening of the aortic valve in ventricular systole when the valve is at its widest opening. This method directly measures the valve area and is dependent on patient anatomy and technician skill. A second method for determining the AVA is the continuity equation. This calculation is a derived number that uses the measurements of the LVOT diameter (in centimeters) and the LVOT velocity time integral, the SV, and the aortic velocity time interval to calculate the area. Two other methods used to calculate the AVA are the Gorlin equation and the Hakki equation. Both these methods use cardiac output to calculate the valve area.[10]

At times, the measurement of the AVA does not tell the whole story. For example, a valve area of 0.8 cm^2 in someone who is 5 feet tall and weighs 45 kg could be less limiting than in someone who is 6 feet tall and 100 kg. For this reason, we can index the valve area to account for BSA. To calculate the indexed valve area, the AVA is divided by the BSA. An indexed valve area of <0.6 is considered severe.[10] Indexing the valve area increased the prevalence of patients meeting criteria for severe AS.[32] Regardless of how the AVA is measured, this value is used as one part of the determinant of severity of AS.

Not every patient has a normal ejection fraction (EF) and gradients in the severe range. In patients with decreased EF (<50%), they should undergo an LS DSE. In this instance, the heart is evaluated for contractile reserve and to determine if the patient has true AS or pseudostenosis.[28] Figure 4.4 highlights the algorithm for evaluating LF/LG AS. In the setting of AVA <1.0 cm^2, EF normal, and gradients <40 mm Hg, this is referred to as paradoxical LF AS.[13] In these patients, the flow state may be due to left ventricular remodeling with impaired filling and reduced strain.[33] In this patient population, other causes of symptoms should be evaluated, including atrial fibrillation, tricuspid regurgitation, and mitral stenosis.[13] If the patient is hypertensive, it is recommended that the patient be treated with antihypertensives and reassessed with echocardiogram when goal blood pressure is reached.[13] Patients with a restricted valve area in the severe category with LF/LG AS had improved survival with valve replacement.[33] When evaluating patient options for potential TAVR, noting low SV and low EF are indicated, as both have poor outcomes regardless of management strategy.

TABLE 4.3. Aortic Valve Classification

Stage	Definition	Valve Anatomy	Valve Hemodynamics	Hemodynamic Consequences	Symptoms
A	**At risk of AS**	• Bicuspid aortic valve (or other congenital valve anomaly) • Aortic valve sclerosis	• Aortic V_{max} <2 m/s	• None	• None
B	**Progressive AS**	• Mild to moderate leaflet calcification of a bicuspid or trileaflet valve with some reduction in systolic motion or • Rheumatic valve changes with commissural fusion	• Mild AS: Aortic V_{max} 2.0-2.9 m/s or mean ΔP <20 mm Hg • Moderate AS: Aortic V_{max}, 3.0-3.9 m/s or mean ΔP 20-39 mm Hg	• Early LV diastolic dysfunction may be present • Normal LVEF	• None
C:	**Asymptomatic severe AS**				
C1	**Asymptomatic severe AS**	• Severe leaflet calcification or congenital stenosis with severely reduced leaflet opening	• Aortic V_{max} ≥4 m/s or mean ΔP ≥40 mm Hg • AVA typically is ≤1.0 cm² (or AVAi ≤0.6 cm²/m²) • Very severe AS is an aortic V_{max} ≥5 m/s or mean ΔP ≥60 mm Hg	• LV diastolic dysfunction • Mild LV hypertrophy • Normal LVEF	• None: Exercise testing is reasonable to confirm symptom status

(Continued)

TABLE 4.3. Aortic Valve Classification (Continued)

Stage	Definition	Valve Anatomy	Valve Hemodynamics	Hemodynamic Consequences	Symptoms
C2	**Asymptomatic severe AS with LV dysfunction**	• Severe leaflet calcification or congenital stenosis with severely reduced leaflet opening	• Aortic V_{max} ≥4 m/s or mean ΔP ≥40 mm Hg • AVA typically ≤1.0 cm^2 (or AVAi ≤0.6 cm^2/m^2)	• LVEF <50%	• None
D:	**Symptomatic severe AS**				
D1	**Symptomatic severe high-gradient AS**	• Severe leaflet calcification or congenital stenosis with severely reduced leaflet opening	• Aortic V_{max} ≥4 m/s or mean ΔP ≥40 mm Hg • AVA typically ≤1.0 cm^2 (or AVAi ≤0.6 cm^2/m^2) but may be larger with mixed AS/AR	• LV diastolic dysfunction • LV hypertrophy • Pulmonary hypertension may be present	• Exertional dyspnea or decreased exercise tolerance • Exertional angina • Exertional syncope or presyncope
D2	**Symptomatic severe low-flow/low-gradient AS with reduced LVEF**	• Severe leaflet calcification with severely reduced leaflet motion	• AVA ≤1.0 cm^2 with resting aortic V_{max} <4 m/s or mean ΔP <40 mm Hg • Dobutamine stress echocardiography shows AVA ≤1.0 cm^2 with V_{max} ≥4 m/s at any flow rate	• LV diastolic dysfunction • LV hypertrophy • LVEF <50%	• HF • Angina • Syncope or presyncope

D3	Symptomatic severe low-gradient AS with normal LVEF or paradoxical low-flow severe AS	• Severe leaflet calcification with severely reduced leaflet motion	• AVA ≤1.0 cm² with aortic V_{max} <4 m/s or mean ΔP <40 mm Hg	• Increased LV relative wall thickness	• HF
			• Indexed AVA ≤0.6 cm²/m² and	• Small LV chamber with low stroke volume	• Angina
			• Stroke volume index <35 mL/m²	• Restrictive diastolic filling	• Syncope or presyncope
			• Measured when patient is normotensive (systolic BP <140 mm Hg)	• LVEF ≥50%	

Reprinted with permission from Nishimura RA, Otto CM, Bonow RO, et al. 2014 AHA/ACC guideline for the management of patients with valvular heart disease. *J Am Coll Cardiol.* 2014. doi:10.1016/j.jacc.2014.02.536.

AR, aortic regurgitation; AS, aortic stenosis; AVA, aortic valve area; AVAi, aortic valve are are indexed to body surface area; BP, blood pressure; HF, heart failure; LV, left ventricular; LVEF, left ventricular ejection fraction; ΔP, pressure gradient; V_{max}, maximum aortic velocity.

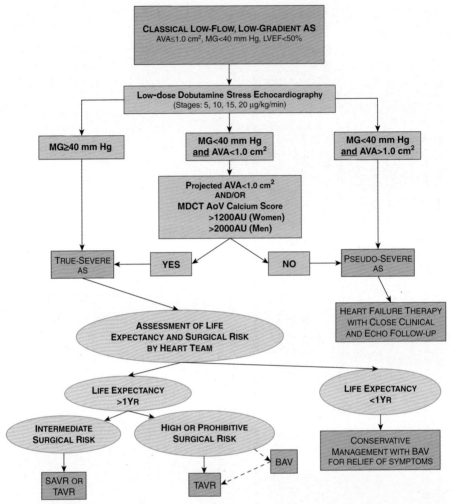

FIGURE 4.4. Algorithm for the management of classical (reduced left ventricular ejection fraction) low-flow, low-gradient aortic stenosis (AS). AoV, aortic valve; AVA, aortic valve area; BAV, bicuspid aortic valve; LVEF, left ventricular ejection fraction; MDCT, multidetector computed tomography; MG, mean gradient; SAVR, surgical aortic valve replacement; TAVR, transcatheter aortic valve replacement. (Reprinted with permission from Clavel MA, Magne J, Pibarot P. Low-gradient aortic stenosis. *Eur Heart J.* 2016;37:2645-2657.)

Some patients undergoing echocardiogram may not meet criteria for severe AS, and in this case, a plan for ongoing surveillance should be established. Patients who fall into this category should be evaluated at specific intervals and advised to notify their provider should they develop symptoms. AS carries a poor prognosis once symptoms are established (Table 4.4).

TTE is a safe procedure with no known risk or side effects. However, TTE is not without technical challenges. Patient habitus and lung disease can limit the ability to obtain adequate images owing to "poor windows." The gradients can be underestimated if the beam is

TABLE 4.4. Frequency of Echocardiograms in Asymptomatic Patients with VHD and Normal Left Ventricular Function

Degree of AS	V_{max}	Echo Interval
Mild	2.0-2.9 m/s	Every 3-5 y
Moderate	3.0-3.9 m/s	Every 1-2 y
Severe	>4 m/s	Every 6-12 mo

If patient has mixed valvular disease he/she may require evaluations at earlier intervals than for single valve disease.
AS, aortic stenosis; VHD, valvular heart disease.
Adapted from Nishimura RA, Otto CM, Bonow RO, et al. 2014 AHA/ACC guideline for the management of patients with valvular heart disease. *J Am Coll Cardiol*. 2014. doi:10.1016/j.jacc.2014.02.536.

not parallel to the velocity jet of the AS.[10] The annulus of the aortic valve is not a circle but an oval. Echocardiogram-determined measurements are an estimation of valve area and not a true measurement.[16] Results of the echocardiogram are used in determining the next course of action for patients. The severity and stage of AS as determined by echo data will determine whether continued evaluation and testing or surveillance and medical management is indicated for the patient. Echocardiographic data can also further quantify risk by evaluating cardiac anatomy if the patient is being considered for intervention.

Transesophageal Echocardiogram
In some instances, TEE is beneficial during the evaluation of AS. The common view used to evaluate the aortic valve is the mid-esophageal long-axis view.[27] There is enhanced resolution and less obstruction in the visualization of the aortic valve. TEE uses a probe placed within the esophagus to obtain images of the heart structures. Images can be gathered in 3 dimensions. This may be especially useful in patients with elevated creatinine levels unable to undergo MDCT owing to the risk of worsening renal failure.[6] Patients must fast for 6 hours before the procedure and 1 hour after the procedure. Risks of the procedure include esophageal tear, sore throat, and complications related to sedation.[34] Because sedation is given for the procedure, the patient should be educated to have someone available to drive them home after the procedure.

Dobutamine Stress Echocardiogram
Low-dose DSE is indicated for the evaluation of patients with LF LG AS in the setting of reduced EF (<50%).[13] This group comprises approximately 10% of patients with severe ASs.[31] Risks of procedure are related to exercise or administration of dobutamine and may include an irregular or rapid heart rhythm, such as atrial fibrillation or ventricular tachycardia. Caution should be used in ordering a DSE in the presence of coronary artery disease (CAD), as this increases the risk of diminished myocardial perfusion during stress and development of arrhythmias. In patients with severe, symptomatic AS using DSE can be dangerous, as nonsustained ventricular tachycardia is observed in 4% to 20% of cases.[35] In rare instances, myocardial infarction can occur. The patient should be monitored for the development of arrhythmias, symptoms, or hemodynamic abnormalities. Careful attention should be given to the evaluation for blood pressure decrease or failure of blood pressure to increase with exercise.[10] The measured AVA may not change with dobutamine infusion, but the mean pressure gradient will increase significantly in severe disease.[13]

Rhythm Assessment

An electrocardiogram should be performed as part of the evaluation process. Common findings on electrocardiogram include left ventricular hypertrophy, which is found in a large number of patients with severe AS.[36] Special attention should be given to pre-existing conduction abnormalities, bifascicular block, left bundle branch block, and PR intervals >200 ms, as these patients are at higher risk for post-TAVR conduction abnormalities requiring pacemaker placement.[37] Post-TAVR pacemaker implantation has been reported in 6% to 28% of patients receiving commercially available valves.[38] Most cases requiring PPM post TAVR are secondary to complete or high-degree AV block.[39] Rhythm predictors of patients at elevated risk for pacemaker post TAVR include pre-existing right bundle branch block.[39] Right bundle branch block has also been noted to be an independent risk factor for mortality post TAVR.[40] Of note, atrial fibrillation is associated with a longer length of stay post TAVR.[5] The monitoring and management of rhythm disturbances have been implicated in increasing critical care requirement, time to mobilization, longer length of stay, and worse outcomes, including heart failure exacerbation and mortality.[37,41]

Radiographic Testing

Unlike surgery, TAVR does not accommodate intraprocedural valve sizing, and extensive preprocedure imaging must occur for proper planning and sizing. Thorough evaluation of annular sizing and valve anatomy is necessary to mitigate complications such as prosthesis embolization, paravalvular leak, and aortic annular rupture.[42]

Computed Tomography

Computed tomography (CT) allows for thorough examination of the heart, including the aortic root, aorta, aortic valve, and peripheral vasculature. The aortic root has specific anatomic characteristics, which can affect clinical outcomes of TAVR.[43] Multiple types of CT can be used to assess aortic valve anatomy for potential consideration of TAVR. There are anatomical differences in the annulus of males and females. Typically, the LVOT, annulus, and sinus of Valsalva are larger in males. The ascending aorta dimensions are similar in males and females.[43]

MDCT is a standard part of the evaluation before TAVR.[6] MDCT, as a single test, can acquire valuable information regarding aortic annulus anatomy, coronary anatomy, as well as vascular access.[44] It is recommended that the MDCT be performed by a CT scanner that is at least 64 detector, with advantages given to 128-, 256-, and 320-slice scanners. The acquisition time is shorter and the contrast volume can be decreased with the faster scanners.[27] At the time of the scan, the patient should be supine and suspend respirations to reduce movement artifact.[45] This is known as a "gated" study, which is imperative to analyze the annulus during various stages of the cardiac cycle.

Images of the chest obtained evaluate the aortic root as noted earlier as well as calcium distribution, which greatly affects procedural planning and may indicate a higher risk of complication during valve deployment. This is also important secondary to increased risk of postprocedural pacemaker owing to LVOT calcification below the right and left coronary cusp.[39] A high-quality preprocedure CT scan can assist with predicting the angle of deployment on fluoroscopy.[39] The thoracoabdominal aorta with ilofemoral branches are evaluated to determine if transfemoral arterial access may be feasible. MDCT measurements are highly reproducible.[47] Iodinated contrast agents used for MDCT are potentially nephrotoxic. There is no consensus regarding the level of serum creatinine (or degree of renal dysfunction) of which the patient should not receive contrast.[46] Risks and benefits of contrast should be thoroughly evaluated by the Heart Team, the patient, and the family. If the patient has an absolute contraindication to MDCT, options such as noncontrast CT, magnetic resonance angiography (MRA), and TEE can be considered.[6]

Cardiac Magnetic Resonance Imaging

Not every patient is a good candidate for CTA. Patients who present with contraindications to ionized contrast, because of either allergy or renal dysfunction can be considered for CMR rather than MDCT.[48] In addition, patients with LF LG AS who are unable to undergo stress echocardiogram are potential candidates for CMR.[48] MRI is noninvasive and radiation-free. Limitations of MRI are multiple breath holds and longer scan time. Contraindications include extreme claustrophobia and certain metal implants.[48]

Coronary Assessment

Currently, there are US guidelines and AUC regarding the use of cardiac catheterization in a patient being considered for valve surgery. It is class I for patients with severe AS who may be surgical candidates to undergo cardiac catheterization for evaluation of coronary anatomy before intervention.[4] There are also AUC for percutaneous coronary intervention (PCI) + TAVR or coronary artery bypass surgery (CABG) + AVR in patients with significant CAD and severe AS.[4] Revascularization of significant coronary disease was required in prior clinical trials for approval of TAVR.[49] The incidence of CAD in patients with concomitant AS older than 50 years has been reported to be approximately 50% to up to 75%[6,10] and has been associated with worsening outcomes post TAVR.[50] Hemodynamic instability during TAVR can induce ischemia in patients with severe AS and CAD.[44] Decision regarding PCI/revascularization before TAVR is guided by the Heart Team decision.[35]

Noninvasive Coronary Evaluation

Noninvasive functional assessments for CAD include nuclear perfusion imaging, CT, MRA, or DSE.[35] Noninvasive assessments for ischemia using positron emission tomography, echocardiogram, or MRI can be performed; however, the specificity of these tests is lower than in patients without valvular diasease.[35] Routinely, patients undergo CTA as part of their TAVR evaluation. This test has the capability of evaluating coronary anatomy.[44] Noninvasive testing appears safe but has a lower sensitivity and specificity than angiography.[51]

Invasive Coronary Evaluation

Invasive coronary angiography remains the gold standard to assess for CAD.[44] The incidence of CAD in patients with concomitant AS older than 50 years has been reported to be approximately 50% to up to 75%.[6,10] Concomitant CAD has been associated with worsening outcomes post TAVR.[50,52] Hemodynamic instability during TAVR can induce ischemia in patients with severe AS and CAD.[44] Aortic valve gradients can also be obtained by an invasive measurement of transaortic gradients, and the valve area can be calculated using the Gorlin formula.[16] This practice has fallen out of favor because of the risk of cerebral embolism and differences in Doppler gradients.[16]

Once the left heart catheterization has been completed, the SYNTAX (Synergy between PCI with TAXUS drug eluting stent and Cardiac Surgery Score) can be generated. SYNTAX is a grading tool used to determine the complexity of CAD.[4] The score was traditionally required as part of clinical trial data and is a field on the NCDR TVT registry data collection form. Decision regarding revascularization is left up to the Heart Team.[6]

Access Evaluation

A variety of access routes are available for TAVR: transfemoral (arterial), transapical, transaortic, transcarotid, transcaval, and subclavian. The transfemoral approach has been shown to have the best outcomes.[15] The diameters of delivery sheaths used during TAVR remain large; however, they have become incrementally smaller with each iteration of the device. Vascular access assessment is critical to ensure safe procedures and optimal outcomes. Evaluation of the entire thoracoabdominal aorta, thoracic arterial vasculature, carotid arteries, subclavian arteries, and iliofemoral vasculature should be performed as part of the evaluation for TAVR.[6]

MDCT is ideal for evaluating the patient for transfemoral access. If MDCT cannot be performed, other methods of assessing the ileofemoral vasculature include ultrasound scan, lower extremity angiogram using a marker pigtail and low-contrast CT, noncontrast CT, or MRA.[6] Intravascular ultrasound imaging is an alternative method with accuracy comparable with that of CT with less contrast usage and less radiation exposure.[53] Potential sources of complication for the transfemoral approach include small luminal diameter, dense or circumferential calcifications, and severe tortuosity. Patients who have this anatomy are at higher risk for stroke and vascular complication.[6]

Pulmonary Assessment

Assessing pulmonary function is recommended as part of the TAVR evaluation.[6] Moderate or severe lung disease, typically diagnosed by PFT, is an independent predictor of mortality after TAVR.[54] Recording the presence of lung disease is a part of the patient evaluation and a component of the STS score. Pulmonary disease may also be noted from the patient's past medical history or as a new finding on radiographic testing. Pulmonary hypertension is a risk factor for increased mortality post TAVR.[55,56] The degree of chronic obstructive pulmonary disease is determined by PFT and further classified by methods such as the Global Initiative for Chronic Obstructive Lung Disease guidelines (Figure 4.5). Pulmonary function is a critical component of accurately assessing surgical risk stratification.

Carotid Ultrasound Imaging

Carotid ultrasound imaging uses sound waves to examine the carotid arteries for stenosis. There is no special preparation required for this procedure. The relationship between internal carotid artery stenosis and AVR is unclear. In a recent study, there was no statistically significant correlation between procedure-related stroke and internal carotid artery stenosis severity.[57] The AUC for evaluation of AS notes that carotid ultrasound imaging may be considered depending on patient history.[6]

Dental Evaluation

The American Heart Association (AHA) guidelines recommend dental evaluation and treatment before surgery to reduce the risk of late prosthetic valve endocarditis.[58] Active dental issues should be addressed before proceeding with TAVR.[6] The dentist or oral surgeon will

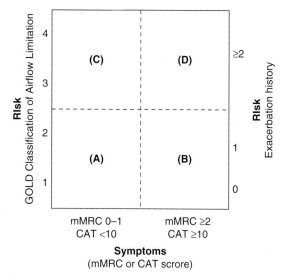

FIGURE 4.5. Chronic obstructive pulmonary disease (COPD) classification using the Global Initiative for Chronic Obstructive Lung Disease (GOLD) guidelines. The severity of COPD can be assessed using GOLD staging (based on FEV1), symptoms (using validated screening questionnaires such as mMRC and CAT), and exacerbation history (0, 1, or greater than or equal to 2 per year). Group A: Low risk, less symptoms. GOLD 1 to 2, 0 to 1 exacerbation/year AND mMRC 0 to 1 or CAT <10. Group B: Low risk, more symptoms. GOLD 1 to 2, 0 to 1 exacerbation/year, AND mMRC >0 to 1 or CAT >10. Group C: High risk, less symptoms. GOLD 3 to 4, >2 exacerbation/year, AND mMRC <0 tov 1 or CAT <10. Group D: High risk, more symptoms. GOLD 3 to 4, >2 exacerbation/year, AND mMRC >0 to 1 or CAT >10. CAT, COPD assessment test; FEV1, forced expiratory volume in 1 second; mMRC, modified Medical Research Council. (From Kollef M. *The Washington Manual of Critical Care*; 2017. Used with permission.)

evaluate for potential sources of infection, including dental caries, gum disease, or abscesses. The dental clearance examination may include x-rays. In patients with dental disease, bacteria in the mouth may be transmitted to the heart valve, placing the patient at risk for infective endocarditis. The patient may also be given anticoagulants after valve replacement. Anticoagulants may put the patient at higher risk for bleeding during dental treatments. Owing to the high mortality of endocarditis, prevention of valvular endocarditis is of concern, and therefore, preprocedure dental evaluation is stressed.[59]

Laboratory Testing

In addition to standard laboratory testing, certain laboratory tests assist in determining physiologic changes secondary to aortic valve disease. The only biomarker testing supported by guidelines is B-type natriuretic peptide (BNP).[60] BNP can be used to predict symptom onset in asymptomatic patients.[61] The heart muscle releases BNP in relation to increased stretch and is useful to determine the severity, prognosis, and management of heart failure.[4]

Kidney function is important to assess before TAVR. Acute kidney injury (AKI) post TAVR has a negative impact on mortality.[62] Effective methods to minimize the risk of AKI before procedure include prehydration, limitation of contrast dye, and avoiding procedural hypotension.[62] Caution needs to be given to patients with CKD, as they are at higher risk for development of post-TAVR AKI.[62] CKD is considered one of the strongest predictors of mortality 1 year post TAVR.[62] In patients with end-stage renal disease, valve calcification can occur 10 to 20 years earlier and can progress at a faster rate than the general population.[63] Abnormal calcium metabolism is common in patients with end-stage renal disease, potentially leading to poorer prosthetic valve longevity.[15]

Albumin levels should be collected as part of the patient evaluation to more thoroughly assess a patient's nutrition status. Malnutrition is defined as faulty nutrition due to inadequate or unbalanced intake of nutrients or their impaired assimilation or utilization.[24] Practically speaking, malnutrition is a BMI <18.5% or unintentional weight loss of >10%, or >5% within the previous 3 months.[24] Assessing nutritional status is an important aspect of the evaluation. Patients who are malnourished have higher morbidity and mortality rates, as well as longer length of hospital stay.[25] Subjective questions to screen for malnutrition include a dietary recall, appetite assessment, and report of altered taste sensation. Patients should be assessed for dysphagia, as this may affect not only their food consumption but also their ability to undergo transesophageal echo (TEE) should screening or procedure require it. Patients should also be assessed for nutrient loss through vomiting and/or diarrhea. The practitioner should also note if the patient has muscle wasting or fragile skin, typical presentations of poor nutrition. Albumin is used as part of a number of tests to assess frailty. Decreased albumin levels are an independent predictor of increased mortality post TAVR.[64]

Functional Assessment

Frailty, physical function, and ability to perform activities of daily living (ADLs) should be included in the patient evaluation.[6] During the patient evaluation for potential treatment of severe AS, the patient should undergo a frailty assessment, physical evaluation, as well as cognitive evaluation.[6] Frailty evaluation should at least include gait speed and nutritional assessment. Physical evaluation should assess gait speed as well as ADL assessment. Cognitive evaluation should encompass evaluations for depression and cognitive status. Based on information gleaned during examination, decisions can be rendered regarding futility.

Frailty

Frailty is a state of vulnerability due to a decreased physiologic reserve when stressors are applied.[65] In this state, the patient can have cumulative declines across multiple organ systems and an increased vulnerability to adverse outcomes. There is no universal definition of frailty, which makes determination difficult. Currently, over 20 various instruments are used to determine frailty. Determining frailty is an important aspect of evaluation, as the recovery post TAVR or SAVR is affected by frailty in the older patient population.[66] The ACC/AHA guidelines recommend use of the Katz ADL index, gait speed, grip strength, and muscle mass as the frailty measurement used for evaluation by the Heart Team.[13] In the extreme-risk population, predictors of lack of symptomatic improvement post TAVR include pre-TAVR wheelchair usage and low serum albumin levels.[67]

One methodology for frailty assessment encompasses evaluation for lower-extremity weakness, cognitive impairment, anemia, and hypoalbuminemia. This scale outperformed other frailty scales and is recommended for use in the evaluation process for AS treatment.[68] One clinical trial, *Safety and Efficacy Study of the Medtronic CoreValve System in the Treatment of Severe, Symptomatic Aortic Stenosis in Intermediate Risk Subjects Who Need Aortic Valve Replacement (SURTAVI)*, included frailty in the screening process.[69] In the PARTNER (Placement of AoRTic TraNscathetER Valves) trial, patient data were collected and assessed for frailty. Data collected included height, weight, albumin, Katz ADL, grip strength, and 5-meter walk test.[70]

Neurologic Testing

Cognitive function should be assessed during the evaluation for potential treatment of AS. This includes screening for prior disabling stroke, cognitive dysfunction, depression, and dementia.[6] Stroke assessment should be completed as part of the AS evaluation. The National Institutes of Health Stroke Scale is an assessment tool designed to provide a quantitative measure of stroke-related neurologic deficit. The stroke scale can gauge the stroke severity. Providers, nurses, or therapists can administer the tool. Other tools that may be used are the Barthel index or the modified Rankin scale.[71]

Dementia

The Mini Mental State Examination (MMSE) is the most common tool used to assess memory issues and mental abilities. It can be used to assess for dementia and cognitive impairment. The tool consists of a series of questions and tests, giving points for correct answers. The MMSE evaluates memory, attention, and language. The maximum score for the MMSE is 30 points. A score of 20 to 24 suggests evidence of mild dementia. Moderate dementia is suggested with scores of 13 to 20. A score of less than 12 is indicative of severe dementia. Lower scores on the MMSE were tied to poorer outcomes post TAVR.[72] An MMSE of less than 24 should be noted as abnormal.[6]

Depression and Anxiety

Depression and anxiety have been implicated in risk for major adverse cardiovascular and cerebrovascular events.[73] Approximately 7% of adults in the United States have had an episode of major depression.[74] Drudi and colleagues evaluated the association of depression and mortality in patients undergoing SAVR or TAVR. The authors note that approximately one-third of patients undergoing TAVR or SAVR had depressive symptoms at baseline and a higher risk of short-term and midterm mortality. Patients with persistent symptoms of depression at follow-up had the highest risk of mortality.[75]

There exist several screening tools for depression. The Center for Epidemiologic Studies Depression Scale is a tool that can assess symptoms of depression. The scale is a part of the Fried Frailty tool assessing exhaustion.[76] Notation of depression or history of depression should be noted on the patient assessment.[6] Other tools that have been validated for depression screening include the Beck Depression Inventory, Patient Health Questionnaire (PHQ), Major Depression Inventory, and the Geriatric Depression Scale. A number of these tools are available in short and long forms.

The PHQ has a 2-question form called the PHQ-2. This questionnaire takes approximately 1 minute to complete and can be used in the clinic setting without additional investment of resources. This form inquires about the frequency of depressed mood and anhedonia over the previous 2 weeks. The purpose of these questions is not to diagnose depression but to identify those who are at risk for having depression. If the patient answers yes to either question, they should be referred for further evaluation.[77]

Delirium

In postprocedure patients, the onset of delirium is associated with worse outcomes in patients undergoing aortic valve procedures.[2] Delirium may be preventable, have a negative impact on patients and their recovery, and lead to increased mortality. It is an acute syndrome that can cause the patient to have confusion or become hyperactive or hypoactive.[78] There is an acute onset of symptoms, which include altered or decreased level of consciousness, inattention, altered mental status, and impaired memory.[78] The risk for this adverse outcome can be mitigated by case selection, procedural considerations, and postprocedure care. Factors that predispose patients to higher risk for delirium include requiring a nontransfemoral approach, preoperative steroid use, increased age, carotid artery disease, current tobacco use, and atrial fibrillation.[78] Procedural-related predictors of postoperative delirium include general anesthesia use, longer procedures, as well as development of AKI postoperatively.[78,79] Following TAVR, delirium can cause prolonged ventilation time, increased hospital stay, as well as increased mortality.[78] Strategies to mitigate the risks for delirium are well established; they include the avoidance of opioids and sedatives; the rapid return to baseline hydration, nutrition, and mobilization; the resumption of diurnal patterns; and the minimal disruption to homeostatic status.[80]

At times, it may be necessary to refer patients to other specialties for consultation. Specialties may include neurology, gastroenterology, or pulmonary or palliative medicine. Occasionally, cancers and other abnormalities are noted on CT and require evaluation. Also, patients with a history of gastrointestinal bleed can be evaluated by gastroenterology to determine if the patient has Heyde syndrome. Palliative care specialists can assist in guiding conversations regarding plan and goals of care if no procedure is to take place. Ensuring a patient's wishes for end-of-life care are respected and honored, palliative care specialists are fantastic partners who can guide these nuanced conversations.

Surgical and Procedural Risk Evaluation

Appropriate treatments for patients are determined by exploring risk versus benefit for each case. The treatment determination is one in which the potential benefits, including survival, health outcomes, and quality of life, exceed the potential negative consequences of treatment.[4]

Surgical Risk Determination

Based on the information gleaned during the patient evaluation, the patient is evaluated for risk of open surgical procedure. Either the EuroSCORE (LES) or the STS score guides risk assessment. Once this information is determined, the patient care plan can be developed. The STS score is designed to calculate a patient's risk of mortality and morbidities for the most commonly performed cardiac surgeries. The calculator incorporates risk models that are designed to function as statistical tools that account for the impact of patient risk factors.[81]

The STS score is largely inaccurate at predicting TAVR outcomes.[82] A number of items are not included in the STS score, which affect clinical outcomes, including porcelain ascending aorta, history of cobalt or other chest irradiation, multiple prior chest surgeries, blood dyscrasias, and liver dysfunction.

Even though the STS risk score may be lower in some patients, anatomical risk factors may increase the risk of surgery. These include chest irradiation, chest abnormalities, and history of previous surgical procedures. Assessment in patients with a history of bypass or fusion to the sternum is warranted as to prevent potentially fatal complications during open surgery. Calculation of the STS score is an important data point in determining surgical risk. This number, in combination with the opinion of the cardiothoracic surgeon, determines the surgical candidacy of the patient. The number is collected by the TVT registry and used to develop predictive models to better identify patient risks and outcomes.

American College of Cardiology Predictive Outcomes

The ACC/AHA guidelines suggest using the STS criteria with 3 additional measures: frailty, major organ system compromise, and procedure-specific impediment.[13] The predictive model categorizes patients into risk groups by using patient characteristics, comorbid conditions, and functional capacity (Table 4.5).[83]

TABLE 4.5. Risk Assessment Combining STS Risk Estimate, Frailty, Major Organ System Dysfunction, and Procedure-Specific Impediments

	Low Risk (Must Meet All Criteria in This Column)	Intermediate Risk (Any 1 Criteria in This Column)	High Risk (Any 1 Criteria in This Column)	Prohibitive Risk (Any 1 Criteria in This Column)
STS PROM	<4%	4%-8%	>8%	Predicted risk with surgery of death or major morbidity (all cause) >50% at 1 y **OR**
	AND	**OR**	**OR**	
Frailty	None	1 index (mild)	2 or more indices (moderate to severe)	
	AND	**OR**	**OR**	
Major organ system compromise not to be improved postoperatively	None	1 organ system	No more than 2 organ systems	3 or more organ systems
	AND	**OR**	**OR**	**OR**
Procedure-specific impediment	None	Possible procedure-specific impediment	Possible procedure-specific impediment	Severe procedure-specific impediment

Adapted from Nishimura RA, Otto CM, Bonow RO, et al. 2014 AHA/ACC guideline for the management of patients with valvular heart disease: executive summary: a report of the American College of Cardiology/American Heart Association Task Force on Practice Guidelines. *Circulation.* 2014;129.

Transcatheter Aortic Valve Replacement–Specific Risk Score for Predicting Patient In-Hospital Mortality

The TAVR risk score has improved reliability to predict TAVR in-hospital mortality over the STS score. Similar to the STS score, the TAVR in-hospital mortality risk score is limited by lack of addressing frailty, disability, or cognitive function.[6] The risk score can be downloaded as an app (TAVR In-Hospital Mortality Risk) for easy use.

Treatment Timeline

AS is a progressive disease. Mortality increases as a patient develops symptoms (Figure 4.6). Given the poor prognosis for patients with symptomatic, severe AS, assessment and treatment should occur in an expeditious time frame (Figure 4.7).

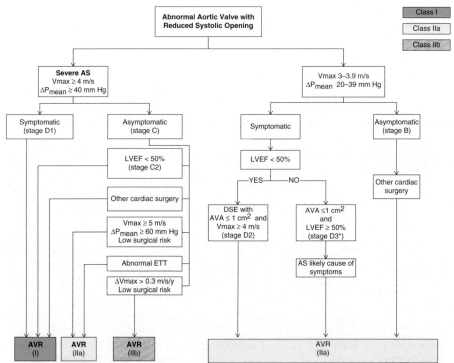

Arrow show the decision pathways that result in a recommendation for AVR. Periodic monitoring is indicated for all patients in whom AVR is not yet indicated, including those with asymptomatic AS (stage D or C) and those with low-gradients AS (stage D2 or D3) who do not meet the criteria for intervention.

*AVR should be considered with stage D3 As only if valve obstruction is the most likely cause of symptoms, stroke volume index <35 mL/m², indexed AVA is ≤0.6cm²/m², and data are recorded when the patient is normotensive (systolic BP 140 mm Hg).

As indicates aortic stenosis; AVA; aortic valve area; AVR, aortic valve replacement by either surgical or transcatheter approach; BP, blood pressure; DSE, doubtamine stress echocardiography; ETT, exercise tredmill test; LVEF, left ventricular ejection fraction ∆P$_{mean}$, mean pressure gradient; and V$_{max}$, maximum velocity.

FIGURE 4.6. Indications for AVR in patients with AS 2014 guidelines indications for aortic valve replacement in aortic stenosis. ∆P$_{mean}$, the mean pressure gradient across the valve; −∆V$_{max}$, change in maximum velocity across the valve on echocardiography. (Reprinted with permission from Nishimura RA, Otto CM, Bonow RO, et al. 2014 AHA/ACC Guideline for the management of patients with valvular heart disease: a report of the American College of Cardiology/American Heart Association Task Force on Practice Guidelines. *J Am Coll Cardiol*. 2014;63:2438-2488.)

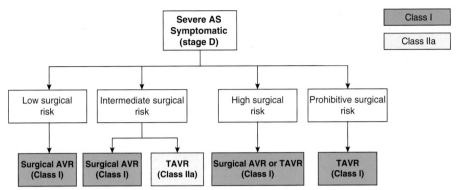

FIGURE 4.7. Choice of transcatheter aortic valve replacement (TAVR) versus surgical aortic valve replacement (AVR) in the patient with severe symptomatic aortic stenosis. (Reprinted with permission from Nishimura RA, Otto CM, Bonow RO, et al. 2014 AHA/ACC guideline for the management of patients with valvular heart disease. *J Am Coll Cardiol.* 2014. doi:10.1016/j.jacc.2014.02.536.)

Device Selection

One function of the Heart Team is to determine the choice of valve. Anatomy and valve size are the 2 main determinant factors regarding valve choice. Currently, there are 2 Food and Drug Administration–approved manufacturers of transcatheter heart valves. One valve, manufactured by Edwards Lifesciences, Irvine, CA, is balloon expandable. This valve is made of bovine pericardial tissue and is mounted in a short, cobalt chromium stent. The second valve, manufactured by Medtronic Corporation, Minneapolis, MN, is self-expanding. The self-expanding valve is made of porcine pericardium and is mounted in a nitinol stent and supra-annular design.[6] Illustration of valve and sizing charts can be found in Figures 4.8 and 4.9.

Anesthesia Assessment

Evolution of the TAVR clinical pathway extends beyond device improvements. Patients can undergo TAVR with general anesthesia, or, in some instances, moderate or conscious sedation. Retrospective and observational studies have evaluated conscious sedation outcomes compared with general anesthesia. Cases using conscious sedation have been associated with fewer inotrope/vasopressor requirements, shorter length of stay, shorter procedural times, and similar outcomes.[84-86]

The goal of conscious sedation is to perform a safe procedure while maintaining patient comfort and promoting rapid recovery. Careful consideration to patient anatomy and evaluation of airway are critical components of anesthesia assessment.[6] Anatomical considerations include coronary height, vascular access, and ease of intubation. Other patient factors include chronic pain, orthopnea, inappropriate mental status, and obesity.[6] Patients should be assessed for potential risks to emergent intubation. Some factors increasing risk include older age, BMI >26, facial hair, edentulous, and snoring history.[87] A Mallampati score should be obtained before use of conscious sedation in case emergent intubation is required periprocedure.

Heart Team Discussion

Incomplete information regarding patient history, physical examination, and imaging assessments can lead to poor outcomes.[43] Goals of the Heart Team include review of patient records

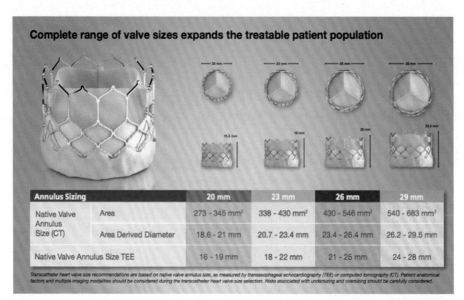

Complete range of valve sizes expands the treatable patient population

Annulus Sizing		20 mm	23 mm	26 mm	29 mm
Native Valve Annulus Size (CT)	Area	273 - 345 mm²	338 - 430 mm²	430 - 546 mm²	540 - 683 mm²
	Area Derived Diameter	18.6 - 21 mm	20.7 - 23.4 mm	23.4 - 26.4 mm	26.2 - 29.5 mm
Native Valve Annulus Size TEE		16 - 19 mm	18 - 22 mm	21 - 25 mm	24 - 28 mm

Transcatheter heart valve size recommendations are based on native valve annulus size, as measured by transesophageal echocardiography (TEE) or computed tomography (CT). Patient anatomical factors and multiple imaging modalities should be considered during the transcatheter heart valve size selection. Risks associated with undersizing and oversizing should be carefully considered.

FIGURE 4.8. Sizing of Edwards SAPIEN 3 Valve. (Used with permission by Edwards Life-sciences LLC, Irvine, CA. (Edwards, Edwards Lifesciences, the stylized E logo, Edwards Commander, Edwards SAPIEN, Edwards SAPIEN XT, Edwards SAPIEN 3, eSheath, PARTNER, PARTNER II, SAPIEN, SAPIEN XT and SAPIEN 3 are trademarks of Edwards Lifesciences Corporation).)

EVOLUT™ TAVR SYSTEM
VALVE SIZE SELECTION CRITERIA PER MSCT

	Valve Size	Aortic Annulus Measurements		Sinus of Valsalva Diameter	Sinus of Valsalva Height
		Diameter	Perimeter		
Evolut™ PRO and Evolut™ R Valves	23 mm	17†/18 mm–20 mm	53.4†/56.5 mm–62.8 mm	≥ 25 mm	≥ 15 mm
	26 mm	20 mm–23 mm	62.8 mm–72.3 mm	≥ 27 mm	≥ 15 mm
	29 mm	23 mm–26 mm	72.3 mm–81.7 mm	≥ 29 mm	≥ 15 mm
Evolut™ R Valve	34 mm	26 mm–30 mm	81.7 mm–94.2 mm	≥ 31 mm	≥ 16 mm

†Measurement for TAV-in-SAV only.
NOTE: The dimensions of SAVs can change in vivo requiring multiple considerations for the physician to make an informed decision of what appropriate Evolut TAVR valve size to use for TAV-in-SAV. These considerations include identification of the SAV, determination of the manufacturer's inside diameter, CT estimated measurement of the SAV's annulus diameter and patient specifics as outlined in the Best Practices.

FIGURE 4.9. Evolut TAVR System. Valve size selection criteria per MST. (Used with permission by Medtronic © 2018.)

and determination of disease severity, determination of appropriate interventions or medical management, and discussion of benefits and risks of proposed interventions.[6] As part of the Heart Team discussion, patients should be examined for risk of postprocedural complications and extended length of stay. Delirium post TAVR is associated with increased mortality.[79] Nontransfemoral approach and preoperative steroid use were associated with higher rates of delirium post TAVR.[79] The most powerful echocardiographic predictors of mortality post TAVR are low left ventricular ejection fraction and LF LG AS.[30] Left atrial enlargement is a predictor of mortality in patients with severe AS.[88] Prior to procedure, the Heart Team investigates anatomic features which may predispose a patient to post-TAVR aortic regurgitation and discusses strategies to minimize the risk. Aortic regurgitation post TAVR blocks reverse remodeling and is associated with poor 1-year survival post TAVR.[89]

Models of Clinic Flow

A number of international societies have recognized the need for specialized valve clinics.[10,13] In the United States, there is no standardized model for structural or valve clinic. Guidelines state the Heart Team is a level I indication for structural heart programs.[10,13] Clinic models are vague in their descriptions and state that the structural clinic comprises a group of health care professionals with an expertise in valvular heart disease.[1] The clinic is dedicated to provide specialized and centralized evaluation for valvular disease.[1] Generally, these clinics are designed to improve patient care, optimize patient evaluation, provide specific valve-related education, reduce morbidity and mortality, improve quality of life, and potentially reduce health care costs.[1]

The structural clinic can differ from a global perspective. Clinics operate differently inside and outside the United States. We even see differences in clinic structure from location to location within the United States. In Europe, the cardiologist involved with the clinic is typically a specialist in imaging and performs the echocardiogram.[1] In the United States, most echocardiograms are performed by the echo sonographer under the auspices of a cardiologist.

Clinic models can vary depending on the organization and physician staffing. The 2 major models include "virtual" clinic and "brick and mortar" clinic. A virtual clinic scenario is where the physicians see patients independently and refer the patient for TAVR thorough the VPC. In these instances, the VPC works to coordinate care by organizing patient evaluation and obtaining patient data. In brick and mortar clinics, the patient is seen in a dedicated space with a goal of joint evaluation by the interventional cardiologist and cardiothoracic surgeon at the same visit.

Conclusion

The delivery of high-quality patient care and attainment of optimal clinical outcomes are priorities for the Heart Team involved in the care of patients undergoing TAVR. A comprehensive evaluation pathway with attention to individualized patient care is of central importance in achieving these goals. The evaluation process should include a thorough history and physical examination, required imaging assessments, and a complete appraisal of social, functional, and cognitive status. Inclusion of the patient and family in the multidisciplinary Heart Team evaluation and decision-making process helps to ensure that their expectations and goals are taken into account.

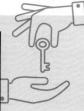

KEY TAKEAWAYS AND BEST PRACTICES

▶ Valve clinic models vary from a global perspective; however, the goal is to use a dedicated group of health care professionals with valvular heart disease expertise to navigate a patient through the evaluation and screening process while offering appropriate and technically feasible treatment options.

▶ Thorough patient history, physical examination, and guideline-directed diagnostic echocardiography are used to diagnose, determine the severity of, and classify AS to ensure that AUC are met before treatment.

▶ The evaluation necessary per patient to determine appropriate interventions to treat severe AS is a resource-intensive process that requires the collection of a number of specific diagnostic, functional, cognitive, and social data components.

▶ Patient experience should be kept at the forefront during the evaluation pathway in attempts to streamline the process and offer swift clinical disposition and treatment plans.

▶ Patient selection requires a multifaceted approach using all data collected to determine surgical and procedural risk stratification via the input of the multidisciplinary Heart Team.

References

1. Lancellotti P, Rosenhek R, Pibarot P, et al. Working group on valvular heart disease position paper–heart valve clinics: organization, structure, and experiences. *Eur Heart J*. 2013;34:1597-1606.
2. Eide LS, Ranhoff AH, Fridlund B, et al. Comparison of frequency, risk factors, and time course of postoperative delirium in octogenarians after transcatheter aortic valve implantation versus surgical aortic valve replacement. *Am J Cardiol*. 2015;115:802-809.
3. He W, Goodkind D, Kowa P. *An Aging World_2015.pdf*; 2015.
4. Bonow RO, Brown AS, Gillam LD, et al. ACC/AATS/AHA/ASE/EACTS/HVS/SCA/SCAI/SCCT/SCMR/STS 2017 appropriate use criteria for the treatment of patients with severe aortic stenosis: a report of the American College of Cardiology Appropriate Use Criteria Task Force, American Association for Thoracic Surgery, American Heart Association, American Society of Echocardiography, European Association for Cardio-Thoracic Surgery, Heart Valve Society, Society of Cardiovascular Anesthesiologists, Society for Cardiovascular Angiography and Interventions, Society of Cardiovascular Computed Tomography, Society for Cardiovascular Magnetic Resonance, and Society of Thoracic Surgeons. *J Am Coll Cardiol*. 2017;70:2566-2598.
5. Arbel Y, Zivkovic N, Mehta D, et al. Factors associated with length of stay following trans-catheter aortic valve replacement – a multicenter study. *BMC Cardiovasc Disord*. 2017;17:137.
6. Otto CM, Kumbhani DJ, Alexander KP, et al. 2017 ACC expert consensus decision pathway for transcatheter aortic valve replacement in the management of adults with aortic stenosis: a report of the American college of cardiology task force on clinical expert consensus documents. *J Am Coll Cardiol*. 2017;69:1313-1346.
7. Brennan JM, Edwards FH, Zhao Y, et al. Long-term safety and effectiveness of mechanical versus biologic aortic valve prostheses in older patients: results from the Society of Thoracic Surgeons Adult Cardiac Surgery National Database. *Circulation*. 2013;127:1647-1655.

8. Cote N, Pibarot P, Clavel MA. Incidence, risk factors, clinical impact, and management of bioprosthesis structural valve degeneration. *Curr Opin Cardiol.* 2017;32:123-129.

9. Rodriguez-Gabella T, Voisine P, Puri R, Pibarot P, Rodés-Cabau J. Aortic bioprosthetic valve durability incidence, mechanisms, predictors, and management of surgical and transcatheter valve degeneration. *J Am Coll Cardiol.* 2017;70:1013-1028.

10. Baumgartner H, Falk V, Bax JJ, et al. Group ESCSD. 2017 ESC/EACTS guidelines for the management of valvular heart disease. *Eur Heart J.* 2017;38:2739-2791.

11. Pibarot P, Weissman NJ, Stewart WJ, et al. Incidence and sequelae of prosthesis-patient mismatch in transcatheter versus surgical valve replacement in high-risk patients with severe aortic stenosis: a PARTNER trial cohort–an analysis. *J Am Coll Cardiol.* 2014;64:1323-1334.

12. Takagi H, Umemoto T, Group A. Prosthesis-patient mismatch after transcatheter aortic valve implantation. *Ann Thorac Surg.* 2016;101:872-880.

13. Nishimura RA, Otto CM, Bonow RO, et al. 2014 AHA/ACC guideline for the management of patients with valvular heart disease: a report of the American College of Cardiology/American Heart Association Task Force on Practice Guidelines. *Circulation.* 2014;129:e521-e643.

14. Nishimura RA, Otto CM, Bonow RO, et al. 2017 AHA/ACC focused update of the 2014 AHA/ACC guideline for the management of patients with valvular heart disease: a report of the American College of Cardiology/American Heart Association Task Force on Clinical Practice Guidelines. *J Am Coll Cardiol.* 2017;70:252-289.

15. Sintek M, Zajarias A. Patient evaluation and selection for transcatheter aortic valve replacement: the heart team approach. *Prog Cardiovasc Dis.* 2014;56:572-582.

16. Margulescu AD. Assessment of aortic valve disease – a clinician oriented review. *World J Cardiol.* 2017;9:481-495.

17. Ross JB, Braunwald E. Aortic stenosis. *Circulation.* 1968;38:61-67.

18. Kadle RL, Phoon CKL. Estimating pressure gradients by auscultation: how technology (echocardiography) can help improve clinical skills. *World J Cardiol.* 2017;9:693-701.

19. Park S-J. Symptomatic presentations of severe aortic stenosis. *Precis Future Med.* 2017;1:122-128.

20. Park SJ, Enriquez-Sarano M, Chang SA, et al. Hemodynamic patterns for symptomatic presentations of severe aortic stenosis. *JACC Cardiovasc Imaging.* 2013;6:137-146.

21. Le VD, Jensen GV, Kjoller-Hansen L. Prognostic usefulness of cardiopulmonary exercise testing for managing patients with severe aortic stenosis. *Am J Cardiol.* 2017;120:844-849.

22. Redfors B, Pibarot P, Gillam LD, et al. Stress testing in asymptomatic aortic stenosis. *Circulation.* 2017;135:1956-1976.

23. Domanski O, Richardson M, Coisne A, et al. Cardiopulmonary exercise testing is a better outcome predictor than exercise echocardiography in asymptomatic aortic stenosis. *Int J Cardiol.* 2017;227:908-914.

24. Cederholm T, Bosaeus I, Barazzoni R, et al. Diagnostic criteria for malnutrition – an ESPEN consensus statement. *Clin Nutr.* 2015;34:335-340.

25. Chermesh I, Hajos J, Mashiach T, et al. Malnutrition in cardiac surgery: food for thought. *Eur J Prev Cardiol.* 2014;21:475-483.

26. Wu W, Masri A, Popovic ZB, et al. Long-term survival of patients with radiation heart disease undergoing cardiac surgery: a cohort study. *Circulation.* 2013;127:1476-1485.

27. Litmanovich DE, Ghersin E, Burke DA, Popma J, Shahrzad M, Bankier AA. Imaging in Transcatheter Aortic Valve Replacement (TAVR): role of the radiologist. *Insights Imaging.* 2014;5:123-145.

28. Baumgartner H, Hung J, Bermejo J, et al. Recommendations on the echocardiographic assessment of aortic valve stenosis: a focused update from the European Association of Cardiovascular Imaging and the American Society of Echocardiography. *J Am Soc Echocardiogr.* 2017;30:372-392.

29. Fedak PWM, Barker AJ. Is concomitant aortopathy unique with bicuspid aortic valve stenosis? *J Am Coll Cardiol.* 2016;67:1797-1799.

30. Capoulade R, Le Ven F, Clavel MA, et al. Echocardiographic predictors of outcomes in adults with aortic stenosis. *Heart.* 2016;102:934-942.
31. Sathyamurthy I, Jayanthi K. Low flow low gradient aortic stenosis: clinical pathways. *Indian Heart J.* 2014;66:672-677.
32. Jander N, Gohlke-Barwolf C, Bahlmann E, et al. Indexing aortic valve area by body surface area increases the prevalence of severe aortic stenosis. *Heart.* 2014;100:28-33.
33. Eleid MF, Sorajja P, Michelena HI, Malouf JF, Scott CG, Pellikka PA. Flow-gradient patterns in severe aortic stenosis with preserved ejection fraction: clinical characteristics and predictors of survival. *Circulation.* 2013;128:1781-1789.
34. Hahn RT, Abraham T, Adams MS, et al. Guidelines for performing a comprehensive transesophageal echocardiographic examination: recommendations from the American Society of Echocardiography and the Society of Cardiovascular Anesthesiologists. *J Am Soc Echocardiogr.* 2013;26:921-964.
35. Danson E, Hansen P, Sen S, Davies J, Meredith I, Bhindi R. Assessment, treatment, and prognostic implications of CAD in patients undergoing TAVI. *Nat Rev Cardiol.* 2016;13:276-285.
36. Rader F, Sachdev E, Arsanjani R, Siegel RJ. Left ventricular hypertrophy in valvular aortic stenosis: mechanisms and clinical implications. *Am J Med.* 2015;128:344-352.
37. Ekeruo IA, Firstenberg M, Mehran R, et al. Timing and algorithm of permanent pacemaker implantation after tavr. *J Am Coll Cardiol.* 2017;69.
38. Fadahunsi OO, Olowoyeye A, Ukaigwe A, et al. Incidence, predictors, and outcomes of permanent pacemaker implantation following transcatheter aortic valve replacement: analysis from the U.S. Society of Thoracic Surgeons/American College of Cardiology TVT Registry. *JACC Cardiovasc Interv.* 2016;9:2189-2199.
39. Siontis GC, Juni P, Pilgrim T, et al. Predictors of permanent pacemaker implantation in patients with severe aortic stenosis undergoing TAVR: a meta-analysis. *J Am Coll Cardiol.* 2014;64:129-140.
40. Auffret V, Webb JG, Eltchaninoff H, et al. Clinical impact of baseline right bundle branch block in patients undergoing transcatheter aortic valve replacement. *JACC Cardiovasc Interv.* 2017;10:1564-1574.
41. Kamioka N, Wells J, Keegan P, et al. Predictors and clinical outcomes of next-day discharge after minimalist transfemoral transcatheter aortic valve replacement. *JACC Cardiovasc Interv.* 2018;11:107-115.
42. Clavel MA, Malouf J, Messika-Zeitoun D, Araoz PA, Michelena HI, Enriquez-Sarano M. Aortic valve area calculation in aortic stenosis by CT and Doppler echocardiography. *JACC Cardiovasc Imaging.* 2015;8:248-257.
43. Buellesfeld L, Stortecky S, Kalesan B, et al. Aortic root dimensions among patients with severe aortic stenosis undergoing transcatheter aortic valve replacement. *JACC Cardiovasc Interv.* 2013;6:72-83.
44. Chieffo A, Giustino G, Spagnolo P, et al. Routine screening of coronary artery disease with computed tomographic coronary angiography in place of invasive coronary angiography in patients undergoing transcatheter aortic valve replacement. *Circ Cardiovasc Interv.* 2015;8:e002025.
45. Achenbach S, Delgado V, Hausleiter J, Schoenhagen P, Min JK, Leipsic JA. SCCT expert consensus document on computed tomography imaging before transcatheter aortic valve implantation (TAVI)/transcatheter aortic valve replacement (TAVR). *J Cardiovasc Comput Tomogr.* 2012;6:366-380.
46. Saade C, Deeb IA, Mohamad M, Al-Mohiy H, El-Merhi F. Contrast medium administration and image acquisition parameters in renal CT angiography: what radiologists need to know. *Diagn Interv Radiol.* 2016;22:116-124.
47. Nguyen G, Leipsic J. Cardiac computed tomography and computed tomography angiography in the evaluation of patients prior to transcatheter aortic valve implantation. *Curr Opin Cardiol.* 2013;28:497-504.

48. Chaturvedi A, Hobbs SK, Ling FS, Chaturvedi A, Knight P. MRI evaluation prior to Transcatheter Aortic Valve Implantation (TAVI): When to acquire and how to interpret. *Insights Imaging.* 2016;7:245-254.

49. Ramee S, Anwaruddin S, Kumar G, et al. Aortic Stenosis AUCWG; Interventional Section of the Leadership Council of the American College of Cardiology. The rationale for performance of coronary angiography and stenting before transcatheter aortic valve replacement: from the Interventional Section Leadership Council of the American College of Cardiology. *JACC Cardiovasc Interv.* 2016;9:2371-2375.

50. Stefanini GG, Stortecky S, Cao D, et al. Coronary artery disease severity and aortic stenosis: clinical outcomes according to SYNTAX score in patients undergoing transcatheter aortic valve implantation. *Eur Heart J.* 2014;35:2530-2540.

51. Hussain ST, Chiribiri A, Morton G, et al. Perfusion cardiovascular magnetic resonance and fractional flow reserve in patients with angiographic multi-vessel coronary artery disease. *J Cardiovasc Magn Reson.* 2016;18:44.

52. Ludman PF, Moat N, de Belder MA, et al. Committee UTS and the National Institute for Cardiovascular Outcomes Research. Transcatheter aortic valve implantation in the United Kingdom: temporal trends, predictors of outcome, and 6-year follow-up: a report from the UK Transcatheter Aortic Valve Implantation (TAVI) Registry, 2007 to 2012. *Circulation.* 2015;131:1181-1190.

53. Essa E, Makki N, Bittenbender P, et al. Vascular assessment for transcatheter aortic valve replacement: intravascular ultrasound compared with computed tomography. *J Invasive Cardiol.* 2016;28:E172-E178.

54. Henn MC, Zajarias A, Lindman BR, et al. Preoperative pulmonary function tests predict mortality after surgical or transcatheter aortic valve replacement. *J Thorac Cardiovasc Surg.* 2016;151:578-585, 586 e1-2.

55. Lucon A, Oger E, Bedossa M, et al. Prognostic implications of pulmonary hypertension in patients with severe aortic stenosis undergoing transcatheter aortic valve implantation: study from the FRANCE 2 registry. *Circ Cardiovasc Interv.* 2014;7:240-247.

56. Lindman BR, Zajarias A, Maniar HS, et al. Risk stratification in patients with pulmonary hypertension undergoing transcatheter aortic valve replacement. *Heart.* 2015;101:1656-1664.

57. Condado J, Jensen H, Maini A, et al. Should we perform carotid doppler screening before surgical or transcatheter aortic valve replacement? *Ann Thorac Surg.* 2017;103:787-794.

58. Wilson W, Taubert KA, Gewitz M, et al. American Heart Association Rheumatic Fever Endocarditis, Kawasaki Disease Committee, American Heart Association Council on Cardiovascular Disease in the Young; American Heart Association Council on Clinical Cardiology, American Heart Association Council on Cardiovascular Surgery; Anesthesia, Quality of Case and Outcomes Research Interdisciplinary Working Group. Prevention of infective endocarditis: guidelines from the American Heart Association: a guideline from the American Heart Association Rheumatic Fever, Endocarditis, and Kawasaki Disease Committee, Council on Cardiovascular Disease in the Young, and the Council on Clinical Cardiology, Council on Cardiovascular Surgery and Anesthesia, and the Quality of Care and Outcomes Research Interdisciplinary Working Group. *Circulation.* 2007;116:1736-1754.

59. Smith MM, Barbara DW, Mauermann WJ, Viozzi CF, Dearani JA, Grim KJ. Morbidity and mortality associated with dental extraction before cardiac operation. *Ann Thorac Surg.* 2014;97:838-844.

60. Redfors B, Furer A, Lindman BR, et al. Biomarkers in aortic stenosis: a systematic review. *Struct Heart.* 2017;1:18-30.

61. Seferovic PM. B-type natriuretic peptide in aortic stenosis: new insight in the era of biomarkers? *J Am Coll Cardiol.* 2014;63:2026-2017.

62. Cheungpasitporn W, Thongprayoon C, Kashani K. Transcatheter aortic valve replacement: a kidney's perspective. *J Ren Inj Prev.* 2016;5:1-7.

63. Hamilton P, Coverdale A, Edwards C, et al. Transcatheter aortic valve implantation in end-stage renal disease. *Clin Kidney J.* 2012;5:247-249.

64. Forcillo J, Condado JF, Ko YA, et al. Assessment of commonly used frailty markers for high- and extreme-risk patients undergoing transcatheter aortic valve replacement. *Ann Thorac Surg.* 2017;104:1939-1946.

65. Thongprayoon C, Cheungpasitporn W, Kashani K. The impact of frailty on mortality after transcatheter aortic valve replacement. *Ann Transl Med.* 2017;5:144.

66. Talbot-Hamon C, Afilalo J. Transcatheter aortic valve replacement in the care of older persons with aortic stenosis. *J Am Geriatr Soc.* 2017;65:693-698.

67. Osnabrugge RL, Arnold SV, Reynolds MR, et al. Health status after transcatheter aortic valve replacement in patients at extreme surgical risk: results from the CoreValve U.S. trial. *JACC Cardiovasc Interv.* 2015;8:315-323.

68. Afilalo J, Lauck S, Kim DH, et al. Frailty in older adults undergoing aortic valve replacement: the FRAILTY-AVR study. *J Am Coll Cardiol.* 2017;70:689-700.

69. Safety and Efficacy Study of the Medtronic CoreValve® System in the Treatment of Severe, Symptomatic Aortic Stenosis in Intermediate Risk Subjects Who Need Aortic Valve Replacement (SURTAVI). 2017;2018:trail information.

70. Medicine USNLo. THE PARTNER TRIAL: Placement of AoRTic TraNscathetER Valve Trial (PARTNER). 2017;2018.

71. Harrison JK, McArthur KS, Quinn TJ. Assessment scales in stroke: clinimetric and clinical considerations. *Clin Interv Aging.* 2013;8:201-211.

72. Arnold SV, Afilalo J, Spertus JA, et al. U.S. CoreValve Investigators. Prediction of poor outcome after transcatheter aortic valve replacement. *J Am Coll Cardiol.* 2016;68:1868-1877.

73. Tully PJ, Winefield HR, Baker RA, et al. Depression, anxiety and major adverse cardiovascular and cerebrovascular events in patients following coronary artery bypass graft surgery: a five year longitudinal cohort study. *Biopsychosoc Med.* 2015;9:14.

74. Health NIoM. Major Depression. 2017;2018.

75. Drudi LM, Ades M, Turkdogan S, et al. Association of depression with mortality in older adults undergoing transcatheter or surgical aortic valve replacement. *JAMA Cardiol.* 2018.

76. Bieniek J, Wilczynski K, Szewieczek J. Fried frailty phenotype assessment components as applied to geriatric inpatients. *Clin Interv Aging.* 2016;11:453-459.

77. Thombs B, Benedetti A, Kloda L, et al. The diagnostic accuracy of the Patient Health Questionnaire-2 (PHQ-2), Patient Health Questionnaire-8 (PHQ-8), and Patient Health Questionnaire-9 (PHQ-9) for detecting major depression: protocol for a systematic review and individual patient data meta-analyses. *Syst Rev.* 2014;3.

78. Abawi M, Nijhoff F, Agostoni P, et al. Incidence, predictive factors, and effect of delirium after transcatheter aortic valve replacement. *JACC Cardiovasc Interv.* 2016;9:160-168.

79. Maniar HS, Lindman BR, Escallier K, et al. Delirium after surgical and transcatheter aortic valve replacement is associated with increased mortality. *J Thorac Cardiovasc Surg.* 2016;151:815-823.e2.

80. Kostas TR, Zimmerman KM, Rudolph JL. Improving delirium care: prevention, monitoring, and assessment. *Neurohospitalist.* 2013;3:194-202.

81. (STS) SoTS. Risk Calculators. 2018;2018.

82. Silva LS, Caramori PR, Nunes Filho AC, et al. Performance of surgical risk scores to predict mortality after transcatheter aortic valve implantation. *Arq Bras Cardiol.* 2015;105:241-247.

83. Minto G, Biccard B. Assessment of the high-risk perioperative patient. *Continuing Edu Anaesth Crit Care Pain BJA Edu.* 2014;14:12-17.

84. Jensen HA, Condado JF, Devireddy C, et al. Minimalist transcatheter aortic valve replacement: the new standard for surgeons and cardiologists using transfemoral access? *J Thorac Cardiovasc Surg.* 2015;150:833-839.

85. Toppen W, Johansen D, Sareh S, et al. Improved costs and outcomes with conscious sedation vs general anesthesia in TAVR patients: time to wake up? *PLoS One.* 2017;12:e0173777.

86. Babaliaros V, Devireddy C, Lerakis S, et al. Comparison of transfemoral transcatheter aortic valve replacement performed in the catheterization laboratory (minimalist approach) versus hybrid operating room (standard approach): outcomes and cost analysis. *JACC Cardiovasc Interv.* 2014;7:898-904.

87. Rosenberg M, Phero J. Airway assessment for office sedation/anesthesia. *Anesth Prog.* 2015;62:74-80.

88. Rusinaru D, Bohbot Y, Kowalski C, Ringle A, Marechaux S, Tribouilloy C. Left atrial volume and mortality in patients with aortic stenosis. *J Am Heart Assoc.* 2017;6.

89. Sato K, Kumar A, Jones BM, et al. Reversibility of cardiac function predicts outcome after transcatheter aortic valve replacement in patients with severe aortic stenosis. *J Am Heart Assoc.* 2017;6.

CHAPTER 5

Understanding Transcatheter Aortic Valve Replacement Diagnostic Imaging

Russell A. Brandwein, MS, PA-C

OBJECTIVES

▶ Highlight the importance of multimodality imaging in TAVR
▶ Review the modalities of TAVR-focused imaging: computed tomography with angiography, cardiac catheterization, and echocardiography
▶ Describe the key assessments in TAVR-focused imaging and their application to patient care

Background

The success of the transcatheter aortic valve replacement (TAVR) is dependent on careful patient selection, optimal performance of a complex and technically demanding procedure, and careful postprocedural care. Unlike traditional surgical aortic valve replacement (SAVR), which is guided by direct visualization via an open chest, TAVR relies on noninvasive imaging to guide therapy. Three-dimensional (3-D) multimodality imaging has emerged as a key component at every level of the evaluation pathway and procedural planning. The goals of multimodality imaging at the preprocedural level include selection of the appropriate device and device size, determination of patient suitability for the proposed access site, and assurance that the proposed device can be safely implanted.[1] Data from diagnostic multimodality imaging is also applied to intraprocedural guidance and postprocedural assessment.[1]

The Role of the Gated Computed Tomography Scan

A single test, computed axial tomography (CAT or CT) angiography (CTA), obtains almost all of the vital information needed to determine the feasibility of performing the procedure. Gated CTA of the chest, abdomen, and pelvis acquires the necessary data to measure the aortic root and aortic valve dimensions for appropriate valve size and selection, aortic valve calcium score (which may help assess the severity of aortic stenosis [AS]), coronary heights, coexisting coronary artery disease (CAD), and the vasculature to determine the appropriate access site.

Key Assessments
Aortic Valve

The aortic annulus is the virtual ring formed where the aortic valve leaflets meet the left ventricular outflow tract (LVOT) and the location where the transcatheter valve anchors and seals. Assessment of this ring is essential in determining if the anatomy is suitable for TAVR and in selecting the most appropriate TAVR valve. The most widely used method for assessing this structure is the CTA.[2] CTA allows for the measurement of aortic annular area and perimeter and helps to determine the appropriately sized valve prosthesis (Figure 5.1).

Accurate evaluation of the aortic valve annulus is crucial to the ability to appropriately size the transcatheter heart valve (THV) and perform the TAVR safely. Undersized devices may lead to paravalvular leak (PVL) or, in extreme cases, device embolization. Oversized devices may result in aortic rupture.[3,4] In the early era of TAVR, annular sizing was performed using two-dimensional echocardiography. The aortic annulus is not a perfect circular structure; advanced 3-D imaging techniques have demonstrated the oval shape of the annulus, which, unlike a circle, has a minimum and a maximum diameter. Two-dimensional echocardiography measurement of the aortic valve provides one diameter of the annulus or LVOT, which may be the smallest diameter, leading to selection of an undersized THV and PVL.

CTA has emerged as the most common method of noninvasive imaging for the aortic annular dimensions. A study from 2012 demonstrated that annular measurements derived from CTA demonstrated a lower rate of "worse-than-mild" PVL when compared with transesophageal echocardiogram (TEE).[5] A more recent comparison between 3-D TEE and CTA showed close approximate measurements between both modalities.[6] Despite the similarities in

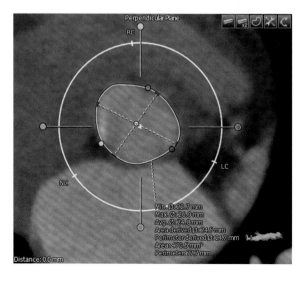

FIGURE 5.1. Gated computed tomography angiography depicting the aortic annular maximum and minimum diameters, area, and perimeter. LC, left coronary; NC, non-coronary; RC, right coronary.

measurements, given its less invasive nature, the CTA is the primary method for annular sizing in most patients who undergo TAVR.

Sizing using 3-D TEE is therefore usually reserved for the patient who cannot undergo a CTA (significant renal dysfunction, prior anaphylaxis to intravenous [IV] contrast, inability to remain still during the test). As with any imaging study, the quality of the measurements depends on the quality of the images. Therefore, reliability on the annular measurements by CTA or TEE may vary, and the factors contributing to the quality of the study must be carefully considered.

A patient's annular measurements by CTA and TEE vary. This large variability is likely related to different methods for measuring the annulus. Studies suggest that the difference may be as high as 9%, which, according to one study, resulted in 50% of patients receiving an inappropriately sized THV.[7] Other studies have shown minimal discrepancies between TEE and CTA measurements.[6]

An institution may consider evaluating the discrepancies between aortic valve measurements obtained by TEE and CTA. In patients who undergo a preprocedural CTA and an intraprocedural TEE, the percent difference between TEE- and CTA-derived annular measurements may be calculated. Thus, the expected percent of discrepancy of the annular measurements between TEE and CTA would be known. In cases relying solely on TEE-guided transcatheter valve sizing, knowledge of the percent discrepancy may contribute to the selection of an appropriately sized THV.

In traditional SAVR, the native aortic valve is removed and replaced with a mechanical or bioprosthetic prosthesis. In the TAVR procedure, the native valve leaflets are displaced into the aortic wall between the aortic wall and the prosthesis and the TAVR prosthesis sits in the aortic root. The confluence of all of these structures requires comprehensive evaluation to increase procedural success. These structures include the LVOT, aortic valve and aortic root, and ascending thoracic aorta.

The LVOT is subannular, or inferior to the aortic valve, and may be evaluated for its size, as well as its relationship to the aortic annulus. CT reveals the extent of the calcification of the LVOT. Significant calcium extending throughout the LVOT (Figure 5.2) is highly predictive of a potential annular rupture.[7]

The LVOT may also be assessed for the anticipated interaction of the THV, thereby guiding THV selection. In this subannular space lies the membranous septum, which is adjacent to critical conduction tissue, including the bundle of His. The prosthesis to LVOT diameter ratio (ie, the larger the implant within a smaller annulus and LVOT) and the depth of the THV implant in relation to the LVOT are associated with a higher risk of conduction abnormalities with TAVR and subsequent permanent pacemaker implantation.[8]

CT is helpful in the assessment of valve morphology, particularly in differentiating between a normal trileaflet aortic valve and a bicuspid valve. TAVR in bicuspid valves has not been studied in a randomized fashion; however, observational data have shown that implantation in bicuspid valves is feasible.[9] Leaflet lengths may be measured and compared with coronary ostia heights to assess the risk of coronary artery obstruction by the native valve leaflets at the time of TAVR. Lastly, aortic valve calcification scoring is also possible on CT and may provide additional data to elucidate the severity of AS.

Evaluation of the aortic root by CTA allows us to measure the sinuses of Valsalva and sinotubular junction and the annulus-to-coronary ostia height and leaflet length. Low coronary height, long and bulky leaflets, and shallow or effaced sinuses have all been shown to increase the risk of coronary occlusion by the native leaflet during the TAVR procedure.[10]

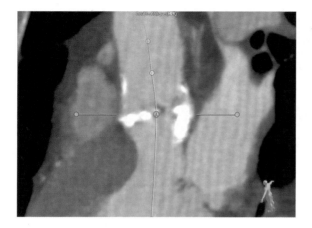

FIGURE 5.2. Significant left ventricular outflow tract calcium.

Another vital piece of information is the distance from the aortic valve to the left main coronary ostium. A review of coronary occlusions post THV implant demonstrated that a left main ostium height of 10.3 ± 1.6 mm increased the risk of coronary occlusion (Figure 5.3).[11]

Other information obtained by CTA, including the ascending aortic width, along with the height and width of the sinuses, helps determine the appropriate THV selection. Patients with aortic root width (or sinus width) of 27.8 ± 2.8 mm were considered to be higher risk for coronary occlusion, as well as women and patients receiving a balloon-expandable valve. The left coronary artery was the most commonly involved artery (Figure 5.4).[12]

Vascular Access

The transfemoral (TF) approach is the preferred access route for the TAVR procedure. This approach is the least invasive and provides the patient with the quickest recovery, compared with transthoracic access sites (transaortic, suprasternal, subclavian, and transapical). Imaging the aortoiliac system via CT scan evaluates whether the patient has

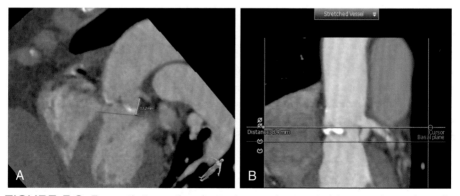

FIGURE 5.3. Transcatheter aortic valve replacement computed tomography angiography demonstrating left main height. A, Height measures 12.2 mm. B, Height measures 8.4 mm.

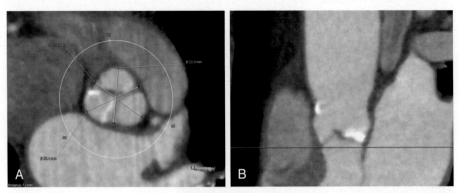

FIGURE 5.4. Assessment of the sinuses via transcatheter aortic valve replacement computed tomography angiography. A, Sinus width measurements. B, View shows effaced sinuses. Notice there is no out-pouching of the sinuses directly above the aortic valve. LC, left coronary; NC, non-coronary; RC, right coronary.

adequate TF access. The sheath sizes of the current THV are considerably smaller than earlier generations, thereby allowing the treatment of a greater number of patients via the TF approach. However, vascular complications remain a major cause of morbidity and mortality in this patient population.

CTA serves to identify known risk factors that increase the chance of vascular injury, including vessel size, tortuosity, and calcification. Current CT workstations have the ability to automatically center-line the vessels (Figures 5.5 and 5.6) and display the vascular system in multiple planes. When needed, they can allow for manual vessel caliber measurements as well. Advanced workstations have the ability to process 3-D volume-rendered images, which can aid in vessel analysis.

Vessel Size
The instructions for use for each of the THV specify the minimal lumen diameter deemed necessary for a TF approach. Historically, the minimal lumen diameter was as large as 8 mm, to accommodate a 24F sheath, and is now as small as 5 mm to accommodate a 14F sheath. A sheath to femoral artery ratio of 1.35 is a significant predictor of vascular complications among patients undergoing TF-TAVR.[13]

Vessel Calcification
Arterial calcification increases the chance of any vascular complications by 3-fold.[14] When assessing vessel size and calcification, it is important to remember that a noncalcified vessel will stretch; therefore, the diameter of the vessel is not an absolute contraindication in proceeding with the TF approach. In addition, vessel calcification that is not completely circumferential, or eccentric, may be less likely to pose difficulty for TF access.

Vessel Tortuosity and Abnormalities
Significant tortuosity and abnormalities such as aortic dissections or large atheromas may also prevent the ability to perform the procedure via the TF approach (Figures 5.5 and 5.6). In these patients with significant peripheral arterial disease, an alternate access site may be more appropriate.

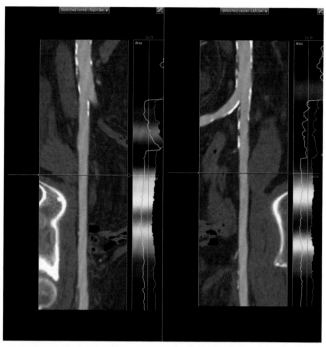

FIGURE 5.5. Straight-line view of iliofemoral arteries. Access is adequate.

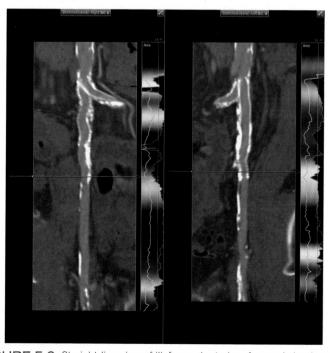

FIGURE 5.6. Straight-line view of iliofemoral arteries. Access is inadequate.

Alternative Access

In patients without TF access, various transthoracic access sites can be assessed for alternative access. A porcelain ascending aorta and prior coronary artery bypass graft surgery are relative contraindications to the transaortic access. As with the TF approach, the subclavian artery should be assessed for calcification, diameter, and tortuosity to determine the feasibility for access. The transapical approach was once the only alternative access used and was extensively studied in the PARTNER (Placement of Aortic Transcatheter Valves) trial.[15] It is associated with a longer recovery than the TF approach, given its lateral thoracotomy access, in which the muscle of respiration between the ribs are affected. Improvements in THV sheath and delivery system technology, along with other viable alternate access approaches, have rendered this approach a last resort.

Coronary Arteries

The TAVR CTA scan can be helpful in assessing the presence of coexisting CAD in this patient population. There is a reported 40% to 70% prevalence of CAD in the TAVR patient population.[16] The CT scan may rule out any obstructive CAD that requires treatment and may save the patient from an angiogram. However, in this patient population, the coronary arteries may be difficult to completely visualize, particularly in the presence of coronary artery calcification. Missing an obstructive, physiologically flow-limiting lesion could complicate the TAVR procedure. Therefore, evaluation of CAD by CTA alone and foregoing cardiac catheterization must be carefully considered. First, coronary arteries and/or bypass grafts must be adequately opacified by contrast and clearly visualized as patent on the CTA. Second, consideration must be given to certain situations in which contrast exposure increases risk. These include patients with renal impairment and patients with a significant allergic reaction to contrast. These factors must be considered in the context of past medical history, clinical presentation, and symptoms. When a CT scan is used in lieu of cardiac catheterization in the preprocedural evaluation of CAD, coronary angiography may be performed at the time of TAVR to confirm patency.

Image Quality

As with most tests in medicine, the ability to interpret the data obtained from imaging depends on the quality of the images acquired. Given the critical decisions stemming from CT imaging, superior image quality must be assured. Factors that influence the quality of the images include the type of CT scanner, experience of the CT technician, experience of the radiologist, amount of contrast given, proper timing of the contrast injection, patient movement, and whether the patient is in atrial fibrillation (AFIB).

Expert consensus on CT data acquisition recommends using a multidetector or multislice CT scanner with a minimum of 64 detector rows, imaging the aortic root with electrocardiogram (ECG) synchronization (gated study), minimizing motion artifact, obtaining slice thickness of less than 1 mm, imaging the aorta and peripheral vessels from the aortic arch to below the groin, and using contrast agents judiciously.[17]

Scanner Type

The accuracy of aortic annular assessment is directly affected by the type of scanner. The number of detector rows determines the volume of the heart covered per gantry rotation. Thus, a larger volume of the heart may be covered with a greater number of detector rows.

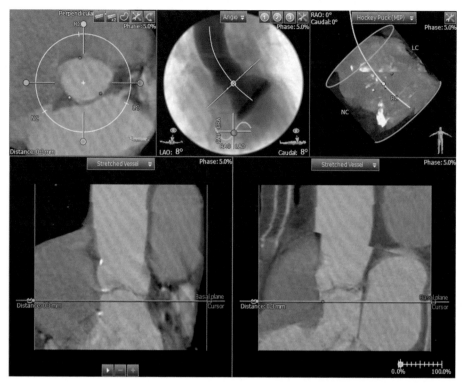

FIGURE 5.7. Images obtained using a 64-slice scanner displaying stair-step artifact.

Notice the difference in image quality in the earlier examples. Figure 5.7, obtained on a 64-slice scanner, appears "pieced" together with obvious artifact. Figure 5.8, on the other hand, acquired from a 320-slice scanner, depicts a much cleaner image owing to the increase in data obtained.

Electrocardiogram Gating

Image acquisition synchronized to the cardiac cycle reduces motion artifact and allows for 3-D reconstruction at any phase. Image quality is affected by the patient's heart rate and rhythm, particularly when the scanner has few detector rows and a slow gantry time. Medications may be used in the setting of CTA to control heart rate; however, typical protocols for this may be unsafe in the patient with severe AS. If and when used, a cardiology imaging expert should be present.

Historically, AFIB was a contraindication to a gated cardiac CT, as image acquisition to the cardiac cycle precluded patients with AFIB from undergoing the scan. This challenge was a common one, as patient eligibility for TAVR is largely driven by surgical risk and AFIB increases the risk of SAVR. In fact, patients who undergo TAVR have been found to have a higher rate of pre-existing AFIB than patients who undergo SAVR. The Society of Thoracic Surgeons (STS)-American College of Cardiology (ACC) Transcatheter Valve Therapy (TVT) registry data show that 41.9% of patients had pre-existing AFIB.[18] With the technology of the

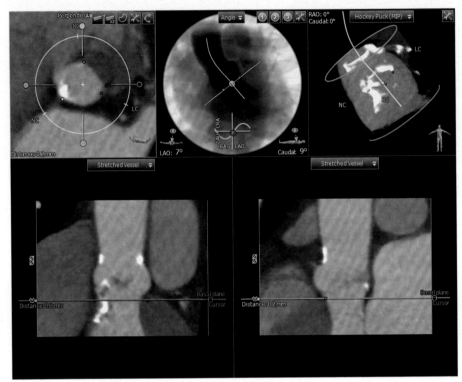

FIGURE 5.8. Images obtained using a 320-slice scanner.

current high-end CT scanners (increased scan speed and/or coverage), the contemporary impact of AFIB on image quality has decreased. AFIB is no longer a contraindication to CTA.

It is critical to understand the relationship of the cardiac cycle and aortic valve measurements. Sizing parameters (area, perimeter, and diameters of the annulus and LVOT) are typically obtained at peak systole, or 40% of the R-to-R interval on the ECG. The largest possible measurements of the aortic valve are obtained at this time, which minimizes the possibility of PVL due to an undersized THV. If image quality is suboptimal in systole, as may be the case with AFIB, measurements may be obtained at other ECG timings in systole or diastole, keeping in mind that early or late systolic or diastolic measurements are likely to underestimate aortic valve sizing. ECG gating ensures that the cardiac structures may be measured and reconstructed at all phases of the cardiac cycle.

Contrast Administration

The IV contrast dose for CTA is determined by patient factors (age, weight, cardiac output, renal function) and CT scanner specifications (scanner type and timing). Using a 128-slice multi-slice CT scanner in a patient with normal renal function, the CT scan may be performed using a contrast volume of 70 to 90 mL (infused at 4-5 mL/s). This dose and infusion rate allow for adequate visualization of the aortic annulus and vascular structures.

Chronic kidney disease (CKD) is a frequently encountered comorbidity in patients with AS who are being evaluated for TAVR. Not only does CKD negatively affect outcomes, but its presence can also complicate the preprocedural assessment of a potential patient undergoing TAVR because of increased risk of contrast-induced nephropathy (CIN).[19,20] Historically, in patients with abnormal renal function, our imaging options were limited to using noncontrast CT and transesophageal echocardiography, or risking CIN. Although there is some debate about the cause of CIN, Ahmed and Newhouse acknowledge its existence.[21] Columbia University Medical Center published a small series using a lower, 20 mL, contrast volume in patients with CKD who required a TAVR CTA. The data obtained from the low-contrast-volume CTA correlated with data from TEE imaging and demonstrated that a lower dose of contrast may be used in patients with CKD.[22]

When there is concern for suboptimal image quality, options may include addressing contributors (heart rate, motion artifact) and repeating the CT scan or using TEE before or at the time of TAVR to obtain these measurements. If a TEE cannot be performed, and available data do not reveal any contraindications to proceeding with TAVR, intraprocedural THV sizing may be accomplished via balloon aortic valvuloplasty immediately preceding implantation of the transcatheter aortic valve.

Special Considerations
Impaired Renal Function

As stated previously, minimizing exposure to contrast using a low-dose contrast protocol is favorable in patients with CKD.[6] However, in patients with significant renal impairment (estimated glomerular filtration rate <20 mL/min or creatinine >2.0 mg/dL), contrast administration may be avoided altogether. In these situations, an alternative preprocedure imaging strategy may include a gated, noncontrast CT scan of the chest, abdomen, and pelvis and intravascular ultrasound scan of the iliofemoral arteries at the time of the cardiac catheterization. The value of assessing the aortic valve and surrounding cardiac structures on a gated noncontrast CTA depends on the type of scanner, and the data obtained are more meaningful if the scanner coverage and speed are high.

Hydration protocols for CTA must be carefully considered in patients with severe AS and impaired renal function. The typical IV hydration protocol may result in iatrogenic CHF, as volume status is precarious in patients with severe AS (or any severe valve lesion), and any added volume may increase the risk of relative hypervolemia. Assurance of euvolemia before the CT scan is paramount. Diuretic or other renally active medications may be held on the day of the scan. Studies using sodium bicarbonate and N-acetylcysteine have been inconclusive, and these have not been recommended.[23]

Contrast Allergy

In general, a prior reaction to IV contrast does not preclude the ability to perform the CTA. Premedication guidelines are set forth in the American College of Radiology Manual on Contrast Media.[24] A prednisone-based regimen is common: 50 mg of prednisone by mouth at 13 hours, 7 hours, and 1 hour before contrast medium administration, plus 50 mg diphenhydramine intravenously, intramuscularly, or by mouth 1 hour before contrast medium administration.[25] In patients with intolerance to prednisone, a methylprednisolone regimen may be used: 32 mg two methylprednisolone by mouth 12 hours and 2 hours before contrast medium administration[26]; 50 mg of diphenhydramine may be added as well.

If a patient is unable to take oral medication, 200 mg hydrocortisone IV may be substituted for each dose of oral prednisone.[27] If a patient is allergic to diphenhydramine, an alternate antihistamine without cross-reactivity may be considered, or the antihistamine portion of the regimen may be dropped. Additional considerations may include whether the patient has reported an allergy to shellfish, previous premedication for contrast allergy, and tolerance of past procedures that required contrast. In patients with normal renal function and a contrast allergy, performing the CTA and cardiac catheterization on the same day allows for premedication on only one occasion.

Radiation Exposure

Considerations for radiation exposure are largely age related. Historically, the bulk of the patients being evaluated for TAVR were in their later decades of life; thus, the risk of radiation exposure was less of a concern. As indications for TAVR expand to a younger patient population, radiation risk may be of some concern. That being said, patients of all ages may have valve disease, and in the evaluation of a younger patient for valve disease (ie, bicuspid versus tricuspid aortic valve), a TEE or magnetic resonance imaging (MRI) may be performed as an alternative to a CT scan and radiation exposure.

Incidental Findings

A near full-body scan in this patient population is sure to identify abnormalities that may require further follow-up.[28] Generally, incidental CTA findings suggestive of a poor prognosis (ie, metastatic lung cancer) warrant further evaluation and may preclude TAVR. The presence of potentially malignant incidental findings on CTA is an independent predictor of long-term all-cause and noncardiovascular mortality but not of cardiovascular mortality.[29]

There is no consensus on which incidental CTA findings preclude a patient from proceeding with TAVR. This decision is left up to the Heart Team of the performing institution. A prognosis of at least 12 to 24 months is a general guideline for TAVR eligibility from clinical trials and government regulatory bodies. Multiple professional societies use a benchmark of a 12-month life expectancy in the appropriate use criteria for the treatment of AS.[30] Payers in the United States will not cover TAVR for patients in whom existing comorbidities would preclude the expected benefit from correction of the AS.[31]

The evaluation and/or treatment of incidental CTA findings, and adjudication of prognosis, may delay or preclude TAVR. Thus, balloon aortic valvuloplasty may be considered for symptomatic relief (palliative care) or as a bridge if another procedure is needed and severe AS precludes that from being performed.[31] Each institution must determine their decision-making criteria and processes pertaining to incidental findings on CTA.

Interpretation and Documentation

Each institution has a site-specific approach to interpretation and documentation of the CT scan, which includes postprocessing software, staff and vendor roles, and documentation. Several software programs for postprocessing TAVR CTA data are used by hospitals and vendors. Staff interpreting and documenting CT scan findings spans radiology technicians, radiologists, cardiology imaging specialists, and Heart Team physicians and clinicians (nurse practitioners, physician assistants, nurses). Vendors may also receive CT scan data and may provide clinical decision support for procedural planning (THV size, access site). Documentation of CT findings may include the study report by radiology and/or cardiology in the patient medical record, the Heart Team's recommendations (consultation, meeting minutes, procedural plan), and the vendor's report. An institution must explicitly define if and how these reports are used, where they are located, how discrepancies are reconciled, and what documentation format serves as the Heart Team's standard.

Each facility should decide on the best way to document the findings, based on their team needs and policies. Documentation of CT findings by the Heart Team must be in the patient medical record; however, not all staff involved in the patient care may be able to access the medical record. Historically, this gap was frequently bridged by assigning documentation and communication responsibilities to the valve program clinician; however, this critical information from CTA must be available to the team at all times and cannot be dependent upon the availability of an individual.

It is strongly recommended that a shared, privacy-compliant system be used for all team members to access the information. All staff involved in patient care should be able to access the team's interpretation of the CTA and the procedural plan (annular/THV size, access site, subsequent anesthesia strategy, invasive lines, emergency considerations). Institutions may use Web-based or mobile applications that require only a Web browser and Internet access, allowing real-time, round-the-clock access to the information. In the United States, the Health Insurance Portability and Accountability Act (HIPAA) regulates how protected health information is used and stored and use of non-HIPAA compliant services (eg, Google, Evernote, Dropbox) is discouraged. Web-based or mobile applications must be evaluated for their adherence to governmental and institutional privacy regulations. Fines have been imposed on institutions and personnel that violate privacy.

The Role of Cardiac Catheterization

Cardiac catheterization in the context of evaluation for valve surgery remains a high-level recommendation from professional societies.[32] As CAD is present in 40% to 75% of patients undergoing TAVR, diagnostic coronary angiography is warranted and recommended,[33] with consideration for special situations as previously described related to CT. Expanded discussion on cardiac catheterization in the evaluation of severe AS is also found in chapter 4.

Key Assessments
Preprocedural Imaging

In addition to assessment of the coronary arteries, cardiac catheterization allows for further evaluation related to procedural planning: assessment of the aorta, aortic root, and vascular access for TAVR. If obtained before a TAVR CTA, fluoroscopy may identify a possible calcified/porcelain aorta, which may aid in the determination of surgical risk. Aortic root angiography may also provide data to determine the adequacy of coronary heights, particularly in patients with a pre-existing bioprosthetic surgical aortic prosthesis. Intravascular ultrasound scan of the iliofemoral arteries may be used to evaluate feasibility of a TF approach in the patient who does not undergo CTA.

Intraprocedural Imaging

At the time of the TAVR, fluoroscopic imaging remains vital, namely, for valve positioning. Accurate positioning of the valve is crucial, as valves positioned too high or too low can result in coronary obstruction, valve embolization, PVL, and/or conduction abnormalities. Fluoroscopy-guided aortic root alignment may be accomplished using the "follow the right cusp rule" (right coronary cusp) as proposed by Kasel et al or by utilizing the fluoroscopic angulation predicted by the TAVR CTA (which reduces contrast volume, procedural time, and radiation).[34] For valve-in-valve TAVR, the pre-existing surgical bioprosthetic valve, if stented and at low risk for coronary artery occlusion, serves as a landmark for deployment of the THV.

Special Considerations

There are times when fluoroscopy or angiography does not suffice and TEE imaging is needed at the time of TAVR. If the valve size based on the TAVR CTA seems to be in the "gray zone" (meaning in-between the recommended size range for a specific THV), TEE imaging may determine the appropriate THV size. TEE imaging is also useful when the TAVR CTA identifies a low left main ostium, extensive valve calcification, or calcification involving the LVOT.[33] Lastly, in valve-in-valve TAVR cases with possible coronary occlusion based on the surgical prosthesis, TEE imaging should be used.[33]

The Role of Echocardiography

Echocardiography remains the mainstay of imaging in diagnosing AS. Echocardiography allows us to image the aortic valve and perform various calculations to aid in determining disease severity. Review of the echocardiographic criteria and the guidelines is provided in a previous chapter; however, it is important to briefly review the criteria for AS severity and how these numbers are obtained via echocardiography, namely, transthoracic echocardiography (TTE).

The echocardiogram assesses many parameters to identify the presence of AS. Morphologically, it can assess whether the valve is bicuspid or tricuspid, the severity of aortic valve calcification, and the aortic valve area (AVA) via planimetry. Hemodynamically, echocardiography can obtain a resting velocity, gradient, and area, as well as under stress (dobutamine or treadmill).

Comprehension of echocardiography is dependent on training and scope of practice. That being said, a basic understanding of how these measurements are obtained and calculated is essential to assess patients with AS.

Key Assessments
Aortic Valve Anatomy

The normal aortic valve is composed of 3 cusps situated in a circular fashion. Bicuspid aortic valves account for 1% to 2% of live births. In patients with AS who are younger than 70 years, 50% will have a bicuspid valve.[35] Although differentiating between a trileaflet and bileaflet valve is sometimes difficult on a regular echo, it certainly is possible (Figure 5.9).

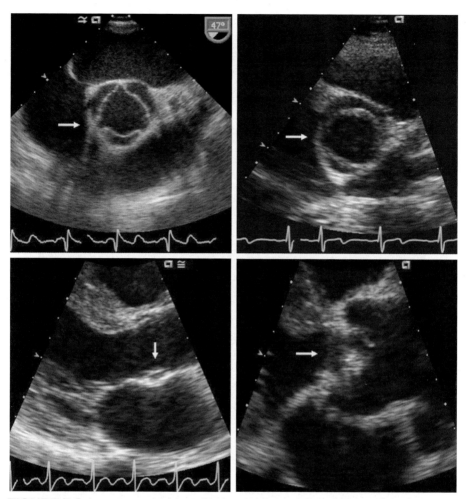

FIGURE 5.9. Images may also be used for imaging the aortic valve/valve leaflets (arrows). Top: Systolic frame of a normal trileaflet aortic valve (left) and a bicuspid aortic valve (right). Bottom: Normal trileaflet aortic valve in systole with the leaflets fully opened (left); a comparison image of a patient with calcific aortic stenosis showing reduced aortic valve leaflet opening in systole (right). (Echo courtesy of University of Washington Medical Center, Seattle, Washington. Reprinted with permission from Woods SL, Sivarajan Froelicher ES, Motzer SU, Bridges EJ. *Cardiac Nursing.* 6th ed. Philadelphia: Wolters Kluwer Health/Lippincott Williams & Wilkins; 2010).

One method to differentiate between a tricuspid and bicuspid aortic valve is the use of continuous wave Doppler (Figure 5.10).

The echocardiogram can also help assess the severity of the calcification, which usually coincides with the severity of the AS (Figure 5.11).

The extent of aortic valve calcification was a strong predictor of subsequent events and event-free survival.[35] Rosenhek et al[36] demonstrated a significant decrease in event-free

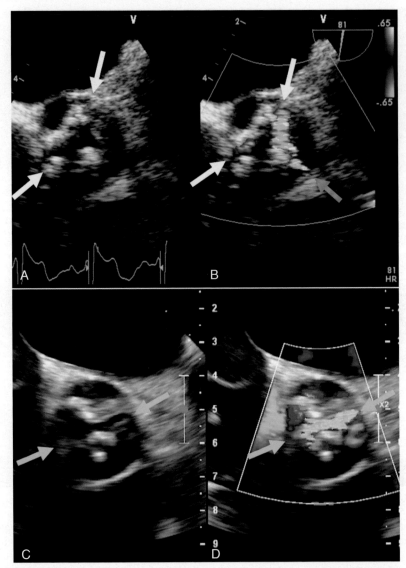

FIGURE 5.10. Flow is clearly seen between all 3 commissures, making the diagnosis of a bicuspid valve unlikely. A, Echo image of aortic valve without doppler. B, Echo image of tricuspid aortic valve with Doppler confirming flow through 3 commissures (arrows). C, Echo image of aortic valve without Doppler. D, Echo image of bicuspid aortic valve with Doppler showing flow only through 2 commissures (arrows). (Reprinted with permission of the American College of Cardiology, 2018).

survival in asymptomatic patients with AS based on their level of calcification. Levels of calcification were graded as none, mild, moderate, or severe. Patients with moderate to severe aortic valve calcification had a significant reduction in event-free survival, compared with patients with no or mild calcification.[36]

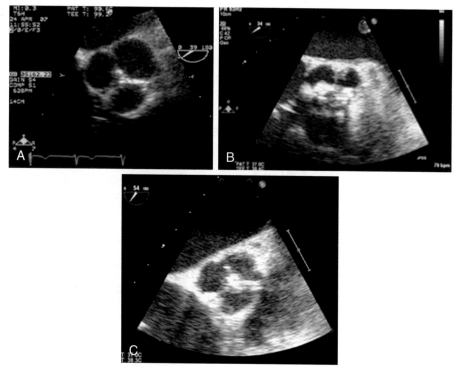

FIGURE 5.11. Various levels of aortic valve calcification obtained via echocardiogram. A, Mild: few areas of dense echogenicity with little acoustic shadowing. B, Moderate: multiple larger areas of dense echogenicity. C, Severe: extensive thickening and increased echogenicity with a prominent acoustic shadow. (Courtesy of Rebecca Hahn, MD.)

Severe AS is defined as a peak velocity greater than 4 m/s, a mean gradient greater than 40 mm Hg, and an AVA less than 1 cm².[35] The AVA is usually obtained using the continuity equation, which utilizes the conservation of mass theory (ie, what comes in must go out) (Figure 5.12).

Like all calculations, there are pitfalls to using the continuity equation. As the equation contains many variables, any error in the measurement of one variable will result in an error in the calculated AVA. Specifically, when measuring the LVOT diameter, any error would be squared and therefore throw off the calculated AVA.

Peak Velocity

AS creates an obstruction to the outflow of blood from the left ventricle, and therefore a pressure gradient exists between the left ventricle and the aorta. This pressure gradient can be measured, using Bernoulli law, by measurement of the maximum velocity across the aortic valve with continuous wave Doppler.

To obtain an accurate measurement, it is crucial to optimize the alignment of the Doppler beam with the jet and to attempt Doppler interrogation from multiple views. Having the probe out of alignment by even a few millimeters can result in underestimated gradients (Figures 5.13-5.15).

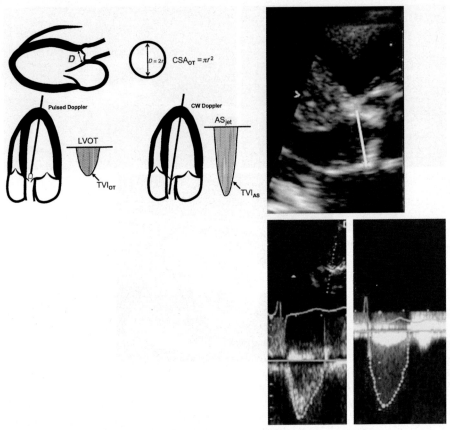

FIGURE 5.12. The measurements needed to calculate aortic valve area using the continuity equation. See text for details. AS, aortic stenosis; CSA, cross-sectional area; D, diameter; LVOT, left ventricular outflow tract; OT, outflow tract; TVI, time velocity integral. (Reprinted with permission from Armstrong WF, Ryan T. *Feigenbaum's Echocardiography.* 7th ed. Wolters Kluwer Health and Pharma/LWW (PE); 2009.)

Measurement of peak velocity is a reliable method to help determine AS severity but has pitfalls to consider. The velocity and gradients ignore the influence of cardiac output and can therefore be influenced by high or low output states unrelated to the severity of the AS. High cardiac output states (usually stroke volume index >58 mL/m^2) that can increase the peak velocity unrelated to AS include aortic regurgitation and hyperdynamic function. Low cardiac output states (usually stroke volume index <35 mL/m^2) that can decrease the peak velocity include low flow/reduced ejection fraction (EF) and low flow/normal EF (such as small left ventricular [LV] cavity, severe mitral regurgitation, and hypertension).

There are multiple methods to calculate AVA using echocardiography, and many variables go into determining the severity of AS. Minners et al demonstrated that "the criteria for the grading of aortic stenosis are inconsistent in patients with normal systolic LV function. On the basis of AVA, a higher proportion of patients is classified as having severe aortic valve stenosis compared with mean pressure gradient and peak flow velocity. Discrepant grading in these patients may be partly due to reduced stroke volume."[37]

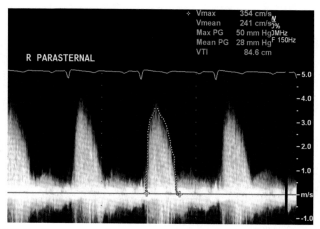

R PARASTERNAL

Vmax	354 cm/s
Vmean	241 cm/s
Max PG	50 mm Hg
Mean PG	28 mm Hg
VTI	84.6 cm

FIGURE 5.13. Continuous wave Doppler tracing obtained in a patient with aortic stenosis from the right parasternal window with the patient in a right lateral decubitus position. This position and view frequently affords the best Doppler alignment with the aortic stenosis jet. Peak and mean gradients are measured on the tracing. (Reprinted with permission from Allen HD, Driscoll DJ, Shaddy RE, Feltes TF. *Moss & Adams' Heart Disease in Infants, Children, and Adolescents.* 8th ed. Wolters Kluwer Health and Pharma/LWW (PE); 2012.)

Dimensionless Index

As mentioned previously, when calculating the AVA, the LVOT cross-sectional area is used. There is great variability in determining the area of the LVOT, given that it is more elliptical than circular, which can therefore lead to errors in the calculation of AVA. Another method to determine AS severity is the dimensionless index (also referred to as velocity ratio). This method eliminates the use of LVOT cross-sectional area. It can be expressed as a simple ratio of velocities (or velocity-time integrals) in the LVOT and across the valve.

$$DI = VTI_{LVOT}/VTI_{AoV} \text{ or } Velocity_{LVOT}/Velocity_{AoV}.$$

A dimensionless index of ≤ 0.25 is consistent with severe AS. Like any method to quantify disease severity, no one method is perfect, and clinical judgment is inherent to the assessment of AS severity.

Low-Flow, Low-Gradient Aortic Stenosis

There are many factors that determine the flow rate through the aortic valve. Most involve the ventricular stroke volume (systolic EF, heart rate, ventricular volume, diastolic filling) or arterial afterload (Figure 5.16).

Now, consider the echocardiogram report that connotes severe AS by AVA, but the peak velocity and mean gradient are below the criteria for severe AS (eg, peak velocity <4.0 m/s and mean gradient <40 mm Hg). Is it truly severe AS? Are patients not being referred because the primary physician or cardiologist believes that the AS is likely not severe, the gradients being low?

Patient A

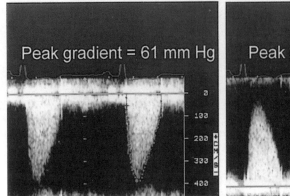 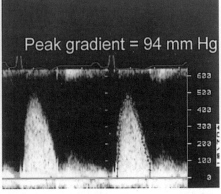

Patient B

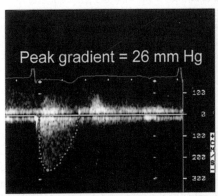 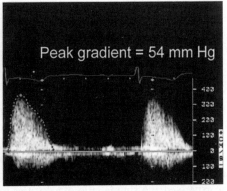

FIGURE 5.14. Two patients with aortic stenosis are included. In both cases, different values for aortic stenosis jet velocity are obtained, yielding different measures of peak gradient. In patient A, the apical view underestimates the true velocity, which is optimally recorded from the right parasternal window. In patient B, the apical window again underestimates true velocity. In this case, the peak gradient was best recorded from the suprasternal notch. (Reprinted with permission from Feigenbaum H, Armstrong WF, Ryan T. *Feigenbaum's Echocardiography.* 6th ed. Wolters Kluwer Health and Pharma/LWW (PE); 2004.)

In this scenario, attention must be paid to the LV EF. Current professional guidelines further differentiate low-flow, low-gradient (LFLG) AS and its management and prognosis according to a preserved or reduced LVEF.

Low-Flow, Low-Gradient Aortic Stenosis With Reduced Ejection Fraction

In patients with LFLG severe AS and an EF less than 50%, a dobutamine stress echocardiogram (DSE) is recommended (maximal dose, 20 µg/kg/min). Patients who respond with an increase in gradients and an AVA that is unchanged or decreased are considered to have severe

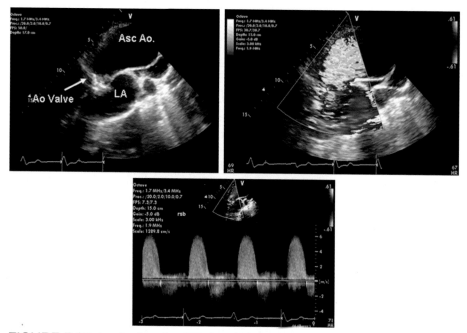

FIGURE 5.15. Imaging from the right sternal window in a patient with severe aortic stenosis. Note the excellent alignment of the Doppler and the direction of the jet. The maximal jet velocity from this window was 6 m/s and only 3.5 m/s from the apical window. Ao, aortic; Asc Ao, ascending aorta; LA, left atrium. (Reprinted with permission from Garcia MJ. *Noninvasive Cardiovascular Imaging: A Multimodality Approach*. Wolters Kluwer Health and Pharma/LWW (PE); 2011.)

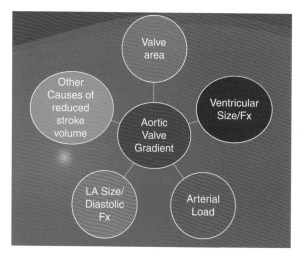

FIGURE 5.16. Factors determining the flow rate across the aortic valve. Fx, function; LA, left atrium.

AS.[35] Caution is advised in performing a DSE with unknown coronary anatomy, as dobuta-mine can potentiate ischemia or an arrhythmia, which is poorly tolerated in the patient with hemodynamically significant AS. To minimize this risk, it is prudent to perform cardiac cathe-terization and exclude obstructive CAD in advance of the DSE.

Low-Flow, Low-Gradient Aortic Stenosis With Preserved Ejection Fraction

There are many causes of paradoxical LFLG states (stroke volume index <35 mL/m^2). An in-depth discussion of all the causes is beyond the scope of this text, but one should be familiar with the list to help determine the underlying cause. These include abnormal LV mechanics (intrinsic myocardial dysfunction, ie, interstitial fibrosis), tachycardia, small LV cavity (hypertrophic/thick LV walls), severe diastolic dysfunction, hypertension, mitral regurgitation, or mitral stenosis. The atrioventricular dyssynchrony associated with AFIB may also contribute to a LF state owing to the loss of atrial kick. These conditions should be considered in the patient with moderate to severe AS, or an AVA of approx-imately 1.0 cm^2 and a peak velocity or mean gradient of less than 4 m/s or 40 mm Hg, respectively.

Pseudosevere Aortic Stenosis

Alternatively, the reduction of flow may be the cause of the low valve area, known as pseudose-vere AS. This is a critical distinction because, in true severe AS, intervention on the aortic valve is likely to result in clinical improvement, whereas if the problem primarily lies at the level of the myocardium, this is less likely. Myocardial dysfunction, due to related secondary causes such as severe multivessel CAD or disease of the myocardium itself, decreases the force of aor-tic valve opening. In this scenario, the AVA is reduced but the disease severity is overestimated because of incomplete opening of the aortic valve.

If the severity of AS is truly in question, particularly with paradoxical LFLG AS, then mul-timodality imaging may further aid in the diagnosis. Quantification by calcium score and visu-alization of calcification on CT scan may be helpful. In some cases, TEE may provide better visualization of the valve, especially in patients with poor transthoracic windows. At times, the data from diagnostic studies may not point in the same direction, but clinical judgment must be combined with multimodality imaging assessment to determine the treatment plan. For example, the treatment approach for the patient with borderline severe AS may differ from that for the patient with LFLG AS and depends on the overall risk, symptoms, and potential benefits from intervention.

Transesophageal Echocardiography

In the prior section reviewing CT, the use of 3-D TEE for assessing the aortic annulus was detailed, especially in cases for which a CTA cannot be performed. In this section, the role of TEE in the diagnosis of AS and other valve lesions and its intraprocedural use are reviewed.

Preprocedural Imaging

TEE is not generally performed in the routine workup of AS. Most patients with high-flow, high-gradient AS do not require a TEE to confirm the AS severity. As mentioned previously, in cases in which the diagnosis is in question (ie, paradoxical LFLG AS, poor acoustic windows), a TEE may be performed to aid in the diagnosis (Figures 5.17 and 5.18).

A preprocedure TEE may serve several purposes in the evaluation for possible valve-in-valve TAVR. The mechanism of failure of a bioprosthetic aortic valve must be assessed, which cannot be readily accomplished by TTE. A bioprosthetic surgical aortic valve may

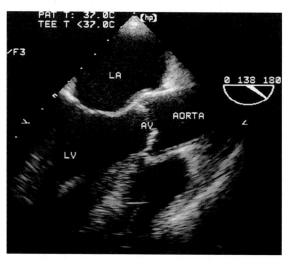

FIGURE 5.17. Transesophageal echocardiogram of the midesophageal aortic valve long-axis view during systole in a patient with aortic stenosis. A multiplane probe at 138° provided this view of an aortic valve (AV) with doming leaflets. Leaflet doming is a qualitative sign of stenosis. The proximal ascending aorta is also imaged in this view. LA, left atrium; LV, left ventricle. (Reprinted with permission from Konstadt SN, Shernan SK, Oka Y. *Clinical Transesophageal Echocardiography.* 2nd ed. Wolters Kluwer Health and Pharma/LWW (PE); 2003.)

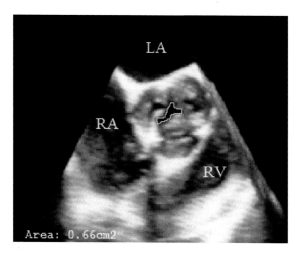

FIGURE 5.18. Three-dimensional transesophageal echocardiogram of the short-axis aortic valve view in the setting of severe aortic stenosis. Aortic valve orifice area is 0.66 cm², determined using planimetry. LA, left atrium; RA, right atrium; RV, right ventricle. (Reprinted with permission from Savage RM, Aronson S, Shernan SK. *Comprehensive Textbook of Perioperative Transesophageal Echocardiography.* 2nd ed. Wolters Kluwer Health and Pharma/LWW (PE); 2010.)

fail owing to stenosis, insufficiency, or both, which may result from a variety of causes including valve degeneration, infective endocarditis, or thrombosis. In this case, a TEE allows for better visualization of the valve leaflets and may reveal the presence of active or healed vegetations, thrombus, or prosthetic leaflet perforation. In bioprosthetic valve insufficiency, the TEE will also differentiate if the regurgitant jets are central or paravalvular. This assessment helps to guide treatment, as central aortic insufficiency may be treated with a valve-in-valve TAVR. PVL is treated with percutaneous PVL closure. TEE may also be used to assess coronary heights, which can be difficult to evaluate by CTA, particularly if artifact is produced by a stented surgical bioprosthetic valve.

TEE may be performed when the evaluation of concomitant valve disease and severity is required before TAVR. For example, a TTE may already confirm that AS is severe and shows moderate to severe mitral or tricuspid valve disease. If warranted, a TEE may provide further clarification of the severity and mechanism of either lesion. This will not only help clarify the lesion severity but also aid in determining if the mitral or tricuspid anatomy is suitable for a transcatheter approach. The aortic valve would also be fully evaluated at the time of the TEE, and measurements for annular sizing would be compared with CT findings. The procedural implication in this specific example is that if the other valve lesions do not require intervention, and the annular measurements by CT and TEE sufficiently guide appropriate THV sizing, then TAVR may be performed without intraprocedural TEE guidance.

The safety and feasibility of TEE must be routinely determined in patients who undergo evaluation for or treatment with TAVR. This screening includes assessment of the airway, dentition, sedation concerns, and dysphagia. If a patient reports dysphagia without a prior workup, an esophogram (barium swallow) may be used to confirm that the dysphagia is not from an obstructive or restrictive cause. As needed, a referral to an ear, nose, and throat specialist or gastroenterologist may be required before performing a TEE. Patients may also be referred to their primary care physician for dysphagia evaluation. If there is a history of evaluation or treatment of dysphagia, then acquisition of relevant medical records and communication with the related consultative specialty occur to ensure that there is no contraindication for the TEE. If TEE is contraindicated in a patient who will undergo TAVR, it must be determined whether TTE is a suitable intraprocedural imaging modality. As TAVR is more frequently performed under moderate or conscious sedation, TTE is increasingly used for intraprocedural imaging.

Intraprocedural Imaging

As discussed in the previous section, there is institutional variability of the imaging modalities used at the time of the TAVR. Each institution should understand its own strengths and weaknesses and proceed with the multimodality strategy that best suits their needs.

If the valve anatomy is appropriate and THV sizing seems adequate by CTA, then a TEE may not be required at the time of TAVR. In this case, the intraprocedural multimodality imaging approach may include TTE and fluoroscopy. If there are insufficient data on THV sizing, left main coronary ostium height, or LVOT calcium on the CT, then an intraprocedural TEE may be performed.

The Role of Magnetic Resonance Imaging

As indicated previously, ECG-gated CTA remains the hallmark for TAVR anatomic procedure planning. Echocardiography (with or without stress) combined with cardiac catheterization and CT scan data all aid in establishing the diagnosis of severe AS. But what if one test can combine both anatomic measurements (annular diameters, perimeter, area) and diagnostic (flow volumes, peak velocities) evaluation?

The noncontrast MRI has the ability to obtain both anatomic and diagnostic measurements. In cases in which contrast CTA is not possible (severe anaphylactic reaction or severe renal impairment) or stress echocardiography cannot be done (inability to exercise, arrhythmias), there may be a role for noncontrast MRI. Chaturvedi et al demonstrated that measurements obtained by noncontrast MRI are similar to those from contrast-enhanced CTA and that noncontrast MRI (Figure 5.19) can also be used to assess the severity of AS.[38]

Some of the advantages of an MRI include noninvasive and radiation-free imaging, anatomic assessment of the aortic valve for identifying congenital valvular abnormalities, planimetry calculation of AVA, visualization of cardiac structures, and characterization of the ventricular mass and function.[38] As discussed previously, noncontrast MRI is frequently the modality of choice in younger patients when trying to identify congenital valve disease, especially when ruling out a bicuspid versus tricuspid aortic valve, and to avoid radiation exposure.

If MRI seems like a "one-stop shop," then why has it not replaced the gated CTA? Some of the disadvantages include multiple breath holds, longer scan time, inability to perform in a patient with non-MRI compatible material in place, and claustrophobia. Also, how well MRI assesses calcified plaques and porcelain aorta is not known. Lastly, semiautomatic analysis software is currently available for CT but not for MRI.[38]

The main reason that MRI has not replaced gated CTA is the long scan time. A busy valve clinic may perform up to 12 gated CTAs per day. This level of access would be impossible to achieve with noncontrast MRI. Therefore, although noncontrast MRI's comprehensive assessment is enticing, its long scan time makes it an inefficient test for all comers and it is generally used on a case-by-case basis. As mentioned previously, each institution must have an expert in the modalities used. Even if cardiac MRI is used infrequently, an expert in cardiac MRI is essential for the interpretation and application of the study findings.

The Role of Imaging for Post–Transcatheter Aortic Valve Replacement Evaluation

New solutions can sometimes create new problems. A historical example of this is the drug-eluting coronary artery stent. The medications used to prevent scar tissue proliferation and in-stent restenosis of bare metal stents produced in-stent thrombosis instead. The TAVR procedure is a tremendous medical breakthrough that has saved thousands of patients with severe AS. But this groundbreaking technology has inevitably led to a new set of problems. Many of these problems are assessed via multimodality imaging.

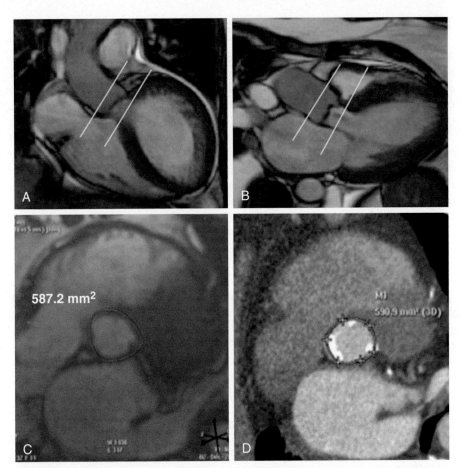

FIGURE 5.19. Acquisition on magnetic resonance imaging for aortic annular plane to measure diameters, area, and perimeter. Aortic root cine stack is prescribed from coronal aorta (A) and left ventricle outflow tract views (B). Systolic image where the luminal diameter is the widest, in a location just below the insertion of the valve leaflets (C), is identified as the annular slice. Corresponding annular image from the same patient obtained from electrocardiogram-gated computed tomography angiography demonstrates similar measurement of annular area (D). (Image reprinted under the Creative Commons Attribution 4.0 International License (http://creativecommons.org/licenses/by/4.0) from Chaturvedi A, Hobbs SK, Ling FS, Chaturvedi A, Knight P. MRI evaluation prior to transcatheter aortic valve implantation (TAVI): When to acquire and how to interpret. *Insights Imaging.* 2016;7(2):245-254.)

Evaluation of the Transcatheter Heart Valve

The initial assessment of the function of an implanted THV is with an echocardiogram. The STS-ACC TVT registry recommends that all THV patients undergo a TTE at discharge and at 30 days post THV implant.[39]

Echocardiographic assessment of the THV is similar to the guidelines for the assessment of a surgically implanted prosthesis,[40] but the THV does have several unique features that need to be evaluated. The echocardiogram should focus on the visual appearance of the THV (stent position, cusp mobility/thickness, color Doppler), hemodynamics (mean gradient, peak velocity, effective orifice area, regurgitation both central and paravalvular), other structures (mitral valve, aorta, coronaries), and cardiac function (ventricular size and function, LV stroke volume).[41] It is important that a member of the imaging team experienced with THV assessment reviews the echocardiograms. Technicians and physicians with limited experience in THV assessment may potentially underestimate or overestimate an issue (eg, PVL of a self-expanding THV) or miss a critical diagnosis (eg, THV thrombus), leading to unnecessary confusion and patient anxiety. For consistent evaluation, the institution that provided the TAVR may prefer to perform follow-up imaging in their facility. Conversely, referring physicians may prefer to have the echocardiogram performed in their facility, which is often more convenient for patients. Thus, education and outreach on the specific considerations of THV assessment on echocardiography, and the sharing of these imaging studies and medical records across mutual providers, is recommended.

Postimplant thresholds for further evaluation of the THV include mean gradient greater than 20 mm Hg (or >50% baseline) or AVA less than 1.0 cm². The Valve Academic Research Consortium-2 published updated guidelines for end-point definitions post transcatheter aortic valve implantation.[42] A patient with a mean gradient greater than 20 mm Hg with associated decreased leaflet mobility, especially with symptoms, should be referred for further evaluation with either CTA or TEE to rule out valve thrombosis.

Bioprosthetic Valve Thrombosis

Bioprosthetic valve thrombosis is a well-known complication of SAVR.[43,44] The first reported case[45] of THV thrombosis was published in 2009, and many case reports followed.[46] The current true incidence is difficult to measure, and the only multicenter systematic review reported a THV thrombosis rate of 0.61% among 4266 patients after a median follow-up of 181 days.[47] The investigators of this review did caution that the rate of THV thrombosis was likely underestimated.

Patients with echocardiographic findings suspicious for THV thrombosis may be referred for gated cardiac CTA. In a report of 140 patients who underwent routine screening with CTA post TAVR, abnormal leaflet thickening was seen in 5 patients (4%) (Figure 5.20).[48]

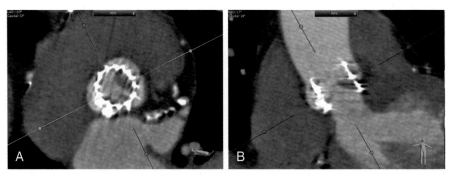

FIGURE 5.20. Gated computed tomography angiography demonstrating thickened leaflet (thrombus) on an implanted transcatheter heart valve. The darkened area within the stent represents thrombus.

A trial of oral anticoagulation has been proven effective for prosthetic valve thrombosis.[46,47] Following a period of therapeutic anticoagulation, THV gradients may be reassessed by echocardiography and gated cardiac CTA may be repeated to confirm resolution of the thrombus.

Bioprosthetic valve thrombosis can frequently go unrecognized, both on TTE and TEE, owing to the lack of awareness of the condition and its evaluation.[49] Pislaru et al suggested diagnostic echocardiographic criteria to identify bioprosthetic valve thrombosis: (1) gradient increase >50% over baseline, (2) increased leaflet thickening, and (3) reduced cusp mobility.[41] When present, prompt evaluation with CTA or TEE is warranted.

A complete review of all aspects of post-THV imaging is beyond the scope of this chapter, but readers can refer to Pislaru et al's paper on the assessment of prosthetic valve function after TAVR.[49]

Conclusions

Technical expertise is needed to perform the TAVR procedure successfully. However, it is demonstrated here that multimodality imaging is a key component at every level. From the initial evaluation process to procedural planning, as well as intraprocedural guidance and postprocedural assessment of the THV and patient outcome, multimodality imaging is integral to the overall success of the procedure and TAVR program development.

The development of the TAVR procedure has allowed multitudes of patients to forego traditional SAVR. Like all aspects of medicine, the team approach to patient care works best. Although the Heart Team may make a treatment decision after extensive review of the available data, including all of the images, we must ensure that the patient is central to the decision-making process. Let us not forget that the patient is the leader of the team.

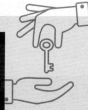

KEY TAKEAWAYS AND BEST PRACTICES

▶ Multimodality imaging is a key component of procedural and program success.

▶ Echocardiography is not the sole modality to determine the severity of AS.

▶ Gated CTAs can be safely performed in patients with contrast allergies and renal dysfunction.

▶ Develop an experienced team with expertise in all imaging modalities.

▶ Establish a systematic approach to documentation and image sharing for the Heart Team.

▶ Identify and address team strengths and challenges in imaging acquisition and interpretation.

▶ Imaging studies help to guide treatment decisions, but patients actually make them—involve the patient in the treatment decision.

References

1. Bloomfield GS, Gillam LD, Hahn RT, et al. A practical guide to multimodality imaging of transcatheter aortic valve replacement. *JACC Cardiovasc Imaging*. 2012;5(4):441-455.

2. Leipsic J, Gurvitch R, Labounty TM, et al. Multidetector computed tomography in transcatheter aortic valve implantation. *JACC Cardiovasc Imaging*. 2011;4(4):416-429.

3. Gilard M, Eltchaninoff H, Iung B, et al. Registry of transcatheter aortic-valve implantation in high-risk patients. *N Engl J Med*. 2012;366(18):1705-1715.

4. Kodali SK, Williams MR, Smith CR, et al. Two-year outcomes after transcatheter or surgical aortic-valve replacement. *N Engl J Med*. 2012;366(18):1686-1695.

5. Jilaihawi H, Kashif M, Fontana G, et al. Cross-sectional computed tomographic assessment improves accuracy of aortic annular sizing for transcatheter aortic valve replacement and reduces the incidence of paravalvular aortic regurgitation. *J Am Coll Cardiol*. 2012;59(14):1275-1286.

6. Khalique OK, Kodali SK, Paradis JM, et al. Aortic annular sizing using a novel 3-dimensional echocardiographic method: use and comparison with cardiac computed tomography. *Circ Cardiovasc Imaging*. 2014;7(1):155-163.

7. Pasic M, Unbehaun A, Buz S, Drews T, Hetzer R. Annular rupture during transcatheter aortic valve replacement: classification, pathophysiology, diagnostics, treatment approaches, and prevention. *JACC Cardiovasc Interv*. 2015;8(1 Part A):1-9.

8. Nazif TM, Dizon José M, Hahn RT, et al. Predictors and clinical outcomes of permanent pacemaker implantation after transcatheter aortic valve replacement: the PARTNER (Placement of AoRtic TraNscathetER Valves) trial and registry. *JACC Cardiovasc Interv*. 2015;8(1 Part A):60-69.

9. Hakeem A, Cilingiroglu M. Outcomes of TAVR in bicuspid aortic valve stenosis. *J Am Coll Cardiol*. 2017;70(13):1684-1685.

10. Vaquerizo B, Spaziano M, Alali J, et al. Three-dimensional echocardiography vs. computed tomography for transcatheter aortic valve replacement sizing. *Eur Heart J Cardiovasc Imaging*. 2016;17(1):15-23.

11. Webb JG, Dvir D. Transcatheter aortic valve replacement for bioprosthetic aortic valve failure: the valve-in-valve procedure. *Circulation*. 2013;127(25):2542-2550.

12. Ribeiro HB, Nombela-Franco L, Urena M, et al. Coronary obstruction following transcatheter aortic valve implantation: a systematic review. *JACC Cardiovasc Interv*. 2013;6(5):452-461.

13. Krishnaswamy A, Parashar A, Agarwal S, et al. Predicting vascular complications during transfemoral transcatheter aortic valve replacement using computed tomography: a novel area-based index. *Catheter Cardiovasc Interv*. 2014;84(5):844-851.

14. Toggweiler S, Gurvitch R, Leipsic J, et al. Percutaneous aortic valve replacement: vascular outcomes with a fully percutaneous procedure. *J Am Coll Cardiol*. 2012;59(2):113-118.

15. Elmariah S, Fearon WF, Inglessis I, et al. Transapical transcatheter aortic valve replacement is associated with increased cardiac mortality in patients with left ventricular dysfunction: insights from the PARTNER I trial. *JACC Cardiovasc Interv*. 2017;10(23):2414-2422.

16. Goel SS, Ige M, Tuzcu EM, et al. Severe aortic stenosis and coronary artery disease—implications for management in the transcatheter aortic valve replacement era: a comprehensive review. *J Am Coll Cardiol*. 2013;62(1):1-10.

17. Achenbach S, Delgado V, Hausleiter J, Schoenhagen P, Min JK, Leipsic JA. SCCT expert consensus document on computed tomography imaging before transcatheter aortic valve implantation (TAVI)/transcatheter aortic valve replacement (TAVR). *J Cardiovasc Comput Tomogr*. 2012;6(6):366-380.

18. Holmes DR, Brennan JM, Rumsfeld JS, et al. Clinical outcomes at 1 year following transcatheter aortic valve replacement. *JAMA*. 2015;313(10):1019-1102.

19. Genereux P, Kodali SK, Green P, et al. Incidence and effect of acute kidney injury after transcatheter aortic valve replacement using the new valve academic research consortium criteria. *Am J Cardiol*. 2013;111:100-105.

20. Saia F, Latib A, Ciuca C, et al. Causes and timing of death during long-term follow-up after transcatheter aortic valve replacement. *Am Heart J.* 2014;168:798-806.

21. Ahmed FS, Newhouse JH. The myth and reality of contrast-induced nephropathy. *Appl Radiol.* 2013;42:16-18.

22. Pulerwitz TC, Khalique OK, Nazif TN, et al. Very low intravenous contrast volume protocol for computed tomography angiography providing comprehensive cardiac and vascular assessment prior to transcatheter aortic valve replacement in patients with chronic kidney disease. *J Cardiovasc Comput Tomogr.* 2016;10(4):316-321.

23. Barbash IM, Dvir D, Weigold WG, Satler LF, Waksman R, Pichard AD. Transcatheter aortic valve replacement in patients with chronic kidney disease: pre-procedural assessment and procedural techniques to minimize risk for acute kidney injury. In: Min J, Berman D, Leipsic J, eds. *Multimodality Imaging for Transcatheter Aortic Valve Replacement.* London: Springer; 2014.

24. https://www.acr.org/-/media/ACR/Files/Clinical-Resources/Contrast_Media.pdf.

25. Lasser EC, Berry CC, Talner LB, et al. Pretreatment with corticosteroids to alleviate reactions to intravenous contrast material. *N Engl J Med.* 1987;317(14):845-849. PMID:3627208.

26. Greenberger PA, Patterson R. The prevention of immediate generalized reactions to radiocontrast media in high-risk patients. *J Allergy Clin Immunol.* 1991;87(4):867-872. PMID:2013681.

27. Mervak BM, Cohan RH, Ellis JH, Khalatbari S, Davenport MS. 5-hour intravenous corticosteroid premedication has a breakthrough reaction rate that is non-inferior to that of a traditional 13-hour oral regimen. *Radiology.* 2017;285(2):425-433.

28. Fathala A, Bin Saeedan M, Zulfiqar A, Al Sergani H. Non-cardiovascular computed tomography incidental findings in patients who underwent transaortic valve implantation procedure. *Cardiol Res.* 2017;8(1):13-19.

29. van Kesteren F, Wiegerinck EMA, van Mourik MS, et al. Impact of potentially malignant incidental findings by computed tomographic angiography on long-term survival after transcatheter aortic valve implantation. *Am J Cardiol.* 2017;120(6):994-1001.

30. Bonow RO, Brown AS, Gillam LD, et al. ACC/AATS/AHA/ASE/EACTS/HVS/SCA/SCAI/SCCT/SCMR/STS 2017 appropriate use criteria for the treatment of patients with severe aortic stenosis. A report of the American College of Cardiology appropriate use criteria task force, American Association for Thoracic Surgery, American Heart Association, American Society of Echocardiography, European Association for Cardio-Thoracic Surgery, Heart Valve Society, Society of Cardiovascular Anesthesiologists, Society for Cardiovascular Angiography and Interventions, Society of Cardiovascular Computed Tomography, Society for Cardiovascular Magnetic Resonance, and Society of Thoracic Surgeons. *J Am Coll Cardiol.* 2017;70(20):2566-2598.

31. Centers for Medicare and Medicaid Services. *National Coverage Determination for Transcatheter Aortic Valve Replacement;* 2012. https://www.cms.gov/medicare-coverage-database/details/ncd-details.aspx.

32. Patel MR, Bailey SR, Bonow RO, et al. ACCF/SCAI/AATS/AHA/ASE/ASNC/HFSA/HRS/SCCM/SCCT/SCMR/STS 2012 Appropriate use criteria for diagnostic catheterization. A report of the American College of Cardiology Foundation appropriate use criteria task force, Society for Cardiovascular Angiography and Interventions, American Association for Thoracic Surgery, American Heart Association, American Society of Echocardiography, American Society of Nuclear Cardiology, Heart Failure Society of America, Heart Rhythm Society, Society of Critical Care Medicine, Society of Cardiovascular Computed Tomography, Society for Cardiovascular Magnetic Resonance, and Society of Thoracic Surgeons. *J Am Coll Cardiol.* 2012;59(22):1995-2027.

33. Otto CM, Kumbhani DJ, Alexander KP, et al. 2017 ACC expert consensus decision pathway for transcatheter aortic valve replacement in the management of adults with aortic stenosis: a report of the American College of Cardiology task force on clinical expert consensus documents. *J Am Coll Cardiol.* 2017;69(10):1313-1346.

34. Kassal AM, Cassese S, Bleiziffer S, et al. Standardized imaging for aortic annular sizing: implications for transcatheter valve selection. *JACC Cardiovasc Imaging.* 2013;6(2):249-62.

35. Nishimura RA, Otto CM, Bonow RO, et al. 2014 AHA/ACC guideline on the management of patients with valvular heart disease. *J Am Coll Cardiol.* 2014;63(22):e57-e185. doi:10.1016/j.jacc.2014.02.536.

36. Rosenhek R, Binder T, Porenta G, et al. Predictors of outcome in severe, asymptomatic aortic stenosis. *N Engl J Med.* 2000;343(9):611-617.

37. Minners J, Allgeier M, Gohlke-Baerwolf C, Kienzle RP, Neumann FJ, Jander N. Inconsistencies of echocardiographic criteria for the grading of aortic valve stenosis. *Eur Heart J.* 2008;29(8):1043-1048.

38. Chaturvedi A, Hobbs SK, Ling FS, Chaturvedi A, Knight P. MRI evaluation prior to Transcatheter Aortic Valve Implantation (TAVI): When to acquire and how to interpret. *Insights Imaging.* 2016;7(2):245-254.

39. Carroll JD, Edwards FH, Marinac-Dabic D, et al. The STS-ACC transcatheter valve therapy national registry: a new partnership and infrastructure for the introduction and surveillance of medical devices and therapies. *J Am Coll Cardiol.* 2013;62(11):1026-1034.

40. Zoghbi WA, Chambers JB, Dumesnil JG, et al. Recommendations for evaluation of prosthetic valves with echocardiography and doppler ultrasound: a report from the American Society of Echocardiography's Guidelines and Standards Committee and the Task Force on Prosthetic Valves, developed in conjunction with the American College of Cardiology Cardiovascular Imaging Committee, Cardiac Imaging Committee of the American Heart Association, the European Association of Echocardiography, a registered branch of the European Society of Cardiology, the Japanese Society of Echocardiography and the Canadian Society of Echocardiography, endorsed by the American College of Cardiology Foundation, American Heart Association, European Association of Echocardiography, a registered branch of the European Society of Cardiology, the Japanese Society of Echocardiography, and Canadian Society of Echocardiography. *J Am Soc Echocardiogr.* 2009;22(9):975-1014; quiz 1082-1084.

41. Pislaru SV, Nkomo VT, Sandhu GS. Assessment of prosthetic valve function after TAVR. *JACC Cardiovasc Imaging.* 2016;9(2):193-206.

42. Kappetein AP, Head SJ, Genereux P, et al. Updated standardized endpoint definitions for transcatheter aortic valve implantation: the Valve Academic Research Consortium-2 consensus document. *J Am Coll Cardiol.* 2012;60(15):1438-1454.

43. Brown ML, Park SJ, Sundt TM, Schaff HV. Early thrombosis risk in patients with biologic valves in the aortic position. *J Thorac Cardiovasc Surg.* 2012;144(1):108-111.

44. Butnaru A, Shaheen J, Tzivoni D, Tauber R, Bitran D, Silberman S. Diagnosis and treatment of early bioprosthetic malfunction in the mitral valve position due to thrombus formation. *Am J Cardiol.* 2013;112(9):1439-1444.

45. Trepels T, Martens S, Doss M, Fichtlscherer S, Schachinger V. Images in cardiovascular medicine. Thrombotic restenosis after minimally invasive implantation of aortic valve stent. *Circulation.* 2009;120(4):e23-e24.

46. De Marchena E, Mesa J, Pomenti S, et al. Thrombus formation following transcatheter aortic valve replacement. *JACC Cardiovasc Interv.* 2015;8(5):728-739.

47. Latib A, Naganuma T, Abdel-Wahab M, et al. Treatment and clinical outcomes of transcatheter heart valve thrombosis. *Circ Cardiovasc Interv.* 2015;8(4).

48. Leetmaa T, Hansson NC, Leipsic J, et al. Early aortic transcatheter heart valve thrombosis: diagnostic value of contrast-enhanced multidetector computed tomography. *Circ Cardiovasc Interv.* 2015;8(4).

49. Pislaru SV, Hussain I, Pellikka PA, et al. Misconceptions, diagnostic challenges and treatment opportunities in bioprosthetic valve thrombosis: lessons from a case series. *Eur J Cardiothorac Surg.* 2015;47(4):725-732.

CHAPTER 6

Frailty, Quality of Life, and Palliative Approach

Sandra B. Lauck, PhD, RN | *Tone M. Norekvål, PhD, RN*

OBJECTIVES

▶ Highlight the importance of the measurement of frailty to inform case selection and support patient care

▶ Discuss why the measurement of quality of life provides pivotal information for TAVR programs

▶ Explore how the integration of a palliative approach can strengthen patient-centered care

Introduction

Careful case selection and patient-centered outcome evaluation are essential components of transcatheter aortic valve replacement (TAVR) program development. In addition to the pivotal question about whether TAVR is anatomically and clinically feasible, there is strong evidence to support the consideration of patients' frailty and self-reported health status when making individual treatment decisions and determining patients' likelihood to derive benefit. Similarly, the incorporation of patient-reported outcomes (PROs) measurement in the evaluation framework of TAVR programs is central to shifting the culture of care from clinician driven to patient focused.

To this end, the purpose of this chapter is to discuss the assessment of frailty in patients undergoing TAVR, the measurement of PROs to inform case selection and clinical evaluation, and the integration of a palliative approach in TAVR program development when treatment is not an option.

Frailty

The word frail originates from the French *frêle*, meaning "of little resistance," and from the Latin *fragilis*, meaning "easily broken."[1] Frailty has become increasingly relevant in TAVR programs because of the raised awareness that age alone is insufficient to characterize the diverse aortic stenosis patient population.[2]

What Is Frailty?

Frailty is different from aging and helps explain the heterogeneity of older adults. There is no universal definition, and multiple criteria have been proposed. Frailty is a complex health state, often defined as an age-related, multisystem syndrome that increases health vulnerabilities and risks of adverse events (eg, significant decline, functional impairment, death) when exposed to stressors (eg, hospitalization, illness), compared with patients of the same age.[3] Clinically, frailty can be conceptualized as a continuous spectrum of impaired resilience.[4] The challenge for patients undergoing TAVR is to maintain the fragile balance between their physical, mental, and social health status reserve; manage their accumulation of deficits and the impact of social determinants of health; and withstand the potential stressors associated with undergoing the procedure (Figure 6.1). Decreased physical activity and impaired walking performance, diminished energy level and endurance (eg, fatigue), weakened strength and balance, poor cognition, depressed mood, impaired nutritional status, and unintentional weight loss further compound the effects of comorbidities, disabilities, and socioeconomic determinants of health (eg, social support, income, education).[5] This reduced reserve affects multiple organ systems and is associated with increased risks, including longer length of stay, delirium and other in-hospital complications, morbidity, and mortality.[6,7] Similar to patients with other cardiovascular disease, the loss of physiological reserves and the progressive accumulation of deficits further worsen the effects of the cycle of frailty in people with aortic stenosis.

Although interrelated, frailty differs and is distinct from disability and comorbidity.[8] These terms are often and erroneously used interchangeably. Disabilities can be broadly defined as

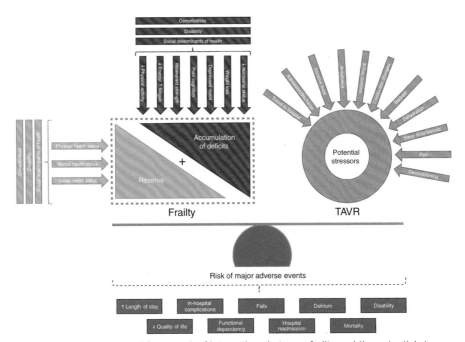

FIGURE 6.1. Conceptual framework of interactions between frailty and the potential stressors associated with transcatheter aortic valve replacement (TAVR).

difficulty or dependency in carrying out activities of daily living or instrumental activities of daily living. In patients undergoing TAVR, disability is often conceptualized as an adverse outcome associated with frailty (eg, a frail patient becomes disabled after TAVR). Comorbidity refers to the burden of illness or disease, defined by the total burden of physiological dysfunction that affects patients' reserve.[9] Although these concepts are interrelated, it is important to understand their distinct features to measure the indicators appropriately and identify opportunities to mitigate risks.[10]

Why Measure Frailty?

The advanced age of most patients undergoing TAVR, and the awareness of many aging-related stressors combine to raise the importance of frailty as an important variable to inform case selection and mitigate risks. Frailty is not captured in the Society of Thoracic Surgeons (STS) predicted risk of mortality score or the European System for Cardiac Operative Risk Evaluation (EuroSCORE) that remain widely used to ascertain the risk for TAVR. Frailty is not a reason to withhold care but rather a means of tailoring care in a more patient-centered fashion.[11] The exposure to the stressors of TAVR, including hospital admission, the insertion of invasive lines, anesthesia, bedrest, and deconditioning, can place frail patients at higher risk for marked and often disproportionate decompensation, adverse events, procedural complications, prolonged recovery, functional decline, delirium, disability, hospital readmission, and mortality.[12-14] Importantly for patients undergoing TAVR, frailty impairs the capacity to recover from disease or iatrogenic stressors due to aging-related impairments.[15]

The predictive value of frailty was highlighted in early clinical trials and continues to play a role in international administrative registries and ongoing studies. In the family of Placement of AoRTic TraNscathetER Valve Trial (PARTNER) trials, the US CoreValve Pivotal trial, as well as the evaluation of other devices, there has been a consistent interest in capturing frailty as a risk factor, albeit with a mixed approach and varying indicators. Similarly, in the US STS/ ACC TVT Registry and other administrative registries, frailty is ascertained with diverse measurements but consistently incorporated in the description of patient characteristics and risk modeling.[16-19] Some studies have found no association between frailty status and outcomes,[20,21] whereas others have reported an association between variables associated with frailty.[2,14,22] There is widespread clinical consensus that the assessment of frailty augments the comprehensive evaluation of patients undergoing TAVR, informs early discharge planning, and supports individualized care to mitigate risks and optimize outcomes.[23]

The effects of frailty may be attenuated, and the syndrome is potentially reversible.[24] Physical therapy and improved nutrition are known to improve slow chair rise times, whereas exercise has also been shown to improve cognitive function. Protein supplementation has measurable effects on improved mortality and morbidity, whereas nutritional supplements are recommended for older adults with low serum albumin, weight loss, and other markers of malnutrition. Last, iron deficiency, deficiency of folate or vitamin B_{12}, or other causes of anemia may be treated. Further research is needed to guide TAVR programs to optimize frail patients' health status before the procedure and inform the development of tailored rehabilitation interventions.[25]

How Is Frailty Measured?

Although widely adopted as a core requirement in clinical trials, the measurement of frailty in clinical practice is often perceived of questionable value and a challenge to consistently and rigorously measure. Upward of 20 frailty assessment tools have been developed, leading to significant confusion and variability in clinical care and research.[11] The absence of consensus surrounding frailty assessment tools, the unstandardized measurements employed in research and clinical care, and the lack of validation in the unique TAVR population have been significant barriers to the seamless integration of frailty measurement in practice.[25] The following are among the most consistently used instruments.

The Fried Scale

This is the most frequently cited frailty scale and has been demonstrated to predict mortality and disability in patients with cardiac disease. The scale captures the core phenotypic domains of frailty and encompasses slowness, weakness, low physical activity, exhaustion, and shrinking (unintentional weight loss), with ≥3 of 5 criteria required for a diagnosis of frailty.[3]

The Short Physical Performance Battery

The scale captures slowness, weakness, and balance and is measured by a series of timed physical performance tests—gait speed, chair rises, and tandem balance, each is scored 0 to 4 (low score = low physical function). A total score ≤5 of 12 is required for a diagnosis of frailty.[26]

The 5-Meter Gait Speed

This measure has been promoted as a single-item measure of frailty that outperforms more complex and time-consuming scales.[27] The short distance and comfortable pace are usually well tolerated by patients with aortic stenosis, whereas there is excellent interrater reliability among clinicians performing the test. The test has been adopted by multiple registries and clinical trials and has been shown to be responsive to change, particularly at a population level.[28] The instructions for the 5-Meter Gait Speed test are outlined in the box. These 3 tools lack measurement of cognitive status and should perhaps be used in conjunction with such an instrument to more comprehensively capture the domains of frailty.

Instructions for the 5-Metre Gait Speed Test
In an Unobstructed area, position the patient with his/her feet behind and just touching the 0-meter start line.
Instruct the patient to "Walk at your comfortable pace" until a few steps past the 5-meter mark (to avoid slowing down before). Walking aids such as canes and walkers may be used if needed.
Begin each trial with the word "Go."
Start the timer with the first footfall after the 0-meter line.
Stop the timer with the first footfall after the 5-meter line.
Repeat three times and record average, allowing sufficient time for recuperation between trials.
Frailty is usually defined as an average time taken to walk the 5-meter course ≥6 seconds.

The Study of Osteoporotic Fractures Index

The Study of Osteoporotic Fractures index was derived using the frailty phenotype in a large prospective study cohort of US women who experienced falls and fractures.[29] The findings confirmed the predictive validity of the phenotype of frailty as defined by Fried and colleagues.[30] The Study of Osteoporotic Fractures index is a composite score of 3 frailty criteria to predict risk:

- Weight loss ≥5% over 3 years (Yes = 1; No = 0)
- Ability to perform 5 sequential chair rises with arms folded on chest (Yes = 0; No = 1)
- Answer to question: "Do you feel full of energy?" (Yes = 0; No = 1)

The score is interpreted as follows: Frail = 2 or 3/3; Prefrail = 1/3; Robust = 0/3.

The Essential Frailty Toolset

The recent publication of the Essential Frailty Toolset (EFT) is poised to give clinicians a pragmatic and reliable tool to improve the integration of the measurement of frailty in TAVR programs, and it is a strong candidate for standardization across registries and clinical trials.[25] The EFT is a simple assessment of 4 easily available indicators.

- Chair rises × 5 (lower extremity strength)
- Cognitive status (short-term memory and orientation): The score obtained on the Mini-Cog measurement of 3-word registration and clock drawing; alternatively, the following questions can be asked: (1) What day of the month is it? (2) What day of the week is it? (3) What hospital are you in? and (4) What floor are you on?
- Hemoglobin (oxygen-carrying capacity and inflammation)
- Albumin (cardiovascular risk, inflammation, sarcopenia)

The 4 indicators generate a score that is associated with a predictive risk of 1-year mortality for TAVR and surgical aortic valve replacement. In a cohort of 1020 patients undergoing TAVR and surgical aortic valve replacement, the EFT outperformed 6 other well-validated scales, including the Fried Scale and the Short Physical Performance Battery, to identify vulnerable older adults who are at higher risk for poor outcomes and predict 1-year mortality after TAVR and surgical aortic valve replacement. It also demonstrated that the objective measurement of frailty adds incremental value above existing risk models to predict midterm mortality and progressive disability after TAVR. Beyond its robust predictive value, the EFT has the advantage of being quick to perform, does not require specialized equipment, and has high interobserver reliability. The EFT is available as a smartphone application ("Frailty Tool," does not require a license, and is free).

Reporting Frailty to Inform Case Selection

The measurement of frailty ought to be considered as a supplemental data report to maximize its value to support case selection. Multidisciplinary agreement supported by all members of the Heart Team is essential to ensure that data are not collected in vain but rather reflects the consensus agreement that frailty is an important variable to consider and that its rigorous measurement is an integrated component of the complex TAVR assessment.

Valve program clinicians have the expertise and competencies to conduct the assessment of frailty, to document findings, and to share their assessment and recommendations with the team. A written report and/or a visual summary can be an efficient and succinct way to present pertinent assessment findings. In addition, multiple programs report using a photograph of the

Date:		Patient Information:	

Centre for
Heart Valve Innovation
St. Paul's Hospital, Vancouver

Essential Frailty Toolset		
Measure	**Score**	**EFT Points**
Chair Rises	13 Sec.	0
Cognition: Items	2	0
Cognition: Clock	Normal	
Albumin	3.0 g/dL	1
Hemoglobin	12.1g/dL	0
EFT Score	**1/5**	
	(Predicted 1-yr mortality: 6% -All access)	

Other Frailty Indicators		
Measure	**Score**	**Rating**
ADLs	5/6	✓
IADLs	4/8	✗
5-Metre Gait	6 Sec.	✓

Overall Nursing Recommendation	
Comments:	✓

Patient photograph guidelines:
- Institutional approval and adherence to clinical documentation protocols
- Patient is told ahead of time that photograph is routine practice (include in patient education resources)
- Patient is encouraged to pretend it is a "family photo" (i.e., not a "passport photo")
- Bulky clothes removed
- Without mobility aid if possible
- Photograph is taken in same setting with consistent approach

FIGURE 6.2. Example of clinical documentation of frailty to Support transcatheter aortic valve replacement case selection. ADL, activities of daily living; IADL, instrumental activities of daily living. (Used with permission by the Centre for Heart Valve Innovation, St. Paul's Hospital, Vancouver, Canada.)

patient taken at the time of assessment in the TAVR clinic to augment the measurement of frailty. Although these data ought to be considered with caution owing to the inherent risk of bias, the visual "look test" can strengthen the patient-centered approach and provide helpful information of the patient's physical status. If this approach adopted, the patient photograph should be taken with a consistent approach in the same setting. Ideally, the patient is photographed in street clothes but without heavy clothing that can mask body habitus and asked to simply look/smile at the camera in a relaxed way. Figure 6.2 displays an example of a report of a patient's EFT score, additional indicators of function, photograph, and the valve program clinician's recommendation about the patient's likelihood to derive benefit from TAVR based on this focused assessment.

Quality of Life

Health status and outcomes have historically been measured and reported in terms of mortality and morbidity. Yet, the way clinicians, researchers, policy makers, and the general public think about health, health care, and the role of patients as partners is changing. Increasingly, multiple stakeholders recognize the importance of physical, mental, and social patient-reported health status, the adverse consequences of illness from patients' perspectives, and that patients are the most important experts of their own health and illness.[31] Most importantly, society acknowledges that clinical outcomes measuring the value of medical interventions and health care programs must account for the quality of people's lives as perceived and reported by those faced with illness.

Research suggests that about one half of people with heart failure would choose enhanced quality of life with a shorter life expectancy over their current quality of life with more years of life expected.[32,33] It is reasonable to extend this priority to patients with valvular heart disease given the significant burden of symptoms associated with degenerative valve disease. To this end, clinicians need to better understand how people experience aortic stenosis and TAVR, whether they report changes in their health status over time, what the rate and direction of change is, and if distinct groups of people experience different patterns of change. This knowledge is key to the development of well-timed and targeted treatment to support care from the time of referral, procedure, and anticipated adaptation and recovery.

Similarly, policy makers and funders have a growing interest in understanding whether societal investment in cardiac innovation yields significant benefits for patients, not just in terms of quantity but also of quality of life. In 2006, the US Food and Drug Administration recommended the standardized inclusion of PROs in clinical trials. This policy is mirrored by the European Medicines Agency, the UK National Health Services, and multiple other regions and jurisdictions. Both the European Society of Cardiology[34] and the US American Heart Association[35] have strongly endorsed the importance of measuring and integrating PROs in practice and research to improve quality of care. This movement prompted the inclusion of quality of life assessment in early TAVR clinical trials and remains the impetus to mandate the collection of similar data in the US ACC/STS TVT and other national registries.

What Are Patient-Reported Outcome Measurements?

Patient-reported outcome measurements (PROMs) is an umbrella term used to capture information obtained *directly from patients* about various aspects of their health and health care, including symptoms, functioning, well-being, quality of life, perceptions about treatment, and satisfaction with care received and with their professional communication with clinicians.[31] A PROM is a precise, reliable, valid, and reproducible measurement of aspects of patients' health status using questionnaires or other scales. PRO data come directly from the patient, without the interpretation of the patient's responses by a physician or anyone else. PROMs capture concepts of disease activity, as reflected by symptoms; physical, mental, and social self-reported health or functional status; and overall quality of life.[36] In addition, patient-reported experiences measures capture indicators of patients' satisfaction with and adherence to treatment. These unique data are distinct from clinician-reported assessments and interpretations and reflect the patient's own perspectives, influenced by internal standards, individual values, and expectations, which are not directly observable by others.[37] Although the more ambiguous terms "quality of life" and "health-related quality of life" remain widely used, the term "PRO" is increasingly adopted by clinicians, researchers, regulatory agencies, and policy makers to better describe the multiple domains of self-reported health status and forefront the patient as the sole source of data.

Why Measure Patient-Reported Outcomes?

The use of PROMs is an essential component of the shift of health care systems to achieve quantifiable and transparent improvement in quality of care, inform individual treatment plans, and manage the performance of health care providers, both in terms of treatment decision and outcomes. The US Food and Drug Administration, the UK National Health Services, and other jurisdictions share a common vision for transforming the culture of health services to measure the impact of health care spending and investment in innovation and reflect patients' perspectives and patient-focused quality.

The purpose of collecting PROs is to augment conventional indicators of treatment decision and outcome evaluation and to strengthen a patient-centered approach to care. PROMs can enable the improvement of the quality of patient care and optimization of resource utilization by:

- Facilitating the early detection and raising awareness of physical or psychological problems and daily functioning and well-being that might be otherwise overlooked;
- Making patients' and family members' concerns more visible;
- Informing the selection and use of therapeutic interventions;
- Monitoring disease progression and response to treatment;
- Establishing common patient-clinician objectives;
- Strengthening care plans;
- Improving communication, patient satisfaction, and adherence;
- Enhancing collaboration among members of the health care team; and
- Monitoring outcomes as a strategy for quality improvement.

Barriers and Challenges

The routine adoption of PROMs in clinical care remains a significant challenge for clinicians and TAVR programs, and their use has not yet been brought to the forefront of crucial discussions on optimizing patient care.[31] Barriers include a lack of familiarity with the instruments, uneven support from physicians and other clinical stakeholders, lack of technological solutions to enable easy and seamless data collection and reporting, costs, and controversy about the evidence.[38] Variations in approaches to measurement, the multitude of available instruments with response options, and the perception of excessive patient burden are problematic. The central problem of interpretability, for example, what changes in score constitute a signal of trivial, small, moderate, or large patient benefit or harm, and how should change over time be gauged, remains highly debated.[31]

Strategies have been proposed to support the successful implementation of PROMs in clinical practice and optimize their contributions to clinicians' capacity to screen patients for previously unrecognized health problems, monitor changes in health status, and stimulate better communication.[39]

Practical and Methodological Considerations When Implementing Routine PRO Assessment in Clinical Practice

1. Identify goals for collecting PROs in clinical practice
2. Select patients, setting, and timing of assessments
3. Determine which questionnaire to use
4. Choose a mode for administering and scoring the questionnaire
5. Design processes for reporting results
6. Identify aids to facilitate score interpretation
7. Identify strategies for responding to issues identified by questionnaires
8. Evaluate the impact of the PRO intervention on practice

Adapted from Snyder CF, Aaronson NK, Choucair AK, et al. Implementing patient-reported outcomes assessment in clinical practice: a review of the options and considerations. *Qual Life Res.* 2012;21(8):1305-1314.

Valve program clinicians often experience firsthand the importance of integrating patients' goals, values, and priorities in the plan of care. They can play an essential role in championing the adoption of PROMs in clinical practice to strengthen patient involvement, promote personalized care in a systematic way, and shift clinicians' thinking that the measurement of patients' perspectives is an essential component of quality of care.

How Are Patient-Reported Outcomes Measured?

The process of PROM development conventionally includes the identification and synthesis of the conceptually driven domains to be measured, followed by validation testing to confirm the robustness of the measures. This rigor is essential to support claims that can be made about outcomes. PRO assessment can be defined as scientifically valid if the outcomes are conceptually defined and operationalized in questionnaires and if the questionnaires can meet established standards of reliability, validity, responsiveness, and sensitivity and withstand the scrutiny of psychometric evaluation.[31]

The selection of PRO instruments should reflect the goals of measurement.[40] Both disease-specific and generic measures can contribute to a comprehensive assessment of patients' health status (Figure 6.3). Disease-specific measurements are more sensitive for clinical use; they capture specific symptoms related to the particular disease (eg, dizziness, dyspnea, and chest pain for aortic stenosis). These scales cannot be used to compare across patient populations.

Generic measurements focus on questions related to general health and can be used to compare between patient populations and the general population. Given these essential differences, instrument selection must be driven by the information that is sought and the specific goals.

There is significant debate about the need for validated and sensitive instruments that are free of charge and enable cross regional/patient population comparisons. High costs and logistics of institutional licensing can be considerable barriers for the measurement of PROs. The early adoption of proprietary instruments in industry-sponsored clinical trials has resulted in the benchmarking of outcomes; this has created expectations and the need for ongoing use

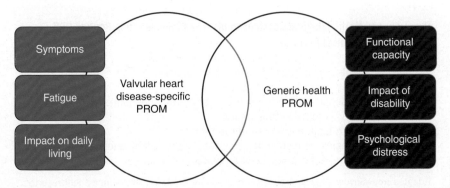

FIGURE 6.3. Examples of domains captured by disease-specific and generic health patient-reported outcome measurements (PROMs).

of costly instruments for individual centers and jurisdictions. There is a need for instrument development and implementation research to create valid measures that are unencumbered by costs and licensing barriers.

The following instruments exemplify proprietary and licensed tools most commonly used in TAVR clinical care, registry-based evaluation, and research.

Disease-Specific Patient-Reported Outcome Measurement: The Kansas City Cardiomyopathy Questionnaire

The Kansas City Cardiomyopathy Questionnaire (KCCQ) is a disease-specific health status survey originally developed to describe and monitor health status in patients with heart failure.[41] The KCCQ has undergone extensive reliability and validity testing in patients with severe aortic stenosis, leading to its adoption in the US ACC/STS TVT and other registries. A 12-item version was developed from the original 23-item questionnaire and found to be psychometrically valid.[42] The questionnaire integrates patients' symptoms, functional status, and quality of life into an overall summary (OS) score and has been shown to predict mortality.

The interpretation of KCCQ scores is well established. Values for all KCCQ domains and the summary score range from 0 to 100, with higher scores indicating less symptom burden and better quality of life. Scores of the KCCQ OS can be categorized as follows:

- Very poor health status: KCCQ <25/100
- Poor: KCCQ 25 to 49/100
- Fair: KCCQ 50 to 74/100
- Good: KCCQ ≥75/100[43]

Prior studies have shown that the KCCQ-OS generally correlates with the New York Heart Association functional class as follows: class I, KCCQ-OS 75 to 100; class II, 60 to 74; class III, 45 to 59; and class IV, 0 to 44.[43] Changes in the KCCQ-OS of 5, 10, and 20 points correspond to small, moderate, or large clinical improvements, respectively.[44] A favorable outcome at 1 year after TAVR can be defined as survival with a reasonable quality of life (KCCQ-OS score ≥60, roughly equivalent to New York Heart Association class I-II symptoms without any meaningful worsening, decrease of ≥10 points in the KCCQ-OS score from baseline to 1 y).[45]

Scoring syntax for multiple data management systems is provided when a license is obtained. Validated translations are available in over 25 languages.

Generic Health Status Patient-Reported Outcome Measurement: The Euro-QOL 5 Domains

The Euro-QOL 5 Domains (EQ-5D) is a generic health status measure consisting of 5 domains: mobility, self-care, usual activities, pain/discomfort, and anxiety/depression. Changes in the score may result from different patterns of impairment across these individual dimensions. The assessment is augmented with a visual analog scale (EQ-VS) that captures patients' perspective on their overall health status based on a scale between 0 (worse possible health) and 100 (best possible health). The EQ-5D summary score can be converted to utilities using an algorithm developed for various populations.[46] Utilities are preference-weighted health status assessments with scores that range from 0 to 1, with 1 representing perfect health and 0 corresponding to the worst imaginable health state.[47] A utility score is an expression of quality-adjusted life-years that is commonly used to conduct cost-effectiveness analyses and inform health policy decisions.

The EQ-5D is available with 3-level (EQ-5D-3L) or 5-level (EQ-5D-5L) responses. The 5-level response has the distinct advantage of better differentiating the population and may have less statistical floor and ceiling effects. Its use requires a fee for service licensing agreement and is available in multiple languages.

Integration of a Palliative Approach

When Transcatheter Aortic Valve Replacement Is Futile

As discussed in previous chapters, clinical trials have demonstrated tremendous survival advantage, symptom benefit, and improved quality of life for many patients undergoing TAVR. In contrast, the treatment of patients who are dying "with" aortic stenosis but not "from" aortic stenosis does little to modify the poor prognosis associated with comorbidities, excessive frailty, and disability.[48] The futility of treatment in patients with excessive comorbidities, functional and cognitive decline, and/or frailty is well established.[49,50] Predictors of poor outcomes include impaired renal function, severe pulmonary disease, severity of aortic stenosis, and excessive frailty indicators, including impaired cognition and slow gait.[22] Although TAVR is not an option for all patients, the adoption of a palliative approach in TAVR programs can help improve continuity of care and support patients' transition to a focus on symptom management.

What Is a Palliative Approach?

The advanced age and health vulnerabilities of patients undergoing TAVR, their procedure-focused clinical trajectories, the complexities of the referral patterns, and the involvement of multiple medical specialties combine to form a "perfect storm" for potentially failing to attend to the important end-of-life requirements of patients presenting with severe aortic stenosis.[51] When TAVR is not a treatment option, programs ought to provide an alternative care plan for the group of patients for whom valve replacement has been deemed clinically futile. The integration of a palliative approach can help attend to end-of-life needs, contribute to continuity of care, and bridge the clinical trajectories for patients unlikely to benefit from treatment.

A palliative approach is a way of caring for those with life-limiting illnesses that focuses on improving patients' and families' quality of life. This holistic, needs-based perspective aims to assess and improve symptom management, communication, advanced care planning, and psychosocial and spiritual needs regardless of prognosis.[52,53] The focus is on meeting a person's and his/her family's full range of needs at all stages of a life-limiting illness. The known natural history and poor prognosis of untreated aortic stenosis matches this mandate. Importantly, this transition ought not be a sudden discontinuation of an aggressive treatment plan followed by a gap in care and/or the start of palliative care. Rather, the integration of a palliative approach can be a parallel process to the pursuit of curative care so that if and when TAVR is not an option, the patient, family and health care team can change the focus of discussions to match

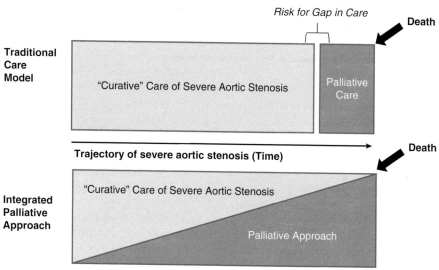

FIGURE 6.4. Conceptual model for the integration of a palliative approach in transcatheter aortic valve replacement program. (Adapted from Jaarsma T, Beattie JM, Ryder M, et al. Palliative care in heart failure: a position statement from the palliative care workshop of the Heart Failure Association of the European Society of Cardiology. *Eur J Heart Fail.* 2009; 11(5):433-443.)

the changing health trajectory.[52,54,55] Figure 6.4 proposes a conceptual model to shift TAVR programs' thinking to the continuous management of aortic stenosis as a life-limiting disease.

A Tailored Palliative Approach for Transcatheter Aortic Valve Replacement Programs

In 2014, the World Health Organization resolved that palliative care should be integrated in all health care settings and by all health care specialties in its member countries.[56] There are many barriers to adopting the philosophy of care in TAVR programs: clinicians may perceive that discussions about end of life may remove hope, cause increased confusion, or be incongruent with previous discussions. The complexity of case selection, prognostic uncertainty, lack of knowledge about palliative care, and confidence to initiate or pursue discussions about end of life further contribute to a lack of clarity of the responsibility of TAVR programs.

To overcome these barriers, the following steps are recommended to identify patients who would benefit from a palliative approach:

- Ask yourself: "Would I be surprised if this patient died in the next 6 to 12 months?";
- Look for one or more general clinical indicators (eg, limited self-care, in chair or bed over 50% of the day, multiple hospitalizations in the past 6 months, requirement for extensive home or residential care); and
- Look for two or more cardiac disease indicators (eg, New York Heart Association functional class III or IV, renal impairment, cardiac cachexia, two or more episodes needing intravenous furosemide and/or inotropes in the past 6 months).

Simple questions such as "Tell me what you understand about your illness," "Tell me what you expect by having the valve procedure," or "What is most important to you?" can help inform patients' goals of care.[55] Additional recommendations for the Heart Team to consider for the integration of best practices are outlined in the box.

Recommendations for the Integration of a Palliative Approach in TAVR Programs
1. Recognize the importance of palliative care in the continuum of the management of aortic stenosis and increase the Heart Team's knowledge about best palliative care practices.
2. Consider establishing a partnership with a palliative care specialist to strengthen the TAVR Heart Team.
3. Provide realistic information to patients and families during the eligibility assessment to outline the process of treatment decision and highlight that TAVR is not an option for all patients.
4. Consider criteria-based early consultation with palliative care during the eligibility assessment to improve symptom management.
5. Consider using the "Ask-Tell-Ask" recommended format of patient-centered communication to ascertain what patients know about their disease progression, the process of TAVI treatment decision making, and their future care planning, followed by clarification of pertinent information and a chance to pursue arising questions.
6. Document patients' symptoms and communicate findings to the primary care provider and community teams.
7. Strengthen communication with the primary care provider; share expertise about disease progression and treatment options.
8. Adopt shared decision-making approaches to incorporate patients' goals, values, and preferences in treatment decision and bridge their understanding of the common goals of procedure-focused and palliative-oriented care.

Adapted from Lauck SB, Gibson JA, Baumbusch J, et al. Transition to palliative care when transcatheter aortic valve implantation is not an option: opportunities and recommendations. *Curr Opin Support Palliat Care.* 2016;10(1):18-23.

Conclusions

There is no single variable, test, or risk score that indicates that TAVR is the appropriate treatment of individual patients. Although the procedure is becoming increasingly routine and less disruptive, case selection in this primarily elderly patient population remains complex. The standardized measurement of frailty and patient-reported outcomes and the integration of a palliative approach can optimize processes of care, contribute to improved outcomes, and strengthen patient-centered care.

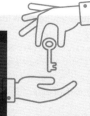

KEY TAKEAWAYS AND BEST PRACTICES

▶ Frailty is an age-related, multisystem syndrome that increases health vulnerabilities and risks of adverse events when exposed to stressors compared with patients the same age. Frailty can be conceptualized as a continuous spectrum of impaired resilience.

▶ The objective measurement of frailty adds incremental value above existing risk models to predict midterm mortality and progressive disability after TAVR. It also informs early discharge planning and supports individualized care to mitigate risks and optimize outcomes.

▶ Frailty is not a reason to withhold care but rather a means of tailoring care in a more patient-centered fashion. Increased frailty is associated with increased risk of in-hospital complications, morbidity, and mortality.

▶ The improvement of quality of life is a priority for patients undergoing TAVR and provides important information to strengthen patient-centered care.

▶ Quality of life can be measured with precise, reliable, valid, and reproducible measurements to capture patients' self-reported health status.

▶ The integration of a palliative approach can help attend to end-of-life needs, contribute to continuity of care, and bridge the clinical trajectories for patients unlikely to benefit from treatment.

References

1. Afilalo J. Frailty in patients with cardiovascular disease: why, when, and how to measure. *Curr Cardiovasc Risk Rep*. 2011;5(5):467-472.
2. Green P, Arnold SV, Cohen DJ, et al. Relation of frailty to outcomes after transcatheter aortic valve replacement (from the PARTNER trial). *Am J Cardiol*. 2015;116(2):264-269.
3. Fried LP, Hadley EC, Walston JD, et al. From bedside to bench: research agenda for frailty. *Sci Aging Knowledge Environ*. 2005;2005(31):pe24.
4. Muscedere J, Andrew MK, Bagshaw SM, et al. Screening for frailty in Canada's health care system: a time for action. *Can J Aging*. 2016;35(3):281-297.
5. Forcillo J, Condado JF, Ko YA, et al. Assessment of commonly used frailty markers for high- and extreme-risk patients undergoing transcatheter aortic valve replacement. *Ann Thorac Surg*. 2017;104(6):1939-1946.
6. Rockwood K, Stadnyk K, MacKnight C, McDowell I, Hebert R, Hogan DB. A brief clinical instrument to classify frailty in elderly people. *Lancet*. 1999;353(9148):205-206.
7. Eide LS, Ranhoff AH, Fridlund B, et al. Comparison of frequency, risk factors, and time course of postoperative delirium in octogenarians after transcatheter aortic valve implantation versus surgical aortic valve replacement. *Am J Cardiol*. 2015;115(6):802-809.
8. Fried LP, Ferrucci L, Darer J, Williamson JD, Anderson G. Untangling the concepts of disability, frailty, and comorbidity: implications for improved targeting and care. *J Gerontol Ser A Biol Sci Med Sci*. 2004;59(3):255-263.

9. Valderas JM, Starfield B, Sibbald B, Salisbury C, Roland M. Defining comorbidity: implications for understanding health and health services. *Ann Fam Med.* 2009;7(4):357-363.

10. Afilalo J, Mottillo S, Eisenberg MJ, et al. Addition of frailty and disability to cardiac surgery risk scores identifies elderly patients at high risk of mortality or major morbidity. *Circ Cardiovasc Qual Outcomes.* 2012;5(2):222-228.

11. Afilalo J, Alexander KP, Mack MJ, et al. Frailty assessment in the cardiovascular care of older adults. *J Am Coll Cardiol.* 2014;63(8):747-762.

12. Shamliyan T, Talley KM, Ramakrishnan R, Kane RL. Association of frailty with survival: a systematic literature review. *Ageing Res Rev.* 2013;12(2):719-736.

13. Instenes I, Gjengedal E, Eide LSP, Kuiper KKJ, Ranhoff AH, Norekval TM. "Eight days of nightmares…" – Octogenarian patients' experiences of postoperative delirium after transcatheter or surgical aortic valve replacement. *Heart Lung Circ.* 2018;27(2):260-266.

14. Eide LS, Ranhoff AH, Fridlund B, et al. Delirium as a predictor of physical and cognitive function in individuals aged 80 and older after transcatheter aortic valve implantation or surgical aortic valve replacement. *J Am Geriatr Soc.* 2016;64(6):1178-1186.

15. Afilalo J. The clinical frailty scale: upgrade your eyeball test. *Circulation.* 2017;135(21):2025-2027.

16. Stub D, Lauck S, Lee M, et al. Regional systems of care to optimize outcomes in patients undergoing transcatheter aortic valve replacement. *JACC Cardiovasc Interven.* 2015;8(15):1944-1951.

17. Holmes DR, Nishimura RA, Grover FL, et al. Annual outcomes with transcatheter valve therapy: from the STS/ACC TVT registry. *Ann Thorac Surg.* 2016;101(2):789-800.

18. Moat NE, Ludman P, de Belder MA, et al. Long-term outcomes after transcatheter aortic valve implantation in high-risk patients with severe aortic stenosis: the U.K. TAVI (United Kingdom Transcatheter Aortic Valve Implantation) registry. *J Am Coll Cardiol.* 2011;58(20):2130-2318.

19. Eltchaninoff H, Prat A, Gilard M, et al. Transcatheter aortic valve implantation: early results of the FRANCE (FRench Aortic National CoreValve and Edwards) registry. *Eur Heart J.* 2011;32(2):191-197.

20. Hermiller JB, Yakubov SJ, Reardon MJ, et al. Predicting early and late mortality after transcatheter aortic valve replacement. *J Am Coll Cardiol.* 2016;68(4):343-352.

21. Edwards FH, Cohen DJ, O'Brien SM, et al. Development and validation of a risk prediction model for in-hospital mortality after transcatheter aortic valve replacement. *JAMA Cardiol.* 2016;1(1):46-52.

22. Arnold SV, Reynolds MR, Lei Y, et al. Predictors of poor outcomes after transcatheter aortic valve replacement: results from the PARTNER (Placement of Aortic Transcatheter Valve) trial. *Circulation.* 2014;129(25):2682-2690.

23. Hawkey MC, Lauck SB, Perpetua EM, et al. Transcatheter aortic valve replacement program development: recommendations for best practice. *Catheterization Cardiovasc Interven.* 2014;84(6):859-867.

24. Ng TP, Feng L, Nyunt MS, et al. Nutritional, physical, cognitive, and combination interventions and frailty reversal among older adults: a randomized controlled trial. *Am J Med.* 2015;128(11):1225-1236.e1.

25. Afilalo J, Lauck S, Kim DH, et al. Frailty in older adults undergoing aortic valve replacement: The FRAILTY-AVR Study. *J Am Coll Cardiol.* 2017;70(6):689-700.

26. Guralnik JM, Ferrucci L, Pieper CF, et al. Lower extremity function and subsequent disability: consistency across studies, predictive models, and value of gait speed alone compared with the short physical performance battery. *J Gerontol Ser A Biol Sci Med Sci.* 2000;55(4):M221-M231.

27. Dumurgier J, Elbaz A, Ducimetiere P, Tavernier B, Alperovitch A, Tzourio C. Slow walking speed and cardiovascular death in well functioning older adults: prospective cohort study. *BMJ.* 2009;339:b4460.

28. Afilalo J, Kim S, O'Brien S, et al. Gait speed and operative mortality in older adults following cardiac surgery. *JAMA Cardiol.* 2016;1(3):314-321.

29. Ensrud KE, Ewing SK, Taylor BC, et al. Comparison of 2 frailty indexes for prediction of falls, disability, fractures, and death in older women. *Arch Intern Med.* 2008;168(4):382-389.

30. Fried LP, Tangen CM, Walston J, et al. Frailty in older adults: evidence for a phenotype. *J Gerontol Ser A Biol Sci Med Sci.* 2001;56(3):M146-M156.

31. Norekval TM, Falun N, Fridlund B. Paktient-reported outcomes on the agenda in cardiovascular clinical practice. *Eur J Cardiovasc Nurs.* 2016;15(2):108-111.

32. Schellinger SE, Anderson EW, Frazer MS, Cain CL. Patient self-defined goals: essentials of person-centered care for serious illness. *Am J Hosp Palliat Care.* 2018;35(1):159-165.

33. Hauber AB, Obi EN, Price MA, Whalley D, Chang CL. Quantifying the relative importance to patients of avoiding symptoms and outcomes of heart failure. *Curr Med Res Opin.* 2017;33(11):2027-2038.

34. Anker SD, Agewall S, Borggrefe M, et al. The importance of patient-reported outcomes: a call for their comprehensive integration in cardiovascular clinical trials. *Eur Heart J.* 2014;35(30):2001-2009.

35. Rumsfeld JS, Alexander KP, Goff DC, et al. Cardiovascular health: the importance of measuring patient-reported health status: a scientific statement from the American Heart Association. *Circulation.* 2013;127(22):2233-2249.

36. Chang S, Gholizadeh L, Salamonson Y, Digiacomo M, Betihavas V, Davidson PM. Health span or life span: the role of patient-reported outcomes in informing health policy. *Health Pol.* 2011;100(1):96-104.

37. Gotay CC, Kawamoto CT, Bottomley A, Efficace F. The prognostic significance of patient-reported outcomes in cancer clinical trials. *J Clin Oncol.* 2008;26(8):1355-1363.

38. Lohr KN, Zebrack BJ. Using patient-reported outcomes in clinical practice: challenges and opportunities. *Qual Life Res.* 2009;18(1):99-107.

39. Snyder CF, Aaronson NK, Choucair AK, et al. Implementing patient-reported outcomes assessment in clinical practice: a review of the options and considerations. *Qual Life Res.* 2012;21(8):1305-1314.

40. Thompson DR, Ski CF, Garside J, Astin F. A review of health-related quality of life patient-reported outcome measures in cardiovascular nursing. *Eur J Cardiovasc Nurs.* 2016;15(2):114-125.

41. Green CP, Porter CB, Bresnahan DR, Spertus JA. Development and evaluation of the Kansas city cardiomyopathy questionnaire: a new health status measure for heart failure. *J Am Coll Cardiol.* 2000;35(5):1245-1255.

42. Spertus JA, Jones PG. Development and validation of a short version of the Kansas city cardiomyopathy questionnaire. *Circ Cardiovasc Qual Outcomes.* 2015;8(5):469-476.

43. Arnold SV, Spertus JA, Lei Y, et al. Use of the Kansas city cardiomyopathy questionnaire for monitoring health status in patients with aortic stenosis. *Circ Heart Fail.* 2013;6(1):61-67.

44. Spertus J, Peterson E, Conard MW, et al. Monitoring clinical changes in patients with heart failure: a comparison of methods. *Am Heart J.* 2005;150(4):707-715.

45. Arnold SV, Spertus JA, Lei Y, et al. How to define a poor outcome after transcatheter aortic valve replacement: conceptual framework and empirical observations from the placement of aortic transcatheter valve (PARTNER) trial. *Circ Cardiovasc Qual Outcomes.* 2013;6(5):591-597.

46. Shaw JW, Johnson JA, Coons SJ. US valuation of the EQ-5D health states: development and testing of the D1 valuation model. *Med Care.* 2005;43(3):203-220.

47. Dyer MT, Goldsmith KA, Sharples LS, Buxton MJ. A review of health utilities using the EQ-5D in studies of cardiovascular disease. *Health Qual Life Outcomes.* 2010;8:13.

48. Leon MB, Gada H, Fontana GP. Challenges and future opportunities for transcatheter aortic valve therapy. *Prog Cardiovasc Dis.* 2014;56(6):635-645.

49. Dharmarajan K, Foster J, Coylewright M, et al. The medically managed patient with severe symptomatic aortic stenosis in the TAVR era: Patient characteristics, reasons for medical management, and quality of shared decision making at heart valve treatment centers. *PLoS One*. 2017;12(4):e0175926.

50. Lindman BR, Alexander KP, O'Gara PT, Afilalo J. Futility, benefit, and transcatheter aortic valve replacement. *JACC Cardiovasc Interven*. 2014;7(7):707-716.

51. Lauck SB, Gibson JA, Baumbusch J, et al. Transition to palliative care when transcatheter aortic valve implantation is not an option: opportunities and recommendations. *Curr Opin Support Palliat Care*. 2016;10(1):18-23.

52. Jaarsma T, Beattie JM, Ryder M, et al. Palliative care in heart failure: a position statement from the palliative care workshop of the Heart Failure Association of the European Society of Cardiology. *Eur J Heart Fail*. 2009;11(5):433-443.

53. Kavalieratos D, Gelfman LP, Tycon LE, et al. Palliative care in heart failure: rationale, evidence, and future priorities. *J Am Coll Cardiol*. 2017;70(15):1919-1930.

54. McIlvennan CK, Allen LA. Palliative care in patients with heart failure. *BMJ*. 2016;353:i1010.

55. Lauck S, Garland E, Achtem L, et al. Integrating a palliative approach in a transcatheter heart valve program: bridging innovations in the management of severe aortic stenosis and best end-of-life practice. *Eur J Cardiovasc Nurs*. 2014;13(2):177-184.

56. Denvir MA, Highet G, Robertson S, et al. Future care planning for patients approaching end-of-life with advanced heart disease: an interview study with patients, carers and healthcare professionals exploring the content, rationale and design of a randomised clinical trial. *BMJ Open*. 2014;4(7):e005021.

CHAPTER 7

Who Is the Right Patient for Transcatheter Aortic Valve Replacement: Complexities of Case Selection

Kimberly A. Guibone, ACNP

OBJECTIVES

▶ Use current indications to present categories of patients who are appropriate candidates for TAVR

▶ Highlight indicators of risk

▶ Discuss best practices for patient selection

Introduction

Transcatheter aortic valve replacement (TAVR) has redefined the population and candidacy for aortic valve replacement (AVR) and definitive treatment to include a wider range of patients with severe aortic stenosis (AS). Significant numbers of patients who were previously considered to be of high or at prohibitive risk, and perhaps denied surgical aortic valve replacement (SAVR) in the past, are now being routinely screened for TAVR. The most common degenerative form of AS presents in later years, therefore increasing the likelihood of concurrent comorbidities. The patient evaluation process becomes more complex when these comorbid conditions are taken into account, especially in view of their potential impact on risk stratification and postprocedure outcomes. Functional and cognitive assessments are integral components of the screening and evaluation process, as anticipated improvement in quality of life is an important determinant of a positive outcome. Since the inception of this technology, we have learned a great deal about who tends to benefit the most and the least from TAVR.[1,2] Patient selection is supported by a multifaceted evaluation process that focuses on technical feasibility as well as reasonability to proceed with definitive therapy as recommended in clinical guidelines.[2] Risk stratification models and factors affecting treatment allocation will be discussed with the intention of providing a balanced overview of individualized patient selection process.

Guidelines

Clinical guidelines are a collectively produced set of practice recommendations based on evidence, research, and expertise. Such guidelines are subject to transparency in development and rigorous review and incorporate a mechanism for change as therapies and evidence progress. Guidelines aim to optimize patient care, improve patient outcomes, and guide clinical decision making while recognizing that certain patients under certain conditions may need to be managed differently.[3]

The 2104 American Heart Association (AHA)/American College of Cardiology (ACC) Valvular Heart Disease guidelines identify AS as occurring in a series of stages grading severity of stenosis, onset of symptoms, and left ventricular dysfunction. Stage A refers to early AS, such as one who may have a known bicuspid valve, although asymptomatic. Stage B refers to mild to moderate AS, whereby there is developing calcification or fusion narrowing the valve, yet the patient remains asymptomatic, such as an incidental finding on a routine echocardiogram. Stage C1 refers to severe narrowing of the aortic valve and some left ventricular hypertrophy, yet the patient denies symptoms and the ejection fraction (EF) is preserved, such as one with known AS followed by serial echocardiograms. Stage C2 is also severe AS in which the patient denies symptoms, but the EF is reduced. Stage D1 is severe AS, with the patient now demonstrating classic symptoms perhaps admitted to a hospital for congestive heart failure and worsening shortness of breath. Stage D2 is severe symptomatic low-flow/low-gradient stenosis in which, although symptomatic, the high gradients are not generated because of the inability of the left ventricle to forcefully contract as is evident in the reduced EF. Stage D3 severe paradoxical low-flow AS refers to the paradox that, although the patient is symptomatic, the peak aortic velocity is less than that quantifying severe owing to the reduced ventricular cavity space because of left ventricular hypertrophy[4] (Figure 7.1).

The classic recommendation is to forego treatment until there is onset of symptoms. However, there are select situations in which AVR should be considered. Although the patient is asymptomatic, it is reasonable to consider AVR in patients with high velocities exceeding 5 m/s who are at low risk for surgery, as the rate of decline with onset of symptoms is rapid at this severe a state. Pathologically, it is also reasonable to consider AVR in

Stage	Definition	Description
A	At risk	Patients with risk factors for development of VHD
B	Progressive	Patients with progressive VHD (mild-to-moderate severity of asymptomatic)
C	Asymptomatic severe	Asymptomatic patients who have the criteria for severe VHD: C1: Asymptomatic patients with severe VHD in whom the left or right ventricle remains compensated C2: Asymptomatic patients with severe VHD, with decompensation of the left or right ventricle
D	Symptomatic severe	Patients who developed symptoms as a result of VHD

FIGURE 7.1. Stages of aortic stenosis. VHD, valvular heart disease. (Reprinted with permission from Nishimura RA, et al. 2014 AHA/ACC valvular heart disease guideline. *Circulation*. 2014;129.)

asymptomatic patients with severe AS who demonstrate rapid disease progression exceeding that of 0.3 m/s increase in velocity per year. Of note, the validation of asymptomatic status may be difficult to ascertain or elicit in patients who have severe AS as often they alter their activity level to compensate for early symptoms or deny symptoms, attributing them to the aging process or other comorbidities. For these patients, exercise testing may expose masked symptoms. If through exercise testing there is a drop in systolic pressure or a failure to increase systolic pressure by at least 20 mm Hg suggesting exercise intolerance, AVR should then be considered[5] (Figure 7.2).

Treatment of severe AS includes medical therapy with possible balloon aortic valvuloplasty (BAV), SAVR, and TAVR. At this time, TAVR is only approved in the United States for patients who are symptomatic and who are at an intermediate or a greater level of risk for SAVR.[6]

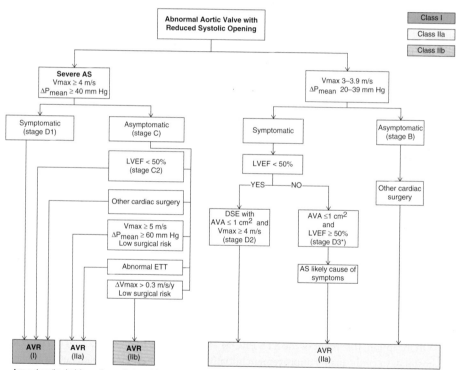

Arrow show the decision pathways that result in a recommendation for AVR. Periodic monitoring is indicated for all patients in whom AVR is not yet indicated, including those with asymptomatic AS (stage D or C) and those with low-gradients AS (stage D2 or D3) who do not meet the criteria for intervention.
*AVR should be considered with stage D3 As only if valve obstruction is the most likely cause of symptoms, stroke volume index <35 mL/m2, indexed AVA is ≤0.6cm2/m2, and data are recorded when the patient is normotensive (systolic BP 140 mm Hg).
As indicates aortic stenosis; AVA, aortic valve area; AVR, aortic valve replacement by either surgical or transcatheter approach; BP, blood pressure; DSE, doubtamine stress echocardiography; ETT, exercise tredmill test; LVEF, left ventricular ejection fraction; ΔP_{mean}, mean pressure gradient; and V_{max}, maximum velocity.

FIGURE 7.2. Abnormal aortic valve with reduced systolic opening. (Reprinted with permission from Nishimura RA, Otto CM, Bonow RO, et al. 2014 AHA/ACC guideline for the management of patients with valvular heart disease: a report of the American College of Cardiology/American Heart Association Task Force on Practice Guidelines. *J Am Coll Cardiol.* 2014;63:2438-2488.)

Percutaneous BAV is a temporizing measure in which a balloon catheter is inflated within the aortic valve to increase the aortic valve area to alleviate some degree of stenosis with effects lasting an average of 6 months.[7] Outside of the TAVR procedure, indications for BAV include bridging hemodynamically unstable patients to TAVR or SAVR as a palliative measure in patients with advanced disease states who are not suitable for TAVR or SAVR or as a measure of therapeutic response to discern benefit from relief of the aortic stenosis in the setting of conflicting comorbidities driving symptoms.[8]

A means of stratifying procedural risk is through use of validated algorithms, such as the Society of Thoracic Surgery-Predicted Risk of Mortality (STS PROM) scoring system.[9] Risk stratification historically has been performed by the cardiac surgeon through use of the "eyeball test." The eyeball test refers to the surgeon's summation of risk through medical reports, physical examination, intuition, and the surgeon's clinical experience. Although reliable, this method lends to variability and decreased reproducibility, as it is dependent on surgeon experience, interpretation, and preference.[10] In addition, certain anatomical conditions such as calcified aorta cannot be captured in the eyeball test. The advent of percutaneous alternatives, including TAVR, and the expansion of patient candidacy, including conditions formerly prohibitive for surgery, support the need for validated risk tools and objective risk measures to predict outcomes.[11]

Defining Risk

Society of Thoracic Surgeons Risk Score

The STS PROM is a validated tool designed to predict risk-adjusted outcomes in patients undergoing specific cardiac surgeries, including isolated AVR. The tool is derived from data collected via the STS cardiac surgery database first established in 1989. Through these data and applied multivariate logistic regression models, predicted probabilities are generated and updated at predetermined intervals.[12] The tool itself is Web-based and elicits input of 34 to 51 points of clinical and demographic data depending on the items answered. The calculated result includes the risk of operative mortality defined as death during hospitalization regardless of length of stay or death within 30 days regardless of location. Morbidity or mortality is the composite end point of risk for permanent stroke, renal failure, prolonged ventilation, deep sternal wound infection, and reoperation for any reason.[13]

On inception, the intent of the STS PROM algorithm was to provide a tool to clinicians and hospitals to guide quality improvement initiatives. The use has since broadened to application in clinical trials, patient-clinician decision collaboration, and pay-for-performance structures. As a widely recognized validated tool of measure, it is now also an active determinant of candidacy for patients undergoing TAVR screening and evaluation.

The STS PROM tool is specific to SAVR and 6 other cardiac surgery procedures, rather than TAVR, and is validated as such. However, certain comorbidities or conditions relevant to surgical candidacy are not captured, including prohibitive anatomy, blood dyscrasias, liver disease, and frailty.

Comorbidities/conditions not captured in STS PROM:

• Liver disease	• Calcified aorta
• Blood dyscrasias	• Prior chest wall radiation
• Cancers	• Hostile chest/severe kyphosis
• Pulmonary hypertension	• Prior graft proximity to sternum
• Failure of the right side of the heart	• Frailty

Currently, the STS PROM risk score remains the standard for cardiac surgical risk stratification and is therefore incorporated into the AHA/ACC guidelines. The AHA/ACC guidelines recognize the limitation of the tool validity as it is specific to the surgical population.
Hence, the guidelines also include measures for frailty, major organ system compromise not
to be improved postoperatively, and procedure-specific impediment in completing the overall
risk assessment[4] (Figure 7.3).

European System for Cardiac Operative Risk Evaluation

The European System for Cardiac Operative Risk Evaluation (EuroSCORE) is a risk predictive tool developed in 1995 and published in 1999 through data extracted from the
European database of patients who underwent cardiac surgery covering 43 countries.
The risk score is derived from assigned weights to risk factors and application of logistic
regression methodology. The resultant single score refers to the patient's predicted operative mortality. The purpose in its development was also to facilitate risk-adjusted quality
monitoring.[14]

The EuroSCORE is available online, in 6 languages, and requires an input of 18 clinical
and demographic points of data. The original EuroSCORE was considered to overestimate the
risk of operative death and was derived primarily from data in patients undergoing coronary

	Low Operative Risk (Must Meet ALL Criteria in This Column)	Intermediate Operative Risk (Any 1 Criterion in This Column)	High Operative Risk (Any 1 Criterion in This Column)	Prohibitive Operative Risk (Any 1 Criterion in This Column)
STS PROM	< 4% AND	4% to 8% OR	> 8% OR	Prohibited risk with surgery of death or major morbidity (all-cause) > 50% at 1 year OR
Frailty	None AND	1 Index (mild) OR	≥ 2 Indices (moderate to severe) OR	
Major organ system compromise not to be improved postoperatively	None AND	1 organ system OR	No more than 2 organ systems OR	≥ 3 organ systems OR
Procedure-specific impediment	None	Possible procedure-specific impediment	Possible procedure-specific impediment	Severe procedure-specific impediment

FIGURE 7.3. Aortic stenosis risk stratification. STS PROM, Society of Thoracic Surgery-Predicted Risk of Mortality. (Reprinted with permission from Nishimura RA, et al. 2014 AHA/ACC
valvular heart disease guideline. *Circulation.* 2014;129.)

artery bypass grafting. This, and the changes in patient risk profile and surgical advancements, led to the development of the EuroSCORE II. The tool is well validated and widely used in Europe, North America, and Asia.[9]

The EuroSCORE II is more general in reference to cardiac surgeries with options for weight of intervention identifying isolated coronary artery bypass versus multiple interventions,[15] whereas the STS PROM delineates predicted risk for select cardiac surgery procedures (isolated coronary artery bypass graft surgery [CABG], isolated AVR, isolated mitral valve replacement, isolated mitral valve repair, CABG with AVR, and CABG with mitral valve replacement or mitral valve repair). The EuroSCORE by design also requires fewer points of data than the STS-PROM, making it easier to use. However, the EuroSCORE refers only to operative risk and does not specify further as in the STS PROM and like the STS PROM does not account for liver disease, hostile chest, or blood dyscrasias. In addition, the EuroSCORE may not have as strongly a predictive power in patients over 70 years, as the data derived population had an average age of 62 to 65 years.[15]

Predictive Risk Models for Transcatheter Aortic Valve Replacement

Patient candidacy for TAVR by surgical risk stratification is supported by risk models such as the STS PROM, the EuroSCORE, and EuroSCORE II. However, as predictive risk models specific to TAVR they are less robust. Most notably, none of the surgical risk models account for frailty, which is a significant determinant of poor outcome at 1 year after TAVR in this elderly population.[16] The STS PROM has also demonstrated a tendency to underscore risk in the transfemoral TAVR group yet overestimate risk in the transapical TAVR group.[17] Notwithstanding, extremely high STS risk scores of >15% do correlate to overall poor outcomes at 2 years likely related to progression of comorbidities, prolonged left ventricular hypertrophy and dysfunction now unreactive to TAVR, or inability to use the benefit of TAVR expressed in improvement in quality of life.[16] The EuroSCORE (based on 1995 data) tends to overestimate risk across all TAVR types, whereas the EuroSCORE II performs similarly to the STS PROM, yet also without capturing indices for frailty and disability.[18]

The TAVR In-Hospital Mortality Risk Calculator can be used to predict in-hospital mortality for the patient under consideration for TAVR. Open to all, it is available online or as a mobile app. Unlike prior AVR risk predictor tools derived from surgical AVR data, the TAVR In-Hospital tool is developed from data extracted from a like-based TAVR population. The Transcatheter Valve Therapies national registry, a compilation of data from all commercial TAVR cases, as a source of clinical information, has propelled the development of this statistical predictive and validated model of in-hospital mortality. The tool consists of entering 13 points of clinical and demographic data, which will produce a risk score for in-hospital mortality for the patient entered as well as provide an updated national average for comparison. Absent from the model are frailty indices, as data volume had not been reached at the time of design and release.[11]

Large European registries are also lending to the development of risk predictor models based on TAVR patient data. The German Aortic Valve Score is a scoring system designed to predict mortality in both surgical aortic valve and TAVR procedures in adults.[19] The Observational Study Of Appropriateness, Efficacy, and Effectiveness of AVR-TVR Procedures For the Treatment of Severe Symptomatic Aortic Stenosis (OBSERVANT) score originating in Italy is a scoring system weighting characteristics of renal function, critical preoperative state, congestive heart failure status, pulmonary hypertension, diabetes, EF, and history of prior balloon valvuloplasty. The FRANCE-2 model identifies predictors of early mortality and assigns a point value to critical state, low body mass, pulmonary disease, end-stage renal disease, and procedural approach.[20] All are effective within their population-derived cohorts but vary when applied externally, indicating the need for broader registry data collection and analysis to improve prediction.[21]

Comorbidities and Considerations

A comprehensive Heart Team evaluation process is essential for appropriate patient selection and optimization of postprocedure outcomes and is supported by the use of the various risk predictive models. Also essential is the recognition of the impact of particular comorbidities on treatment allocation and expectations for postprocedure recovery and quality of life, all of which are important components for discussion with patients and families as part of the shared decision-making process.

Mitral Valve Disease

Up to one-third of patients with severe AS have concomitant moderate to severe mitral valve regurgitation (MR).[22] Moderate to severe MR is associated with both short-term and long-term adverse outcomes in patients undergoing SAVR and TAVR. Significant MR is depicted here (Figure 7.4). Patients deemed of acceptable surgical risk may be better treated with a combined surgical valve procedure. However, surgical risk is nearly 3-fold for combined valve surgeries as opposed to isolated AVR leading some to redirect to TAVR.[22]

The cause and progression of mitral regurgitation may adversely affect the likelihood of improvement post TAVR. Mitral regurgitation is classified as organic, functional, or both. Organic MR is valve dysfunction due to an abnormality of the valve itself, including the leaflets, chordae tendineae, papillary muscles, or annulus. This may be due to myxomatous disease as in mitral valve prolapse of one of the leaflets or due to buildup of annular calcification as is associated with aging. Functional mitral regurgitation refers to an intact mitral valve with dysfunction of surrounding structures. This can include annular stretching due to dilated cardiomyopathy preventing coaptation of leaflets, ischemic injury to the papillary muscles, or hypertrophic cardiomyopathy.[22] Progression of the disease can eventually cause dilation of the left ventricle and left atria to compensate, with the prolonged state leading to left ventricular systolic and diastolic dysfunction, reduced left atrial compliance, and elevated left atrial pressure causing pulmonary hypertension and eventual impairment of the right ventricle.[23] Significant mitral regurgitation can increase procedural risk as an occurrence of hemodynamic instability and may not be as well tolerated with greater risk for decompensation and cardiogenic shock.[22]

TAVR has been shown to improve some degree of mitral regurgitation in up to 60% of patients by removing the left ventricular outflow tract obstruction thereby decreasing the pressure in the left ventricular cavity.[22] However, the overall effect is limited. The effect is more notable in patients with functional mitral regurgitation than with organic mitral regurgitation.[22] Patients with functional mitral regurgitation are more likely to gain some improved left ventricular function, as the disorder is not due to the valve itself. Both, however, are associated with a significant increase in mortality in short-term and long-term follow-up.[22]

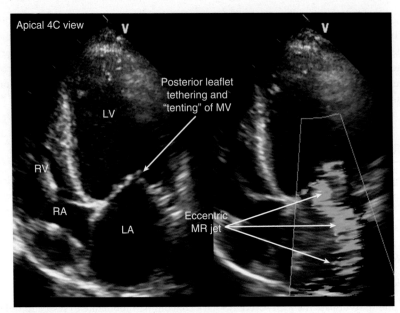

FIGURE 7.4. Mitral regurgitation. Tenting of the posterior mitral valve (MV) leaflet with apical and lateral displacement of leaflet coaptation resulting in eccentric posteriorly directed mitral regurgitation (MR). LA, left atrium; LV, left ventricle; RA, right atrium; RV, right ventricle. (Reprinted with permission from Quader N, Makan M, Perez J, eds. *The Washington Manual of Echocardiography*. 2nd ed. Philadelphia, PA: Wolters Kluwer; 2017.)

Patients undergoing TAVR with significant mitral regurgitation at baseline have a higher risk for perioperative instability, longer length of stays, and more frequent readmissions.[24] Patients with functional mitral regurgitation may show some improvement in left ventricular function more so than in patients with organic mitral regurgitation, but overall, patients with moderate to severe mitral regurgitation after TAVR have significantly increased short-term and long-term mortality rates.[24]

Mitral stenosis, a narrowing of the mitral valve, has been found to occur in 10% of patients with aortic valve disease in the surgical population.[25] Mitral stenosis most commonly is secondary to rheumatic heart diseases as a sequela to rheumatic fever. Rheumatic fever damages the valve endothelium in varying degrees to all of the heart valves, although more significantly in the mitral valve.[26] The process can cause the leaflets of the mitral valve to fuse near the edges and the chordae to distort contributing to a subvalvular obstruction to flow.[27] This causes the left atrium to enlarge and increase pulmonary pressures, which can strain the right side of the heart, causing failure.[27] TAVR with mitral stenosis has a higher incidence of readmission for heart failure and long-term adverse events[25] (Table 7.1).

Pulmonary Disease

Chronic lung disease exists as a comorbidity of approximately one-third of patients with AS and has been associated with a higher risk of short- and long-term mortality post TAVR.[28] Chronic lung disease is a known contributor to mortality following overall cardiac surgery,[29]

TABLE 7.1. Mitral Valve Disease: Points of Consideration and Patient Discussion

Points of Consideration	Points of Patient Discussion
1. Heart Team review to determine surgical risk stratification for combined aortic and mitral valve surgery 2. Patients with significant MR at baseline are at increased risk for perioperative instability, longer length of stays, and more frequent admissions[25]	1. TAVR may or may not improve mitral regurgitation (MR) 2. Symptoms may not dramatically improve or resolve after TAVR 3. Ongoing CHF management will be necessary 4. Diuretic therapy is unlikely to be weaned completely post procedure

CHF, congestive heart failure; TAVR, transcatheter aortic valve replacement.

and, for patients requiring definitive therapy for severe AS, especially those with moderate to severe lung disease, a less invasive procedure such as TAVR may be desirable.

Chronic obstructive pulmonary disease (COPD) is the inflammatory chronic lung disease resulting in poorly reversible airflow obstruction. Although the condition is manageable, it is irreversible and likely progressive. Chronic inflammation and mucoid excretion narrow and clog the small airways allowing air to enter on inhalation, then become trapped by the airway narrowing on exhalation. The consequence is a hyperinflation of the small airways. The process is compounded by alveolar destruction over time, impairing elastic recoil, further limiting the ability to expel air. Existence of this hyperinflation decreases the inspiratory capacity in inhalation and reduces the functional residual capacity. These anatomical changes impair gas exchange. The overt symptoms of this translate as breathlessness and limited capacity to exercise.[30] COPD occurs in stages with coinciding worsening prognosis. The BODE index is a scoring system to predict long-term outcomes for patients with COPD. The model is base on Body mass index, airflow Obstruction, Dyspnea, and Exercise (BODE). Items are assigned points that when tallied have an associated predicted survival rate of the patient with COPD at 4 years.[29]

Patients with COPD who undergo TAVR have a 1.5-fold higher risk of death at 6 months.[31] A moderate or greater degree of COPD (FEV1<80% on pulmonary function testing) has been correlated to complications post TAVR.[31] Many of these patients developed respiration-related complications during the perioperative period, requiring a longer length of hospital stay.[28,31] Multiple studies have shown oxygen-dependent lung disease as an independent predictor of poor outcomes post TAVR, with nearly a third dead at 1 year.[28,31]

Despite the presence of COPD, most surviving patients report an improvement in their New York Heart Association (NYHA) functional heart class, although in patients with more severe COPD, not to the level of NYHA class I or II. Those reporting improvements were likely experiencing significant symptoms related to their AS. On the contrary, those who reported little improvement and with lower gradient AS were more likely experiencing symptoms related to their lung disease.[32]

For patients with severe AS and moderate to severe chronic lung disease, it is recommended that pulmonary function be optimized before TAVR to reduce perioperative complications. This may include multidisciplinary collaboration with a pulmonary specialist in titrating oral and inhaled medications. Pulmonary rehabilitation, muscle strengthening, and nutritional support are also beneficial. For patients with advanced lung disease, lower exercise capacity, and muscle wasting, a thorough evaluation is necessary to assess for futility. If futility

TABLE 7.2. Pulmonary Disease: Points of Consideration and Patient Discussion

Points of Consideration	Points of Patient Discussion
1. Pulmonary function testing should be performed within 1 y 2. BODE score calculation 3. Collaboration with pulmonologist is advantageous to medically optimize lung function 4. Pulmonary rehabilitation 5. In the case of advanced lung disease, balloon aortic valvuloplasty can be used to ascertain clinical benefit versus futility	1. TAVR will not treat underlying lung disease 2. Shortness of breath may not dramatically improve or completely resolve after TAVR 3. Post-TAVR hospitalization may be longer 4. If severe COPD, clinically may improve only minimally post TAVR[27]

COPD, chronic obstructive pulmonary disease; TAVR, transcatheter aortic valve replacement.

versus benefit remains unclear, BAV should be considered to determine if alleviation of stenosis improves patient status[28,31] (Table 7.2).

Pulmonary hypertension (pulmonary artery pressure >25 mm Hg) secondary to AS is also associated with a higher mortality rate in TAVR. Left ventricular remodeling due to AS is associated with subsequent increased left ventricular pressure. Pulmonary hypertension occurs in greater than 50% of patients with left ventricular diastolic dysfunction related to AS. Severe pulmonary hypertension due to pressure overload can change the structure of the pulmonary arterial vascular bed, leading to right ventricular overload and eventual failure.[33] Some patients undergoing TAVR have been shown to demonstrate a 15-mm Hg decrease in pulmonary arterial pressure in the short term. Those who do not may be indicative of prolonged advanced pulmonary hypertension less likely to resolve carrying with that an increased risk for mortality.[34] Pulmonary hypertension therapies should be optimized before proceeding with TAVR[34] through pharmacotherapy and exercise training.[35]

Kidney Disease

Chronic kidney disease (CKD) is defined as a glomerular filtration rate (GFR) <60 mL/min/1.73 m^2 persisting more than 3 months.[36] Among a host of causes causing kidney damage, GFR, based on serum creatinine, is the most accurate measure of kidney function.[36] Normal GFR in healthy young persons ranges around 125 mL/min/1.73 m^2. Less than half of normal GFR <60 mL/min/1.73 m^2 reflects decreased kidney function, and GFR <15 mL/min/1.73 m^2 is indicative of kidney failure. CKD is associated with an increased risk for all-cause cardiovascular mortality, kidney failure, acute kidney injury (AKI), and progression of renal dysfunction.[36]

There is a high incidence of CKD observed in the patient population suffering from AS. Age, gender, smoking, hypertension, and hyperlipidemia have been associated with coronary artery disease (CAD) and calcific aortic disease. Most patients with these characteristics also later develop CKD. Renal dysfunction can alter vitamin D levels, parathyroid hormone, and serum phosphate, which are early markers for impaired mineral metabolism and correlate to increased calcific aortic valve disease.[37]

Up to 75% of patients with AS have been found to have some degree of kidney disease.[35] Advanced or end-stage kidney disease is an independent predictor of increased mortality post

TAVR.[38] Patients with advanced kidney diseased have been demonstrated to have a 2-fold increase in in-hospital mortality and all-cause mortality at 1 year.[38] A large-scale review of patients has identified that patients with advanced CKD when compared with patients with no CKD have significantly higher incidence of cardiovascular events, pacemaker need, and bleeding complications.[39] Patients already with CKD have a greater risk for renal disease progression. Periprocedural events can be deleterious should high contrast load, hypotension, or bleeding complications occur further affecting renal function. Bleeding incidence is elevated in this patient population as impaired platelet function and drug interactions amplify risk.[39] AKI post TAVR in patients with preexisting advanced CKD occurs 7-fold more than those without pre-existing CKD, with a 15-fold greater incidence of AKI requiring renal replacement therapy (RRT), including hemodialysis, peritoneal dialysis, intermittent dialysis, or continuous renal replacement therapies.[39] Patients with CKD tend to require prolonged hospitalizations and discharge to rehabilitation facilities.[39]

RRT, such as hemodialysis, and the accompanying symptom burden in the elderly patient is comparable with cancer. The need for RRT may be initiated in the acute care setting when the patient is under duress and subject to the guidance of the medical team and family without the advantage of full understanding of the implications and effect on quality of life. Patient shared decision making and elaboration on the impact of RRT should be included in the patient selection process for patients at elevated risk for kidney failure. Although RRT has been shown to prolong life in the elderly, such advantage is significantly reduced in patients with other comorbidities, notably heart disease.[40] In elderly patients older than 84 years, hemodialysis has been shown to have a 30% mortality at 90 days and a 50% mortality at 1 year.[40] In the patient with concomitant heart disease or dementia, the likelihood of survival worsens, with a predicted time to death of 1 year and a survival rate of 24% at 2 years.[40] It is necessary to include the nephrologist in the Heart Team and patient selection (Table 7.3).

Considerations

Low-Flow-Low-Gradient/Normal or Reduced Ejection Fraction

Patients with low-flow low-gradient AS and normal or reduced EF are associated with poorer outcomes and increased early and long-term mortality.[41] Low-flow low-gradient is defined as severe AS with a low gradient due to a small ventricular cavity from invading left ventricular hypertrophy allowing for only a small stroke volume that cannot generate a gradient or a low gradient due to a weakened heart muscle and reduced EF unable to contract with strength to reveal a gradient. Compensatory measures in the setting of AS include left ventricular remodeling and myocardial hypertrophy resulting in temporary preservation of EF. This hypertrophy maintains a normal EF. However, prolonged hypertrophy can result in distortion of the left ventricle and an increase in the relative wall thickness due to hypertrophy by >50%.[42] This distortion causes an elongated narrow cavity capable of containing only a small amount of blood. Therefore, despite a normal EF, only a low stroke volume is produced, stroke volume index <35 mL/m defining low flow, and inadequate volume to produce a more robust gradient in the setting of true AS.[42]

Reduced EF is indicative of myocardial weakening or absence of contractility, versus preserved contractility constrained by the severity of the obstruction caused by the AS. Diagnostic

TABLE 7.3. Kidney Disease: Points of Consideration and Patient Discussion

Points of Consideration	Points of Patient Discussion
1. Risk stratification for AKI 2. Collaboration with nephrologist preprocedure may be beneficial 3. Procedure planning to reduce risk for AKI (reduced contrast load, consideration to alternatives for general anesthesia, renal protective therapies, avoiding nephrotoxins) 4. Combined comorbidities compound likelihood of poor outcome and futility of TAVR	1. Realistic understanding of current renal function 2. Risk for AKI or HD 3. Implication of HD on symptom burden and survivability 4. Conduct a goals of care discussion 5. Potentially longer hospitalization and need for rehabilitation facility at discharge

AKI, acute kidney injury; HD, hemodialysis; TAVR, transcatheter aortic valve replacement.

testing by low-dose dobutamine stress echocardiography can provide some data to delineate. Administration of the inotrope dobutamine at doses up to 20 μg/kg/min with an increased augmentation of flow velocity and >20% increase in stroke volume indicates the contractile reserve of muscle function. If the aortic valve area increases with the addition of an inotrope to help myocardial force, the likelihood is cardiomyopathy rather than severe AS. If there is no change in EF or no increase in transvalvular gradient, the cause is weighted toward cardiomyopathy, although AS may still be present.[43]

Patients with reduced EF yet with contractile reserve are more likely to experience greater symptomatic improvement and improved EF once the obstruction (AS) is removed. In addition, patients with severe diastolic dysfunction that may be sensitive to excessive pressure forces related to obstruction may improve function post TAVR. Patients with reduced EF due to cardiomyopathy are less likely to demonstrate dramatic improvement post TAVR with overall poorer outcomes short and long term. More recent studies correlate low-flow, low-gradient to negative outcomes post TAVR, as this carries a greater component of myocardium disease that is less likely to improve significantly in symptoms or function. Patients with low-flow, low-gradient AS have a higher 1-year mortality and higher incidence of heart failure post TAVR.[41] Subsequently, hospital length of stay is longer and the necessity for rehabilitation facility at discharge more likely. Patients with low-flow, low-gradient AS have a higher rate of mortality with TAVR than those with non–low-flow, low-gradient AS but better than that of medical therapy alone[44] (Table 7.4).

Anatomy

Detailed anatomical evaluation including various imaging modalities is necessary for TAVR procedure planning and patient selection. The Heart Team must be intimately familiar with imaging protocols and criteria for technical feasibility of the TAVR procedure. Heart Team review of anatomical findings can predict procedure complexity and guide patient discussion of risk for procedural complications. Complex imaging via multidetector computed tomography has become a standard portion of TAVR evaluation for potential candidacy.

TABLE 7.4. Low-Flow, Low-Gradient AS: Points of Consideration and Patient Discussion

Points of Consideration	Points of Patient Discussion
1. Evaluation of stroke volume index 2. Dobutamine stress echocardiography may be used 3. Collaboration with Advanced Heart Failure team 4. Postdischarge follow-up and ongoing CHF management 5. Consideration of futility of TAVR with low-flow, low-gradient AS without contractile reserve and with significant additional comorbidities	1. TAVR may or may not improve heart muscle function 2. Symptoms may not completely resolve after TAVR 3. Ongoing CHF management will be necessary 4. Diuretic therapy is unlikely to be weaned completely

AS, aortic stenosis; CHF, congestive heart failure; TAVR, transcatheter aortic valve replacement.

Concerning anatomy revealed by computed tomography may include heavily calcified or tortuous access vessels at greater risk for vascular complication or various anatomical anomalies associated with greater risk if considering alternative access options. For further discussion please see chapter 5.

As the Food and Drug Administration approved indications for TAVR will likely move to include lower-risk patient populations, close attention to annular calcium burden and distribution should be reviewed and discussed by the Heart Team. A low-risk patient may benefit from SAVR as opposed to TAVR in situations in which paravalvular leak may be present post TAVR secondary to calcium distribution. Multidetector scanners and 3-dimensional reconstruction allow precise measurements and analysis of calcium distribution. Positioning of large deposits of calcium at the annulus level can prevent full expansion of the valve, increase the risk of annular rupture with excessive force, and result in paravalvular leak as the valve cannot conform to the large protrusion. Calcium extending into the lumen >4 mm should be reviewed to determine if risk versus benefit would show preference to SAVR and avoidance of paravalvular leak.[2] Similarly, large calcium burden throughout may also increase risk for paravalvular leak with calcium laden leaflets potentially obstructing coronary ostium with TAVR deployment[2] (Figure 7.5). Situations such as these mandate comprehensive review to ascertain acceptable risk for optimal outcome.

Coronary angiography is the standard means of assessing for the presence of CAD. The decision to treat coronary lesions is based on current guideline recommendations and expertise of the Heart Team. In patients who are of acceptable surgical risk with multivessel CAD, the recommendation is for combined SAVR with coronary artery bypass grafting.[4] In patients with single vessel disease or at high or extreme risk for SAVR, the decision is less clear. Limited data exist as throughout the major clinical trials, patients with significant CAD were excluded from trial participation.[45] Recommendations from the Interventional Section Leadership Council of the ACC for patients having TAVR are to treat major coronary arteries with significant proximal disease (>70%) before TAVR.[46]

Various iterations of transcatheter valves and improved operator technique and experience have resulted in a reduction in the risk for permanent pacemaker placement after TAVR; however, the possibility still exists. Conduction abnormalities post TAVR can include new-onset left bundle branch block, bradycardia, first degree atrioventricular block, complete heart block, and others. The proposed mechanism is temporary or permanent

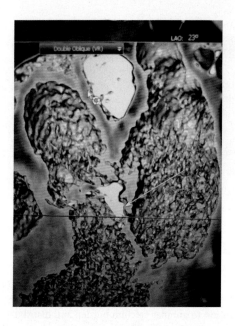

FIGURE 7.5. Heavily calcified leaflets at risk for coronary occlusion. (Courtesy of Jeffrey J. Popma, MD, Beth Israel Deaconess Medical Center, MA.)

trauma to the atrioventricular and infranodal regions during valve placement causing conduction disturbances and can be elicited by implantation of both surgical and transcatheter valves in the aortic position. Pre-existing conduction abnormalities, notably right bundle branch block, are associated with a higher incidence of bradydysrythmia and need for pacemaker post TAVR.[47] Right bundle branch block is also correlated with an increased overall mortality after TAVR.[47] Data suggest that the larger valve sizes may also have an increased incidence of pacemaker need post TAVR.[48] Patients with electrocardiograms showing right bundle branch block or requiring larger valve sizes should be provided additional education regarding potential pacemaker need and long-term implications at the time of procedural consent (Table 7.5).

Frailty

The advent of TAVR and patient screening for candidacy have spawned a burst of inquiry into frailty. The focus has grown from risk stratification for surgery to prognostic indicator of outcomes. Frailty is a critical component of patient selection with a need for objective measure and link to causality. Earlier readings in this handbook expand on the evaluation, indications, and implications of frailty.

Recognition of frailty and its impact has been well described in early transcatheter valve clinical trials.[16] Frailty identifiers of serum albumin, hand grip strength, gait speed, and Katz activity of daily living survey have been correlated to a frailty state. Clinical data outline that patients with high frailty scores have a nearly 2-fold greater risk of poor outcomes than those with low frailty scores.[16]

Frailty is not currently a component of the STS Risk Calculator, EuroSCORE, or TAVR In-Hospital Mortality Risk Calculator yet is recognized as a predictor of morbidity and mortality and referenced in the current guidelines. Several frailty scoring tools are available varying in

TABLE 7.5. Anatomy: Points of Consideration and Patient Discussion

Points of Consideration	Points of Patient Discussion
1. Use imaging to identify concerning anatomy, eg, vascular access, annular calcium distribution, coronary heights	1. Detailed discussion regarding potential risks associated with anatomical findings
2. Consideration for percutaneous coronary intervention	2. Elevated possibility of pacemaker with pre-existing RBBB
3. Consider electrophysiology involvement in Heart Team review	3. Consideration weighing pros and cons for SAVR vs TAVR
4. Consider SAVR vs TAVR in the lower risk population with adverse calcium burden	4. Long-term implications of PPM implantation

PPM, permanent pacemaker; RBBB, right bundle branch block; SAVR, surgical aortic valve replacement; TAVR, transcatheter aortic valve replacement.

single versus multiple component measure. Commonly used is the 5-m gait speed, a measure of time it takes for the patient to walk 5 m, with greater than 6 seconds indicating frailty correlating to a 2- to 3-fold risk of major morbidity or mortality in the patient undergoing cardiac surgery.[49] This frailty measure was used in TAVR clinical trials and is now a necessary data point for the Transcatheter Valve Therapy registry.

For patients with moderate to high frailty scores, a complete geriatric review should be initiated for more thorough evaluation of risks versus benefits and the likelihood of improvement of quality of life. A more comprehensive geriatric review may also better assess cognitive functioning and the degree of dependency. Patient and family members may underestimate the degree of existing frailty masked by the compensatory frameworks of caretakers and patient denial, which a geriatric evaluation can discern. For patients with high frailty scores compounded by multiple system disorders, medical therapy is advised, including consideration for BAV to alleviate advanced AS symptoms. Palliative care should be considered.

On the contrary, although frailty is a dynamic process often progressive, recognition of the prefrail state, demonstrating only 1 or 2 frailty criteria,[50] can allow opportunity for strengthening, improving nutritional status, and optimization before TAVR. Prehabilitation is the concept of active conditioning before a surgery or treatment plan such as chemotherapy. Patients participate in a formalized plan for endurance training, aerobic capacity, and stabilizing frailty. Evidence suggests that proactive prehabilitation reduces postoperative complications, length of stay, and postdischarge services.[50] Prehabilitation programs are rapidly being implemented in a variety of surgical and medical specialties. Additional benefits include patient engagement, positive sense of control, and an increased likelihood of continuing a higher activity level post discharge[51] (Table 7.6).

Dementia

Dementia presents a challenge in evaluating for potential TAVR benefits and anticipated improvement in quality of life. Symptoms of severe decompensated AS and progressive dementia can be similar. Best practice is to determine which is the driving cause of functional decline. Gerontology or neurology input is often necessary to decipher underlying processes.

TABLE 7.6. Frailty: Points of Consideration and Patient Discussion

Points of Consideration	Points of Patient Discussion
1. Frailty testing 2. Prehabilitation for prefrail, frail patients 3. Gerontology collaboration for moderate to severe frailty and potential futility 4. For patients with severe frailty, the Heart Team must initiate a goals of care discussion, consideration for medical therapy, and palliative care	1. Frailty testing, perceived frailty 2. Candid input from family members of patient's current baseline functional status 3. Elicit patient and family goals and expectations 4. Gauge willingness to participate in prehabilitation 5. Define goals of care in case of adverse events

Cognitive impairment in patients undergoing procedures is associated with an increased rate of complications, prolonged hospitalization, and greater long-term mortality. All forms of dementia have a reduced life expectancy.[52]

There are several main types of dementia, all characterized by worsening memory, cognitive function, and behavior. Most patients with dementia have Alzheimer disease (AD). AD is a progressive neurodegenerative disorder and one of the leading causes of death in the United States.[49] Stages progress from short-term memory loss to advanced disease in which all activities require assistance; there is verbal loss, incontinence, immobility, and physical decline susceptible to infection or injury.

Vascular dementia occurs in 15% to 20% of adult patients with dementia and is related to cerebrovascular disease impairing blood flow. Hypertension is a cause in approximately half of the patients. Vascular dementia is also known as multi-infarct dementia in which cerebrovascular disease results in small vessel narrowing, embolic or thrombotic vascular occlusions, and cell death. Symptomatology and deficits are specific to the areas of infarct. A portion of patients who have vascular dementia will also have AD.[53]

Lewy body dementia is related to Parkinson disease and Parkinson dementia. Aberrancy in Lewy body protein production and replication alters chemical function, causing synapse disruption and neuronal destruction. The resulting symptoms include parkinsonism, altered reasoning, hallucinations, sleep disorders, and depression. Lewy body dementia is progressive and with no known treatment or reversal.[54]

The Mini-Mental State Exam (MMSE) is a screening tool for dementia and cognitive function. A 30-item questionnaire is administered including recall, math, drawing, and writing. Points are attached to the correct answers totaling up to 30. A score of less than 24 is suggestive of dementia and should be followed up with further evaluation. Additional data support that, in patients with a college or higher level of education, a score less than 27 should be investigated.[55] MMSE scores fall 2 to 4 points yearly in patients with AD. The Mini-Cog is an alternative screening tool. The advantage is its ease of use with only 5 items, including repeating, clock drawing, and memorization each with an assigned point up to 5. A score of less than 3 suggests the need for further evaluation. The Mini-Cog is a simple tool less influenced by education level or culture.[56]

If through expert review it is determined that dementia is not the primary cause of the patient's current state, the decision remains as to whether to proceed. In the patient with mild dementia who is functionally independent with a support system and stating desire,

TAVR is reasonable. In the patient with profoundly advanced dementia, it is unlikely that TAVR would improve quality of life. Commonly this is apparent to family and clinicians. However, if needed, application of the MMSE and neurology or gerontology evaluation may provide more objective findings to clarify the likelihood of recovery and establish goals of care.

The challenge presents in the patient with mild to moderate dementia who has severe AS. The ethics of autonomy supports the patients right to decide yet discussion of risks and implications may not truly be understood. Informed consent may be of issue. In cases of dementia impairing judgment, a proxy may advocate greatly for TAVR under the premise of "he always said he wants everything done" feeling responsible to carry forth wishes regardless of outcomes. Alternatively, the challenges of ongoing care for the patient with dementia warrants discussion of burden, as the progressive nature of dementia will continue despite TAVR. These types of discussions need to be fully vetted with the Heart Team, patient and family, and additional resources such as social workers or ethics teams to best decide individualized care and treatment goals (Table 7.7).

Medical Therapy and Futility

TAVR is not recommended for patients with multiple organ system dysfunction, severe frailty, advanced malignancies, or other comorbidities with less than 1-year life expectancy, as it is unlikely to benefit the patient clinically or improve quality of life. The decision-making process to forego definitive therapy should include discussion with the patient and family to ensure that all perspectives are adequately represented and that all relevant information is communicated with clarity. These are complex, and often emotional, decisions, and the Heart Team must be able to facilitate appropriate care pathways for these patients (Table 7.8).

A referral to a palliative care program may be considered, as these clinicians have a specialized focus on addressing the needs of patients with life-limiting illnesses for whom definitive therapy is not an option. They can work in conjunction with the Cardiology team with a primary focus on quality of life and employ supportive measures for comfort and symptom management. The needs of the caretakers are also addressed, and improved communication and discussion of goals of care are facilitated.[57]

TABLE 7.7. Dementia: Points of Consideration and Patient Discussion

Points of Consideration	Points of Patient Discussion
1. Evaluation of cognitive function (MMSE, Mini-Cog) 2. Rule out reversible causes (infection, metabolic disturbance, delirium) 3. Collaboration with Neurology 4. Collaboration with Gerontology 5. Candid conversations about anticipated improvement in quality of life especially in the patient with "moderate" dementia	1. Evaluation of patient's wishes 2. Evaluation of family/caretaker/social support 3. Evaluation of patient and family expectations 4. TAVR is unlikely to affect underlying progressive disease process and cognitive decline will likely be ongoing

MMSE, Mini-Mental State Exam; TAVR, transcatheter aortic valve replacement.

TABLE 7.8. Medical Therapy and Futility: Points of Consideration and Patient Discussion

Points of Consideration	Points of Patient Discussion
1. Balanced consideration of risk vs benefit of proceeding with TAVR 2. Reasonable expectation of improved quality of life post procedure 3. Overall life expectancy 4. Role of concomitant comorbities in symptomatology 5. Heart Team consensus to not offer TAVR secondary to futility 6. Mechanisms to involve palliative care 7. Comprehensive handoff to medical therapy	1. Ensure patient and family understand all aspects of the case were explored in detail and specialists were consulted 2. Consensus of the Heart Team is the risk of undergoing the procedure likely outweighs any potential benefit 3. Offer support and palliative care services to assist the patient and family with transition to comfort measures to maintain focus on quality of life

TAVR, transcatheter aortic valve replacement.

Case Scenarios

Case 1—Dementia and Frailty

An 85-year-old woman presented to the emergency department with shortness of breath, weakness, and confusion. She had been experiencing increasing fatigue, malaise, and worsening shortness of breath for several days at home. Her family brought her to the emergency department when they noted her becoming increasingly confused. She was afebrile, with blood pressure 106/57, heart rate 77 in atrial fibrillation, and oxygen saturation of 94% on room air. Chest x-ray demonstrated pulmonary edema, laboratory testing showed an elevated white blood cell count, and urinalysis suggested infection. She was oriented to person only. Antibiotics were initiated; she was dosed with intravenous diuretics and admitted to the cardiology stepdown unit for congestive heart failure (CHF) and confusion in the setting of urinary tract infection (UTI). Her past medical history included known AS for 2 years, atrial fibrillation, diabetes, hypertension, gait disorder, CKD, recurrent urinary tract infections, dementia, and falls.

A transthoracic echocardiogram was obtained. Findings included aortic valve area of 0.5 cm², mean gradient 60 mm/s, peak gradient 99 mm/s, and EF 45% to 50% with mild aortic regurgitation, mild mitral regurgitation, and mild tricuspid regurgitation. After several days of antibiotics, the mental status was mildly improved, and she was able to recognize family. She required persons to assist her from bed to chair. Family was aware of the AS and had discussed pursuing evaluation for TAVR with her primary cardiologist in the past. A Heart Team consult was initiated.

The patient underwent cardiac catheterization with findings of 50% left anterior descending artery stenosis with plans for medical management. She was evaluated by 2 cardiac surgeons and deemed high risk for SAVR. TAVR was discussed with patient and family, all of whom agreed to evaluation. Computed tomography angiography scan confirmed procedural candidacy.

On Heart Team review, it was noted that, although the patient was robustly agreeable to TAVR with family members present, she demonstrated limited recall of discussions when met with alone. Family members stated that the present mental status was below her baseline. Per the family, before admission, the patient had lived alone for many years without the need for assistance from home health aide, visiting nurses, or the like. The family very much wanted the patient to undergo TAVR to resume prior quality of life.

Given Heart Team concern and discrepancy in clinical versus family assessment of baseline mental status, an MMSE was performed. Patient score was 15/30. Geriatrics was consulted for further evaluation for dementia versus delirium.

A complete geriatric evaluation was performed with family members present. The patient scored poorly on frailty testing, including zero on sit to stand test, low on mini-nutritional testing, and a Katz score of 2/6. Cognitive function testing was suggestive of moderate to severe dementia. On focused interview with family it was determined that, although the patient lived alone, she was never unsupervised. Family members scheduled around-the-clock coverage to "keep her company." Family members expressed initial surprise at the objective findings but later endorsed that over the last 6 months she had demonstrated rapid cognitive decline and increasing near falls.

An extended discussion was had with the patient and family including Heart Team members and a geriatrician. It was explained that, although the patient may have a reduction in heart failure symptoms, it was unlikely that TAVR would significantly improve the quality of life. Limited benefits of TAVR were weighted against worsening delirium, expected progressive cognitive and functional decline, and the likely need for skilled nursing placement. The family was grateful for the thorough review and opportunity to participate in the evaluation and discussion and opted for medical therapy and ongoing geriatric care.

Case 2—Pulmonary Disease

An 87-year-old man with a history of transient ischemic attacks, carotid disease, atrial fibrillation, and hypertension was referred to the valve clinic for severe AS. He had been under treatment for 2 years prior for atrial fibrillation and diastolic heart failure. He developed pulmonary fibrosis likely secondary to amiodarone toxicity[58] and was given home oxygen. In addition, he had a remote history of smoking 2 packages of cigarettes per day for many years. He had 2 recent hospital admissions for congestive heart failure. On presentation, he had dyspnea, orthopnea, and New York Heart class III symptoms.[59] He had severe AS by echocardiogram, with aortic valve area 0.7 cm^2, mean gradient 38 mm Hg, peak gradient 68 mm Hg, EF 55%, moderate mitral regurgitation, and moderate tricuspid regurgitation. A cardiac catheterization showed minimal CAD. He was frail in appearance in a wheelchair and unable to ambulate greater than 20 feet due to shortness of breath. The STS risk score was 12.4%. He was evaluated by 2 cardiac surgeons and deemed extreme risk for SAVR primarily owing to his poor lung function.

Differential diagnoses for the primary cause of his shortness of breath included his pulmonary fibrosis versus severe AS. He was referred to a pulmonologist. Pulmonary function tests showed a restrictive ventilatory defect and severe gas exchange defect. He was subsequently readmitted for hypoxemia and CHF. He was relatively unstable and hypotensive. A BAV was done as bridge to TAVR and to assess for therapeutic response in symptoms.

Post BAV, the patient was hemodynamically stable and reported feeling improved despite ongoing oxygen requirement. The Heart Team consensus was to move forward with TAVR, as the BAV demonstrated symptomatic relief. A TAVR was performed without complication, and the patient was discharged to a rehabilitation facility. He continued to require oxygen; however, he maintained that he felt an improvement in his clinical symptoms as well as overall quality of life.

Conclusions

The TAVR patient selection process is dependent on a comprehensive Heart Team evaluation pathway, clearly defined measures of success, and the incorporation of patient and family expectations in the decision-making process. It is essential to take into account factors associated with technical feasibility as well as the potential impact of comorbid conditions and decline in functional or cognitive status. Although there are certainly predictors of poor outcomes that have been collected over the last decade by means of clinical trial data and cumulative clinical experience, each case deserves a dedicated and thorough Heart Team evaluation and discussion. There are clinical conundrums involving cognitive impairment and functional decline, which may greatly affect the recovery potential and must be brought to the table for candid consideration. There are prognostic indicators and tools that may be used to determine if the patients' functional or cognitive reserve may make them a better candidate for intervention. Although there is no failsafe prediction model, the Heart Team must rely heavily on clinical data, past experiences, and educated speculation about the procedural impact on a patient's overall health status. Proper patient selection is integral to the growth and success of a TAVR program, but most importantly, the goal of the Heart Team is to focus on anticipated improvement in the quality of life for each patient.

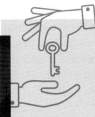

KEY TAKEAWAYS AND BEST PRACTICES

▶ Consult the clinical guidelines to determine the classification and severity of AS. Embedded within these guidelines are algorithms for patients who are asymptomatic but demonstrate abnormal aortic valve opening during systole.

▶ Assessing procedural/surgical risk and exploring case selection is a multifaceted process. The Heart Team must evaluate all diagnostic data and candidly share the potential risk-benefit ratios with the patient and family.

▶ Functional and cognitive assessments via formalized screening processes are recommended as standard practices during the evaluation of a patient for TAVR and factor into defining risk, recovery potential, and futility.

▶ All comorbid conditions and concomitant disease processes should be explored to ensure that a patient's symptoms are indeed stemming predominately from AS. BAV can be a beneficial tool in deciphering the cause of symptoms.

▶ All factors that may negatively affect the recovery potential should be taken into consideration when the Heart Team is formulating treatment options and discussed openly with the patient and family to set realistic expectations.

References

1. Puri R, Iung B, Cohen DJ, et al. TAVI or no TAVI: identifying patients unlikely to benefit from transcatheter aortic valve implantation. *Eur Heart J.* 2016;37(28):2217-2225.
2. Cocchia R, D'Andrea A, Conte M, et al. Patient selection for transcatheter aortic valve replacement: a combined clinical and multimodality imaging approach. *World J Cardiol.* 2017;9(3):212-2229.
3. Shekelle P, Aronson MD, Melin JA. *Overview of Clinical Practice Guidelines.* UpToDate; 2017. Retrieved from www.uptodate.com.
4. Nishimura RA, Otto CM, Bonow RO, et al. 2014 AHA/ACC guideline for the management of patients with valvular heart disease: a report of the American College of Cardiology/American Heart Association Task Force on practice guidelines. *Circulation.* 2014;129:1-235.
5. Rashedi N, Otto CM. *When Should We Operate in Asymptomatic Severe Aortic Stenosis?* American College of Cardiology CardioSource Plus for Institutions; 2015. Retrieved from http://www.acc.org/latest-in-cardiology/articles.
6. Nishimura RA, Otto CM, Bonow RO, et al. 2017 AHA/ACC focused update of the 2014 AHA/ACC guideline for the management of patients with valvular heart disease: a report of the American College of Cardiology/American Heart Association Task Force on Clinical Practice Guidelines. *J Am Coll Cardiol.* 2017;70:252-289.
7. Kogoj P, Devjak R, Bunc M. Balloon aortic valvuloplasty (BAV) as a bridge to aortic valve replacement in cancer patients who require urgent non-cardiac surgery. *Radiol Oncol.* 2014;48(1):62-66.
8. Keeble T, Khokhar A, Akhtar MM. Percutaneous balloon aortic valvuloplasty in the era of transcatheter aortic valve implantation: a narrative review. *Open Heart.* 2016;3:e000421.
9. Kirmani BH, Mazkar K, Fabri DM, Pullan DM. Comparison of the EuroSCORE II and Society of Thoracic Surgeons 2008 risk tools. *Eur J Cardiothorac Surg.* 2013;44(6):999-1005.
10. Jain R, Duval S, Adabag S. How accurate is the eyeball test? A comparison of physician's subjective assessment versus statistical methods in estimating mortality risk after cardiac surgery. *Circ Cardiovasc Qual Outcomes.* 2014;7(1):151-156.
11. Edwards FH, Cohen DJ, O'Brien SM, et al. Development and validation of a risk prediction model for in-hospital mortality after transcatheter aortic valve replacement. *JAMA Cardiol.* 2016;1(1):46-52.
12. Puskas JD, Kilgo PD, Thourani V, et al. The Society of Thoracic Surgeons 30-day predicted risk of mortality score also predicts long-term survival. *Ann Thorac Surg.* 2012;93(1):26-35.
13. *STS Adult Cardiac Surgery Database Risk Model Variables – Data Version 2.81*; 2014. Retrieved from www.sts.org.
14. Roques F, Michel P, Goldstone AR, Nashef SA. The logistic EuroSCORE. *Eur Heart J.* 2003;24(9):1-2.
15. Poullis M, Pullan M, Chalmers J, Mediratta N. The validity of the original EuroSCORE and EuroSCORE II in patients over the age of seventy. *Interact Cardiovasc Thorac Surg.* 2015;20(2):172-177.
16. Green P, Arnold SV, Cohen DJ, et al. Relation of frailty to outcomes after transcatheter aortic valve replacement (from the PARTNER Trial). *Am J Cardiol.* 2015;116(2):264-269.
17. Durand E, Borz B, Godin M, et al. Performance analysis of EuroSCORE II compared to the original logistic EuroSCORE and STS scores for predicting 30-day mortality after transcatheter aortic valve replacement. *Am J Cardiol.* 2015;111(6):891-897.
18. Wendt D, Thielmann M, Kahler P, et al. Comparison between different risk scoring algorithms on isolated conventional or transcatheter aortic valve replacement. *Ann Thorac Surg.* 2014;97(3):796-802.
19. Kottig J, Schiller W, Beckmann A, et al. German aortic valve score: a new scoring system for prediction of mortality related to aortic valve procedures in adults. *Eur J Cardiothorac Surg.* 2013;43(5):971-977.

20. Ribiero HB, Rodes-Cabau J. The multiparametric FRANCE-2 risk score: one step further in improving the clinical decision-making process in transcatheter aortic valve implantation. *Heart.* 2014;100(13):993-995.
21. Martin GP, Sperrin M, Ludman PF, et al. Inadequacy of existing clinical prediction models for predicting mortality after transcatheter aortic valve implantation. *Am Heart J.* 2017;181:97-105.
22. Nombela-Franco L, Ribiero HB, Urena M, et al. Significant mitral regurgitation left untreated at the time of aortic valve replacement. *J Am Coll Cardiol.* 2014;63(4):2643-2658.
23. Rubenfire M, Patel H, Desai M, Tuzcu EM, Griffin B, Kapadia S. *Pulmonary Hypertension in Mitral Regurgitation Ten Points to Remember*; 2014. Retrieved from www.acc.org.
24. Vollenbroich R, Stortecky S, Praz F, et al. The impact of functional vs degenerative mitral regurgitation on clinical outcomes among patients undergoing transcatheter aortic valve implantation. *Am Heart J.* 2017;184:71-80.
25. Joseph L, Bashir M, Siang Q, et al. Prevalence and outcomes of mitral stenosis in patients undergoing transcatheter aortic valve replacement. *JACC Cardiovasc Interv.* 2018;11(7):693-702.
26. Kumar RK, Tandon R. Rheumatic fever and rheumatic heart disease: the last 50 years. *Indian J Med Res.* 2013;137(4):643-658.
27. Holmes K, Gibbison B, Vohra HA. Mitral valve and mitral valve disease. *BJA Edu.* 2017;17(1):1-9.
28. Mok M, Nombela-Franco L, Dumont E, et al. Chronic obstructive pulmonary disease in patients undergoing transcatheter aortic valve implantation. *JACC Cardiovasc Interv.* 2013;6(10):1078-1084.
29. Cote CG, Celli BR. BODE index: a new tool to stage and monitor progression of chronic obstructive pulmonary disease. *Pneumonol Alergol Pol.* 2009;77:305-313.
30. MacNee W. Pathology, pathogenesis, and pathophysiology. *BMJ.* 2006;332(7551):1202-1204.
31. Dvir D, Waksman R, Barbash I, et al. Outcomes of patients with chronic lung disease and severe aortic stenosis treated with transcatheter versus surgical aortic valve replacement or standard therapy. *J Am Coll Cardiol.* 2014;63(3):1072-1084.
32. Crestanello JA, Popma JJ, Adams DH, et al. Long-term health benefit of transcatheter aortic valve replacement in patients with chronic lung disease. *JACC Cardiovasc Interv.* 2017;10(22):2283-2293.
33. Kiefer TL, Bashore TM. Pulmonary hypertension related to left-sided cardiac pathology. *Pulm Med.* 2011. 2011:381787. doi:10.1155/2011/381787.
34. Tang M, Liu X, Lin C, et al. Meta-analysis of outcomes and evolution of pulmonary hypertension before and after transcatheter aortic valve implantation. *Am J Cardiol.* 2017;119(1):91-99.
35. Galie N, Manes A, Palazzini M. Exercise training in pulmonary hypertension: improving performance but waiting for outcome. *Eur Heart J.* 2016;37:45-48.
36. Chapter 1: Definition and classification of CKD. *Kidney Int Suppl.* 2013;3(1):19-62.
37. Masuda C, Dohi K, Sakurai Y, et al. Impact of chronic kidney disease on the presence and severity of aortic stenosis in patients at high risk for coronary artery disease. *Cardiovasc Ultrasound.* 2011;9(31).
38. Codner P, Levi A, Gargiulo G, et al. Impact of renal dysfunction on results of transcatheter aortic valvel replacement outcomes in a large multicenter cohort. *Am J Cardiol.* 2016;118(12):1888-1896.
39. Gupta T, Goel K, Kolte D, et al. Association of chronic kidney disease with in-hospital outcomes of transcatheter aortic valve replacement. *JACC Cardiovasc Interv.* 2017;10(20):2050-2060.
40. Thorsteinsdottir B, Swetz KM, Feely MA, et al. Are there alternatives to hemodialysis for the elderly patient with end-stage renal failure? *Mayo Clin Proc.* 2012;87(6):514-516.
41. Baron SJ, Arnold SV, Hermann HC, et al. Impact of ejection fraction and aortic valve gradient on outcomes of transcatheter aortic valve replacement. *J Am Coll Cardiol.* 2016;67(20):2349-2358.
42. Bartel T, Muller S. Preserved ejection fraction can accompany low gradient severe aortic stenosis: impact of pathophysiology on diagnostic imaging. *Eur Heart J.* 2013;34(25):1862-1863.
43. Yavagal ST, Deshpande N, Admane P. Stress echo for the evaluation of valvular heart disease. *Indian Heart J.* 2014;66(1):131-138.

44. Clavel MA, Magne J, Pibarot P. Low-gradient aortic stenosis. *Eur Heart J.* 2016;37:2645-2657.

45. Leon M, Smith C, Mack M., et al. Transcatheter aortic-valve implantation for aortic stenosis in patients who cannot undergo surgery. *N Engl J Med.* 2010;363(17):1597-1607.

46. Ramee S, Anwaruddin S, Kumar G, et al. The rationale for performance of coronary angiography and stenting before transcatheter aortic valve replacemet. *JACC Cardiovasc Interv.* 2016;9(23):2371-2375.

47. Watanabe Y, Kozuma K, Hioki H, et al. Pre-existing right bundle branch block increases risk for death after transcatheter aortic valve replacement with a balloon expandable valve. *J Am Coll Cardiol Interv.* 2016;9(21):2210-2216.

48. Fadahunsi O, Olowoyeye A, Ukaigwe A, et al. Incidence, predictors, and outcomes of permanent pacemaker implantation following transcatheter aortic valve replacement. *JACC Cardiovasc Interv.* 2016;9(21):2189-2199.

49. Hansen DV, Hansen JE, Sheng M. *Microglia in Alzheimer's Disease*; 2018. Retrieved from doi:10.1083/jcb.201709069.

50. Afilalo J, Eisenberg MJ, Morin J, et al. Gait speed as an incremental predictor of mortality and major morbidity in elderly patients undergoing cardiac surgery. *J Am Coll Cardiol.* 2010;56(20):1668-1676.

51. Waite I, Deshpande R, Baghai M, et al. Home-based preoperative rehabilitation (prehab) to improve physical function and reduce hospital length of stay for frail patients undergoing coronary artery bypass graft and valve surgery. *J Cardiothorac Surg.* 2017;12(12):1-7.

52. Ries E. *Better Sooner and Later: Prehabilitation*; 2016. Retrieved from http://www.apta.org/PTinMotion/2016/2/Prehabilitation/.

53. Chapman DP, Williams SM, Strine TW, et al. Dementia and its implications for public health. *Prev Chronic Dis.* 2006;3(2):1-13.

54. Dohaghy PC, McKeith IG. The clinical characteristics of dementia with Lewy bodies and a consideration of prodromal diagnosis. *Alzheimer's Res Ther.* 2014;6(46).

55. O'Bryant SE, Humphreys JD, Smith GE, et al. Detecting dementia with the mini-mental state examination (MMSE) in highly educated individuals. *Arch Neurol.* 2008;65(7):963-967.

56. Doerflinger C. *Mental Status Assessment of Older Adults: The Mini-Cog*; 2018. Retrieved from https://consultgeri.org.

57. Dharmarajan K, Foster J, Coylewright M, et al. The medically managed patient with severe symptomatic aortic stenosis in the TAVR era: patient characteristics, reasons for medical management, and quality of shared decision making at heart valve treatment centers. *PLoS One.* 2017;12(4). doi:10.1371/journal.pone.0175926.

58. Wolcove N, Baltzan M. Amiodarone pulmonary toxicity. *Can Respir J.* 2009;16(2):43-48.

59. Yancy CW, Jessup M, Bozkurt B, et al. 2017 ACC/AHA/HFSA focused update of the 2013 ACCF/AHA guideline for the management of heart failure: a report of the American College of Cardiology/American Heart Association Task Force on Clinical Practice Guidelines and the Heart Failure Society of America. *J Am Coll Cardiol.* 2017;70:776-803.

CHAPTER 8

Decision Support and Education: Strategies for Patient-Centered Care

Roseanne Palmer, MSN, RN

OBJECTIVES

▶ Outline patient and family educational needs for treatment support and early discharge planning

▶ Review key components of shared decision making and its application for TAVR

▶ Discuss strategies to optimize patient-centered education and treatment support

Background

Transcatheter aortic valve replacement (TAVR) is now mainstream therapy for patients whose options may have previously been suboptimal or nonexistent. As clinicians, the foundational premise of patient education is that, when we give people knowledge, we also give them power. The more information provided to patients regarding their disease, its expected trajectory, possible treatment strategies, and associated risks, the better prepared they will be to advocate for themselves and make their own health care decisions.

However, as many more treatment options with ever increasing complexity become available, it is clear that simply providing information in a single, perhaps rushed, clinical encounter with one physician provider is insufficient to truly give patients the necessary power and permission to make health care decisions that align with their values and goals. Assuredly, the Heart Team, and particularly the valve program clinician (VPC), strives to take every opportunity available to provide education to our patients and families by clarifying confusing information, helping them understand what they read or just heard from their physician, walking them through periprocedural expectations, and providing the literature and websites.

Despite all this, the giving of information alone may not be enough for patients to understand that they do have the power to be an active participant in choosing the best course of action. Joseph-Williams et al[1] dispel the belief that patients do not wish to actively participate in decision making but rather cannot because of power inequities that still remain in today's patient-clinician relationships. Perhaps because of the patient's belief system, or perhaps because of the milieu fostered in health care, there may be an expectation that the provider will make one recommendation based on their expert medical knowledge and the patient will defer to that strategy. In essence, the only option or choice offered to the person is whether to opt in or out.

Fortunately, with current research as well as guidance from the Institute of Medicine and the Center Medicare Services, the trend has been to move away from a paternalistic model of care in which a single physician recommends a preferred and perhaps biased treatment option to a more patient-inclusive, team-based approach that uses shared decision making (SDM) for the care of people with aortic stenosis (AS). Alston, Brownlee, et al[2] describe SDM as a model whereby treatment decisions are guided by patient preferences in combination with clinical evidence through collaborative discussions between the patient and the provider. Clayman, Gulbrandsen, and Morris[3] take this concept further by suggesting a shift from patient-centered to person-centered decision making to incorporate who the individual is in the world, his/her experiences and values, and how he/she affects decisions rather than being a patient with its implied limitations. Clayman and colleagues propose that health care decisions should be made in the context of the person's lived experience rather than a more structured, cookbook approach that captures just one moment in time.

In navigating this new and evolving paradigm of care, the obvious emerging challenge is whether clinicians are prepared to communicate, educate, and practice in this unfamiliar domain. The technological advances in cardiovascular devices have given rise to the development of structural heart programs in institutions across the globe. Although the services offered by these programs and the configuration of multidisciplinary team members may differ across facilities and over time, the groundwork in how we approach communication, education, and decision making has been solidified by the learnings and leadership of the pioneers of the early TAVR teams. Among the TAVR teams, now frequently referred to as the Heart Team, VPCs have a pivotal and unique role and skill set. They are generally the first point of contact following the referral for evaluation and remain the patient's constant along their health care journey. As such, VPCs are perhaps best positioned to create the trusting relationship and environment necessary to elicit patient preferences and values that are essential elements for successful outcomes and decision making.

Shared Decision Making

Meaningful Conversations in a Complex Paradigm

Without intervention, AS has an unforgiving trajectory. Although the timing of the disease progression may be unpredictable, once symptomatic, the patient's life expectancy is grim. Current research projects a mortality rate of 50% at 1 to 2 years once symptoms of heart failure develop.[4]

As patients enter the health system, it may be the first time they are actually hearing these statistics and emotions may be raw as they come to terms with the health care decisions at hand, thus making it difficult to absorb the depth and level of detailed information they are about to receive. They come to our clinics with varying degrees of knowledge, anxiety, and understanding about AS and the disease progression. Some have misguided fear that any exertion beyond minimal activities of daily living will result in sudden cardiac death. Conversely, they may be unaware of how AS affects their functional status and what to expect next. Because the disease progression and its symptoms are generally insidious, patients often compensate over time so that they are unaware of the decline in their activity tolerance, or they may believe the symptoms to be a natural part of growing older rather than from a physiological condition. Likewise, their expectations about the management and treatment options for AS may be unfounded or unrealistic based on misinformation, out-of-date statistics, or historical surgical experiences from family and friends.

Added to this is the complex and evolving nature of treatment options for AS. There are treatment options that are commercially available and others that are available only as part of a research trial. The inclusion and exclusion criteria for either of these options are dynamically moving targets, which makes it difficult for referring providers to remain current so as to adequately inform their patients.

This emerging field may indeed prompt as many questions as the science provides answers. For example, where along the spectrum of options from asymptomatic, to low risk, to inoperable or prohibitive risk does this particular person fit, and how do these options best align with their values and goals? How do we explain and how do they choose when there is equipoise among options, risks, and benefits? Should they get treatment before they have recognizable symptomatology or wait until they feel debilitated? What happens when there is an incidental finding discovered during diagnostic evaluation or they do not fit into an expected set of criteria such as a young patient whose AS is a result of an irradiated heart secondary to cancer treatments years ago? Suppose the patient has comorbid conditions, interstitial lung disease, for example, that make symptom relief from aortic valve replacement less promising or less predictable. Perhaps the patient is at significant risk for renal failure; should he/she proceed with diagnostics and intervention? When should palliation be introduced, in the beginning as one of the viable options or later should something go awry? How is decision making confounded by patients who have cognitive decline or by families and support persons whose goals differ from those of the patient? Is there an arbitrary age bias for surgical aortic valve replacement versus TAVR versus palliative or medical management choices? What if patients believe in life-sustaining measures at all costs even when options are futile? How do you tease out whether their decision is a choice and not a default because they believe they have no alternatives? How do a nonagenarian's values and goals regarding treatment differ from that of a baby boomer? How do cultural, socioeconomic, and spiritual variances play into patient choice, and how do we alter the conversation to align with the patient's frame of reference?

Added to this list of complexities is the notion of provider bias. Are they providing information with sufficient depth and substance, or is the information inadvertently colored by their own lens as a surgeon or as an interventionalist or even as a researcher? Does the provider paint a picture that favors patient enrollment in a research arm? Is the interventionalist able to help a patient recognize when a less invasive option may not be in their best interest? Suppose the provider has an allegiance with an organization that performs only open-heart surgery or only has limited transcatheter options. In this scenario, would the provider be willing to risk losing case volume by referring the patient to an alternate facility in an attempt to optimize viable options and ethical decision making? And, if so, is the provider willing to explore, if given the choice, the patient's willingness to travel and whether or not he/she has the financial resources, physical capability, or necessary family support to do so? Is there a relationship between the numbers of referrals that go on to TAVR versus surgery that parallels fluctuating surgical volumes? How do we balance confusing and competing interests so that the patient is at the forefront of all clinical decision points? And, how do we accomplish this in a way that is respectful, timely, efficient, and embraced by all members of the Heart Team?

Certainly, the skill set for the level of communication required in today's structural heart world is neither inherent nor adequately addressed in medical school. As health care providers, we may consider ourselves to be exquisite communicators, thinking that we are indeed already engaging in rich dialogue with our patients' representative of SDM. The reality is that many of us actually have little insight into how inadequately and ineffectively we are approaching patient conversations despite the best of intentions. As leaders in SDM continue to peel back the communication layers and explore in real time how providers present information to patients, it is evident that training, guidance, and mentorship are needed to eliminate unintended roadblocks and pitfalls so that patients are not inadvertently left with unrealistic expectations, false hope, or misguided clinical decisions. We have a responsibility to ensure that our patients have the necessary meaningful information about their options to make informed decisions and that our clinicians have the crucial skills needed and that they are indeed supported in the use of SDM models of care.

As key members of the Heart Team, VPCs are in the ideal position to guide practice in this arena. They have the capacity to quickly evaluate the patient's baseline understanding as well as their concerns and to draw from them that which is most important in determining treatment options that best support individual values and goals of care.

Posing the Question

The manner in which patients are referred into the health care system varies as does the severity of their AS and intensity of their symptoms. For some, a new murmur may be identified during a routine examination, which prompts a referral from a primary care provider. Other patients may be encountered for the first time during a hospitalization for an acute event such as heart failure. No matter where on this spectrum the patient perches, it is essential that the first encounter leaves them with a sense of trust, a feeling of connection, and an understanding of what to expect next.

Whether the initial interaction is with a patient on the phone, in a clinic examination room, or in a hospital bed, the conversation must be meaningful for the patients and their support persons. As Matthias, Salyers, and Frankel[5] point out, clinicians should adopt 4 behaviors while interacting with patients. These behaviors include empathy, seeking the patient's perspective, and, most interestingly, investment in both the beginning and in the end. This profound thinking on a conscious act of investing in the patient from the start and committing all the way through to the end point may seem obvious for health care providers; however, it may, in fact, be an element of SDM that begs further attention. The dialogue on the first encounter should begin by asking patients what they understand about why they have been referred to the program and what their goal is in coming. Resonating throughout this work is the single question: "What is your goal?" This goal should be considered the guiding principle across the continuum of care.

Optimizing Patient-Centered Treatment Decisions

Although it is more than 10 years now that the Institute of Medicine's groundbreaking work, Crossing the Quality Chasm,[6] defined patient-centered care to be one of the key elements of quality care, true SDM remains rather illusive in today's practice. We continue to struggle with how to best communicate so that patient preferences and values guide all clinical decisions throughout all phases of care. Despite the overwhelming evidence that SDM and, to some degree, the use of decision aids (DAs) result in an increased knowledge and understanding of the risk to benefit ratio as well as a reduction in internal conflict, indecision, passivity, and undue burden on health care resources, these strategies are not yet widely used.

According to Oshima and Emanuel,[7] a Cochrane Collaborative review revealed that in one study only an abysmal 10% of the 1000 office visits reviewed met the expected standards for SDM. Of those patients, only 41% believed that their treatment plans aligned with their preference for palliation rather than aggressive treatments. Similarly, Pollard et al[8] note that most providers recognize the value that SDM holds in gleaning patient preferences especially when risks and benefits have ambiguous outcomes related to quality of life. Unfortunately, however, their literature review suggests that fewer than 40% of physicians globally use a process whereby provider and patient collaboratively decide treatment plans together. Rather, they adhere to a paternalistic model of decision making particularly when the physician feels there is a superior recommendation for one treatment over another. They believe this is perhaps influenced in part by provider specialty, urgency of treatment, and an ownership of the responsibility to ensure that the right decision is being made.

The Agency for Healthcare Research and Quality[9] also concurs. In their publication, Strategy 61: Shared Decision-Making, it is noted that physicians' affinity to recommend one particular treatment option may be less influenced by the scientific evidence than it is by their prior experience or where they happen to practice. We are certainly well aware of the phenomenon of making clinical decisions based on our last worst case. To elaborate, if a sound treatment decision, such as using an alternate access for valve delivery, for example, ultimately results in an untoward or devastating outcome, when faced with a similar clinical picture next time, a provider may be less likely to recommend the same treatment option to the patient, even though it may indeed be the superior choice based on research evidence and best practice.

If we are to fully consider our patient population knowing that they are generally at an advanced age with life-limiting disease, it is essential that providers among the TAVR team relinquish their stronghold. Tulsky et al[10] suggest that anything short of an SDM model can actually contribute to unwarranted suffering at end of life. The authors postulate that communication that fails to adequately elicit patient preferences actually results in an increased number of invasive therapies performed every year and ultimately has negative downstream outcomes and poor quality of life for the individual patients. Furthermore, Tulsky proposes that reliance on advanced directives is insufficient to satisfactorily assess patients and their support persons' understanding of the disease trajectory and the goals of care for the specific choices at hand.[10]

In further evaluating roadblocks to effective communication, Ubel, Scherr, and Fagerlin[11] highlight that it is extremely important for patients to feel that they are not alone in their decisions. They acknowledge that even when clinicians are making valiant attempts at unbiased dialogue, they may fail to recognize when patients are overwhelmed with excessively detailed or obfuscatory information or when they are emotionally unprepared to translate what they heard into meaningful decisions. In addition, attempts at transparency may actually unwittingly act as subtle influence over patient choice. Using cancer as an example, Ubel et al[11] note that the decision points from active surveillance to surgery have different positive and negative implications for the patient. In the spirit of true SDM, some surgeons will disclose their bias as a surgeon. Interestingly, that gesture of honesty and integrity actually solidified trust in their provider and the patients subsequently opted for surgery over alternate choices.

Lastly, fiscal imperatives as well as environmental distraction have the potential to impede the necessary rapport building between patients and their providers that is crucial for SDM. Consider the constraints placed on physicians in facilities that mandate that providers increase their relative value units by increasing the number of patients seen in an 8-hour clinic. Although the need to be more productive and efficient is certainly a reasonable expectation in today's health care environment, it may inadvertently create a gap in care that is ultimately costlier to the system. Providers rushing to get through their busy patient load may not be inclined to adequately present information in an SDM model.

In their review of patient-reported barriers, Joseph-Williams et al[1] specifically identify insufficient clinic time as notably affecting patients' perception of SDM. Even something seemingly inconsequential as a busy waiting room can influence the patient's comfort in taking up what they perceive as too much of their physicians' valuable time. As a result, patients may not feel comfortable posing questions or initiating dialogue.

Joseph-Williams and colleagues propose this as further evidence of the power inequities that remain in physician-patient relationships. They suggest that the introduction of DAs for the purpose of leveling the playing field with unbiased information may be a developing practice and caution that DAs used in isolation are not the sole solution in bridging gaps. Coylewright, Mack, Holmes, and O'Gara[12] agree that simply providing information does not compare with an unequivocal invitation to the patient to participate in decision making. They also note that SDM done in the context of the Heart Team model provides effective resource utilization and cost reduction through more expeditious clinical decisions for the patients with complex conditions. Expanding on this concept, as SDM is considered across the continuum of care, the ability to bring the patient's preferences and goal to the discussion table during team meetings as well as incorporating the SDM techniques within the group can only result in patient-centered recommendations for treatment strategies and hopefully sidestep some of the roadblocks previously described.

As the team members deliberate over complex or controversial case presentations, it is important to also invite each member to bring his/her worldview, expertise, and concerns to the discussion for consideration. As with the patient encounter, the team meetings should embrace the sharing of knowledge, which includes, of course, the clinical picture as well as patient preferences, the sharing of provider preferences, and discussion leading to decision.

Influencing Clinical Practice

Irrespective of the evidence favoring SDM, the question that remains is this: How are nurse clinicians and providers best supported in adopting this model of care and gaining the skills necessary for successful implementation? Although there is a great deal of literature available on the numerous barriers to the application of SDM as it is intended in practice, there is an obvious gap in providing guidance in how to best incorporate this philosophy into every clinical encounter. Realizing benefit from small practice changes over time that allow for conversations more conducive to collaborative models of care may indeed be the answer. Perhaps the simplicity of a single question, "What is your goal?" is where practice change can and should begin.

When presented with the question, "When thinking about the problem with your heart valve, what is your goal?" or alternately, "In thinking about your aortic valve, what do you hope to accomplish?" patients are provided the opportunity and are singularly able to easily and quickly articulate their hopes, values, preferences, and fears. They are consistently clear about what they desire and are able to formulate their answer without a single moment of hesitation. It is rare, if ever, that a patient is unable to provide an immediate and precise answer.[13]

The details of their responses are described later; however, it is important to highlight that this one question can actually help to focus the conversation on what is most important and make the clinical encounter more effective and efficient. This question, or some variant of it, helps to frame the patient's point of reference and provides the clinician with the opportunity to expand on knowledge, allay fears, dispel misconceptions, and set the groundwork for sound clinical choices that include the deliberation of medical expertise and patient preference.

Once identified, the patient's goal statement can be embedded into the medical record and into the team discussions, thus providing transparency and consistency throughout their course of care. Referring to the goal statement as the guiding principle is essential in navigating decisions when unexpected findings emerge, when changes in course occur, or when the patient or their family is at a crossroads for decisions. It is equally important to invite the patient to clarify that the goal or goals continue to be consistent with their wishes as they proceed through this journey.

Surprisingly, there is little variability in the categories that patients have globally identified as most important goals of therapy. In exploring the themes of what patients have identified as goals that align with their preferences and values, it is evident that quality of life is most valued. Although some certainly give voice to not feeling ready to die and prefer life-extending choices, most express a desire to maintain or improve their current level of independence. For others, valve therapy is a means to accomplish another more urgent goal, such as being able to proceed with surgery for tumor debulking.

Commonly, patients describe concern that their symptoms have already or will soon impinge on their ability to continue to live independently, maintain their own home, or to be able to perform their usual activities of daily living. They are fearful of becoming a burden to family and support persons. For most patients, the relief of symptoms as a means to improve their quality of life is paramount. They verbalize feeling as though they no longer have energy to accomplish simple chores or participate in the activities that bring them joy. They describe wanting to be able to continue to work, resume volunteer activities, spend quality time with family, dance just one more dance. For some, their functional decline is rapid, and for others it is insidious or perhaps it is inevitable in the foreseeable future.

In weighing all the risks of proceeding with TAVR, even when those risks are significant, most patients are clear that they prefer taking the risk over facing living at the current level of function or worse. Equally as important is that the process of stating their goal helps them to illuminate what quality of life means from their own perspective, which for a small number of patients may ultimately move them toward choosing medical management and palliation. For some patients, this is the first time they have ever been asked to explore their goal of therapy and this activity helps to solidify and make known their intention. When the family is present, the goal statement serves to provide clarity when the patient's choice differs from that of loved ones. In this way, the family has the opportunity to align their thinking with the patient's preferences and values so that the entire team, patient, family, and providers can approach decision making with a common goal and the with same end game in view. By seeking to understand what matters most to the patient as they make decisions about their disease trajectory, we are reminded that, from the very first encounter, this journey belongs to the patient and all subsequent choices for treatment must be guided by their values and goals.

Shared Decision Making in Practice

Patient 1

Patient 1 is a gentleman in well into his 90s. He is widowed and lives independently in the home where he and his wife raised their family. Until recently, he cut his own wood to heat his home, maintained his property, including mowing in the summer and shoveling in the winter, and participated in social activities in town. He has a supportive family; however, they live almost 200 miles away. In months before his referral to the TAVR team he has had significant decline in activity tolerance because of critical AS. He has had multiple admissions for heart failure, and each time there is documentation that the patient is agitated and cries out with the same phrase, "Please just let me go."

Despite his repetitive cries, he has also verbalized to his primary care providers that he wants to be considered for life-extending therapy. Some documentation would suggest he had moments of intermittent cognitive decline, although his family did not support this thinking. The family felt at odds with how to proceed, given what he was verbalizing and yet feeling that he still had life in him. Likewise, there was disparity among the TAVR team, with some members suggesting palliation to be the only option and others recommending moving forward with transcatheter therapy.

When meeting patient 1 for the first time during an acute heart failure admission, the question is posed to him by the VPC as follows: "Sir, I see that you have been asking the nursing staff to let you go. Can you please help me understand what you mean by that and also what your goal is in thinking about your heart disease today?" Without hesitation and with solid eye contact he said, "If I have to live my life like this, where I can't do things for myself, then I want God to take me, but if you tell me you have something to offer that could possibly give me back my energy so I can stay in my own house and not be a burden to my kids, then I want a shot at trying it."

For the family and the provider team alike, this one question instantly and completely changed the course of action for this person. Without exploring this patient's goal and understanding what was most important to him, the discussions with him would have defaulted to a paternalistic recommendation for medical management and palliative care rather than giving him the option of moving forward with transcatheter intervention. As he wished, he was able to return to independent living following his TAVR and had no further readmissions. Sadly, he eventually sustained a mortal injury while doing his chores, but his family relayed his gratitude in having his wishes honored. They said that he was happy and passed while doing the things he most enjoyed in life.

Patient 2

Patient 2 is an 80-year-old gentleman with valvular heart disease and newly diagnosed heart failure with an ejection fraction of 35%. He has no other comorbidities. Notable is his body mass index of 17 kg/m^2 (54 kg and 175 cm); he appears emaciated, frail, and withdrawn. He presents to clinic with a 50-lb weight loss over the prior 8 weeks, which is thought to be secondary to his critical AS. He ascribes to living an active life until the previous few months at which time he developed what he reports as a sudden decline in activity tolerance and exertional dyspnea. He was so fatigued that the simple act of preparing breakfast of toast and coffee would necessitate him having to rest before he could actually consume it, and it would generally take over an hour to eat. When asked about his goal of care, he became animated. He replied that he wanted his energy back; he wanted to dance just a few more dances. He went on to describe that in his retirement, he discovered that he loved to dance. He spoke of how sad it made him knowing he just could not finish a single dance any longer. He felt his quality of life had significantly declined as a result. The ensuing dialogue included the concern that he was thought to be at high risk for surgery given his age, significant frailty, and malnutrition, and therefore, a DA was used that focused on medical management versus TAVR.

When presented with the 1-year mortality data for medical management, the patient said immediately, "Toss that out. I don't want that option. What else do you have to offer?" Following dialogue in which the specific choices available to the patient were called out and then considered in relation to the patient's values and stated goal, it was decided that the patient's preference was to proceed with TAVR and he subsequently went on to dance more dances.

Patient 3

Patient 3 is a retired business executive who now volunteers in the community and manages a nonprofit organization. She enjoys hiking, swimming, and exercising at the gym 3 to 4 times a week. She is well known to her primary care provider who has been following her AS with serial echocardiograms for the past several years. Her medical history also included hypertension and newly diagnosed Parkinson's disease. She presented recently with new dyspnea on exertion, profound fatigue, and lower extremity edema. Echocardiography confirmed progression from moderate to severe AS.

From the first telephone introductions and throughout her evaluations, she was noted to be well informed about AS. Her questions were well thought out, systematic, and intelligent, and she expressed a clear desire to proceed with diagnostics and evaluation. At her first clinic visit, she was accompanied by her daughter, who had also done considerable research on the disease and treatment options. Together, with the provider, they began to engage in conversation around the choice between surgical and transcatheter intervention. However, when asked about her goal of therapy, she became quiet and introspective. Her daughter began to fill the space of silence but the patient stopped her. She responded by reflecting that she had not thought about this previously and realized that what was important to her was to be as functional and as comfortable as possible in the time she has left. She most feared a long and steady decline from Parkinson disease. She voiced that she did not want to fix her heart valve only to then go on to suffer a long and debilitating functional decline from her neurological disorder. She had substantial research on both disease entities and said she would rather die sooner from heart failure than suffer over many years with loss of function.

Although she came to clinic fully expecting to proceed with intervention, the inquiry about her goal of therapy surprisingly captured feelings and concerns that she had not previously been able to process. Palliative care was quickly brought into the discussion to further explore her understanding of both diseases as well as her hopes and expectations and also to work with her daughter who was having difficulty accepting her mother's thinking. It was made clear to the patient that her decisions would be fully supported by the team and that we would explore a change of course if at any time her situation or preferences changed. She was followed over time and remained steadfast in her resolution for medical management.

Patient 4

Patient 4 was thought to be at prohibitive risk for surgery. The concern was two fold. Her valvular heart disease included a mitral and tricuspid component, and she also had lung disease requiring home oxygen. Her oxygen demand shifted from nocturnal and intermittent use to a continuous requirement. In light of this, her provider was not convinced that TAVR would result in anything more than marginal symptom relief insufficient to justify the risk of further diagnostic testing or TAVR procedure. On examination, she was notably short of breath at rest. Her pulmonologist was included in the discussion, and it was deemed in her best interest to proceed with a palliative balloon valvuloplasty (BAV). The hope was to perhaps provide some small, albeit temporary, symptom relief and to also act as proof of concept to better define how symptomatic she might continue to be post valve intervention. In this case, it was thought that the BAV would support the decision to medically manage symptoms rather than move on to TAVR.

Surprisingly, on her post-BAV follow-up visit, she had improved remarkably. Her demeanor was bright and cheerful, and she walked in without using oxygen. She had her portable tank with her "just in case" but did not need to turn it on. She reported that she was back to her baseline of using oxygen only at night, performing all her own activities of daily living and getting out to socialize. She was hopeful and wanted to discuss moving forward with TAVR; however, her provider remained cautiously reluctant. Her goal of therapy was to proceed with a more permanent solution before her symptoms returned. They agreed to a brief period of watchful waiting but within a few months she began to notice subtle recurrence of symptoms. On her return visit she restated her original goal. A detailed discussion ensued about the general risks of procedure and the risks that were specific to her. A transfemoral approach was not an option owing to small, tortuous, calcific vessels so she would require general anesthesia. The concern for her ability to wean from ventilatory support was paramount. In addition, she had high potential for compromised kidney function.

At this point, the provider's communication was heavily weighted in favor of medical management; however, when the VPC asked the question about goals, the conversation focused on and shifted toward intervention. She asked the patient to consider what her goals of therapy are in the face of such significant risks. The patient stated that she did not want to go back to feeling like she did before she had the BAV. She was unwavering in her belief that risking it all was superior to slipping back to the poor quality of life she experienced before BAV. Taking her lead and investing in the end game as previously described, the surgeon on the team walked her through the possible various scenarios from extremely optimistic to the catastrophic. He trusted the process to take the conversation through to the very end so that patient could fully understand what she might be facing and was better able to articulate how each possible outcome should look for her. At the end of the conversation, her preferences were clear for every stop point and they were communicated to the team. She was willing to consider time-limited ventilatory support as long as there was evidence of progress and would entertain a short rehabilitation stay if needed. She would not want to go to the operating room nor would she agree to dialysis. Her preference would be palliative care in the setting of renal failure.

Post procedure she experienced two episodes of respiratory compromise requiring intubation. Her goals were revisited with her and her family. She declined further reintubation, choosing comfort measures instead. With her last decision she took her interventionalist's hand and told him she was happy with her decisions. She wanted him to understand that she went into the TAVR procedure with her eyes wide open and that they both "gave it a good run." In the days that followed, her family also shared that they were at peace knowing that she made her choice fully aware of the possible outcomes. They said she made this choice the same way she lived her life: she was always all-in.

The patient stories are used as a means to illustrate of how easily SDM can be incorporated into every day practice no matter the setting. Every aspect of care and stop point along the way should be considered an opportunity to use the SDM model. Consider the way in which we schedule the patient's evaluation as an example. Do we simply provide them with a date and a predetermined schedule of events wherein the patient arrives at a certain time, moves through various diagnostic and frailty testing and meets with providers? If so, is there an opportunity to understand if their preference is to complete the testing in 1 day versus splitting the evaluation into multiple, perhaps more manageable, visits for them?

Without question, opportunities for SDM present themselves regularly along the patient's course of care when we are open to the concept. These case scenarios used minor variations of the same question to initiate important conversation and suggest how effortless it is to engage even the most reluctant providers. The tool used is less important than the commitment to true SDM. Its value is worthy of reiteration. Through hundreds of similar conversations with patients of varying degree of intellectual capacity, physical stamina, age, disease progression, support systems, and a multitude of other variables, it is evident that when communication roadblocks are avoided and providers are on a path that marches along with the patient toward their stated goal, and when the goals are revisited at every juncture, there is more overall satisfaction and less disparity. To walk away as an active participant is far more desirable to patients than feeling as though they were just sold a product. A successful outcome is when patients feel that their voices are heard and their decisions were supported and honored throughout the course of their care.

Patient-Stated Goal as a Quality Indicator

In an age of outcomes data and reporting transparency, it is reasonable to consider the use of the patients' stated goal as a quality indicator. It may no longer be sufficient to look at quality outcomes in terms of 30-day and 1-year mortality rates alone. Perhaps as this science progresses, it makes sense to also examine how frequently we are meeting the patients' goals of therapy or how often we are falling short and why. Was the patient able to resume the thing that was important to them, did their end of life have dignity and quality in the way they defined good life, did they dance the last dance?

Patient and Family Education Needs

Patient and Family Education Needs for Treatment Support and Early Discharge Planning

For the VPC on the Heart Team, the underpinning of practice is exemplary communication, patient and family education, and advocacy. As the first interactions with patients are the gateway to setting the stage for their postprocedure expectations, the practice of quickly building rapport is essential. Just as with SDM for clinical decisions, taking the time and asking poignant questions to best understand the specific educational needs of the patient and their support persons will focus all future conversations into meaningful dialogue. The challenges faced by this subset of patients often compound their ability to process the amount and level of detailed information they will receive over the course of their treatment plan for AS.

Owing to the typical age of this patient population, they may be facing physical concerns that weigh heavily on them. To elaborate, they may be hearing impaired, making phone contact near impossible. They may be experiencing debilitating symptoms. Fatigue or dyspnea from their AS or chronic pain from osteoarthritis, for example, may make the thought of traveling long distances and lengthy clinic visits seem insurmountable. Likewise, worries about incontinence or the need to medicate with insulin or analgesics may be a burdensome concern as they think about how they can possibly get though their evaluation.

Socioeconomic constraints may also be at the forefront of patients' thoughts. Social isolation may be a factor in their ability to find transportation if they no longer drive. It may also affect their ability to have the necessary support to help them understand information or navigate through the complicated health system. Or they may have a chronically ill partner who needs care and supervision while they are away from home. Some may be still working and need to juggle work responsibilities, or they may be of an age that they have minor children at home who need them. For those who continue to live an active, social, and civically responsible lifestyles, they may be preoccupied with the things that need to be accomplished on their busy calendars or are looking toward a future endeavor for which they have no tolerance for being held back by AS.

In making that first contact with the patient, the ability to tease out their baseline knowledge and most pressing concerns is the cornerstone of communication. With that in mind, clinicians need to keep the goalpost in view, seek to understand what the patient needs most, and how we can best get our patients as close as possible to their stated goal.

Globally, TAVR programs will differ in their structure, available resources, and approaches to how patients are processed through the system, as will the programs' educational paradigms. There will obviously be variances in methodology and preferred tools; however, the basis for treatment support focuses attention on knowledge of AS, its trajectory, treatment options, and associated risks, as well as expectations around preprocedural evaluation, periprocedural processes, and posttreatment reentry. Certainly, attention also needs to be given to real-time and "just-in-time" information that may arise specific to the individual.

Implications for Nursing Practice

Initiating Dialogue

We now understand that people can be overwhelmed by the impact of what they are facing and the vast amount of information that follows. The most important educational element you can initially provide, therefore, is the name and contact information for the nurse clinician whom they can trust to support them throughout the continuum of care.

Second, initiating dialogue that invites patients to describe what they know about their referral to the TAVR program and what they understand about AS will efficiently lay the groundwork for educational needs specifically targeted for the individual. In revisiting the work of Ubel, Scherr, and Fagerlin,[11] the relevance to allowing the patient to frame the conversation on all levels throughout the continuum of care is apparent. They caution that the use of rote scripts describing, for example, disease and risks and benefits of each therapy may impinge on effective communication because some of the elements may not be of any value or concern to that particular patient.

As an example, patients may not have a clear understanding of why they have been referred for evaluation so that diving into a description of what to expect on an initial visit may not be the best place to start, whereas someone with more clarity about the consultation may have different needs at the onset. To further elaborate, consider the patient who understands that the decisions ahead of him/her have significant mortality and morbidity implications. It may likely be the first time the patient has had to think about the uncertainty of the choices that exist between quality versus quantity of life. The patient may be unconcerned about the specifics of the clinic visit and would rather learn about procedural timelines and specific data about the program's outcomes.

The fallout from missteps has the potential to unnecessarily complicate or shut down communication, and ultimately education altogether. Open-ended questions and comfort using them to help to ascertain the patient and family educational needs may be the most valuable thing in the clinician's toolkit. Questions such as "Tell me what you understand about this referral," "Help me to understand what is most important to you," or "Help me understand what would be most important for you to know about your visit with us" can often capture the essence of the patient's initial educational needs. Ask the open-ended question, state the obvious, and reiterate the invitation for further communication. Once the most compelling and pressing needs are uncovered and addressed, patients or their support person will need the pertinent details of what to expect depending again on their frame of reference and familiarity with the organization: the date and time of the visit if available, where to park, how to navigate the building, who and what they should bring with them, how long they can anticipate being in the building, who they will meet with, whether or not they will need a driver following any of the anticipated diagnostics, provisions for overnight stays such as local hotels or hostels if needed, how long before they can expect a call with dates, and what are the anticipated next steps in the process.

Concluding the first introductory meeting with contact information and the assurance that they or their support persons may call at any time with further questions or concerns opens the door to the opportunity to provide more robust education as they progress through the process. If relevant, they should be made aware that the phone lines are nonemergent business hours lines so that they are not awaiting call back for urgent issues requiring rapid response. It is also an opportune time to recommend that they seek medical care should their symptoms progress while waiting for upcoming evaluations. It is not uncommon in this population that patients begin to experience worsening symptoms but do not contact their provider because they feel they will be evaluated in the near future and they unfortunately continue to clinically decline while waiting.

Navigating Expectations and Educational Goals

Health systems have a longstanding history of attempting to set discharge plans early in the course of care. Not surprisingly, the earlier patients are educated about what to expect at the end of their course the better prepared and aligned they will be to be able to accomplish what is expected. To date, many facilities have developed solid educational tools based on best practice that provide patients with detailed information to guide them through procedure and home care. The information can be altered to capture individual organizational preferences and also as practice guidelines change. The general intent of these educational tools is to outline details of what to expect the morning of TAVR procedure and during the hospital stay, postprocedural activity and activity restrictions, how to assess incision sites, when to contact a provider, follow-up care, medication changes, anticoagulation plan, pain management, and dental follow-up.

Just as with DAs, the education tools and pamphlets are best used as part of an active discussion with patients and their support persons. The utilization of heart models and computer simulations are typically appreciated by patients as they attempt to better understand the disease process and TAVR procedure. It is impressive to see their understanding of the workload of the heart shift when they can actually put their finger through a model of a normal versus stenotic valve. There are also ample Web-based programs that provide up-to-date information designed specifically for patient education. In addition to the aforementioned materials, there are key elements of patient education worthy of highlighting. These include providing information in the form of dialogue that includes managing patient and family expectations and preparing them to verbalize their concerns and preference.

By nature of the valve clinic design, the VPC is center stage in understanding the patients' expectations and assisting them when necessary to reset realistic expectations. The first visit is a favorable opportunity to explore aspects of patient's home situation. Early education may evolve around investigating available resources and the capacity to return to their current level of living assuming the plan is to proceed with intervention. Commonly, patients and their families believe that, following TAVR, patients will require inpatient rehabilitation stay or at the very least visiting nurses to come into the home. They are generally surprised to learn they will return to their own living situation, typically without additional services, unless there is an unforeseeable complication. Their misconception can be based on the lack of knowledge of what to expect, what they have been told, or experiences with older models of care maps related to open-heart surgery.

Nonetheless, when their beliefs are such that going home following the procedure is unexpected, it may require a shift in the approach to education that includes exploring their worries about discharge. In many cases, they simply do not want to burden their children or family by asking that someone accompany them for the first few days at home. For patients living alone, planting the seed early provides them with the opportunity to consider options and make appropriate arrangements. Discussing this element up front also allows the providers to maintain consistent messaging about discharge planning over time.

On the reverse, some patients believe they will be able to immediately engage in activities such as driving, resuming work, weight lifting, and extended travel. It is equally important to understand their frame of reference and provide education that honors their concerns while setting realistic parameters that they can align with. To highlight this with an example, imagine the patient in clinic has signs of NYHA class III heart failure and has reported a significant recent decline in activity tolerance due to dyspnea. He is anxious to talk about the next steps in the evaluation and set a date for procedure in hopes that he can air travel and attend his grandchild's graduation from medical school. The timeline for travel would be approximately 1 week following the anticipated procedure.

In this case, providing education that centers on what matters most to the patient will serve to guide the treatment strategy in terms of procedural timing. When patients fully understand the predicted postprocedural recovery and its restrictions, the possibility of complications, and the implications of postponing their procedure or missing a grandchild's graduation, they are best able to weigh options in how to proceed in a manner that is consistent with their values and preferences.

Situations in which patient expectations are not clarified or validated have the potential for negative downstream results. Consider, for example, the immediate postrecovery phase. Patients whose preprocedure education failed to include information about how they might expect to feel clinically during the days following procedure may become anxious, alarmed, bewildered, defeated, or depressed about not progressing as quickly as they had imagined they would. Their concern may conceivably result in unwarranted clinic visits, phone calls, and undue stress to the patients and care providers. If instead, they understood that, although some people feel remarkably better immediately, others progress slowly over time taking days or even weeks to experience clinical improvement, then they are psychologically better prepared to allow themselves to take the necessary time to recover.

Another equally important educational element to emphasize with patients is the concept that they are in the driver's seat for the entire course of their care. When we consider the number of stop and start points along the patient's course from decision to disposition, it is imperative that the patients understand that they can stop the plan, change the course, or pause for clarity at any time. The significance of this is multifactorial. To begin, patients need to know that they can opt out at any time. It should be unequivocally clear that their decisions will be supported and they should not be fearful that they will be left without a plan for an alternate strategy. There are situations in which no matter the time invested and the level of education and understanding, the patient decides against moving forward with TAVR. Without explicitly providing them with the knowledge that they can and should be comfortable voicing their change of heart, the results could be tragic. When patients remain silent in their choice, when they are fearful of appearing to question a provider's judgment or insulting them or thinking they have wasted the clinician's time, they may proceed reluctantly into a treatment strategy that least suits their desired goal and could lead them to less than optimal outcomes. Imagine the patients whose instincts are telling them to get off the symbolic bus but they do not feel empowered to put voice to their concerns. Instead, they proceed on to TAVR and subsequently have an unexpected, untoward outcome that affects their quality of life.

Consider the patient who decided against invasive procedure and opted instead for medical management. Suppose after a period of time, AS progressed to the point that symptoms were becoming burdensome and debilitating and the management extremely challenging but the patient had not been given unequivocal permission to reach out for reevaluation of the decision. Perhaps because the patient had not received information to indicate that his/her decisions were not irrevocable, the patient never feels comfortable coming back into the system or may eventually do so in the setting of an acute heart failure admission at which time markedly reduced ventricular function precludes anything but palliation.

There are a number of other situations and decision points along the course of care that have similar implications. Take, for example, the patient who made the decision to proceed with TAVR knowing fully well that the patient's lung disease could possibly be a limiting factor in his/her recovery. The patient's decision for ongoing life-sustaining treatments, including intubation, was made based on the patient's worldview at the time; it was made post BAV when the patient experienced significant improvement in symptomatology. The patient was euphoric and hopeful at that time. However, during the days following TAVR when the outcome looked less promising, the patient's preference was no longer aimed at life-extending interventions but turned instead to comfort measures. Certainly, the patient's clinical picture would not likely have changed significantly; however, without the initial education that ultimately empowered the patient to articulate his/her shifting goals of therapy, undoubtedly the patient's final days would not have aligned with his/her wishes and values.

There are endless examples of how this phenomenon plays out in practice, particularly when there is equipoise, and we must remain vigilant in seeking the cues that will help us understand the individuals' intent.

Conclusions

Over time, AS will dramatically alter an individual's quality of life. The ability to perform the usual activities of daily living, the activities that bring joy, and one's social network are typically affected in a negative way. For most people, even at advanced ages, the ongoing decline in their quality of life is an unacceptable option so that even when faced with substantial risk, they often will choose a chance at a better quality over a steady deterioration. The choices they face are difficult given their stage in life and the complexities of therapies available today.

As VPCs, we are likely the person on the team who will spend the greatest amount of time with the individuals and their support persons and build the trusting relationship necessary for them to navigate through their health care journey. It is imperative that our education focuses on setting the stage so that patients are fully informed, armed with the information they need to navigate through the process, and clearly understand that there is no right or wrong decision. The only decision is the one that has significance for them at that moment in time, speaks to their quality of life, and is grounded in their preferences and goals.

KEY TAKEAWAYS AND BEST PRACTICES

▶ Seek to understand what matters most to patients as they make their health care decisions. Ask the open ended, state the obvious, invite further dialogue.

▶ Engage every conversation with intention so that patients and families have full disclosure of all viable options.

▶ Ensure that patients fully understand the trajectory with and without treatment, and determine how their values align with proposed options.

▶ Take conversations with patients all the way to the very end points. They need to know what they may be facing, and we need to know how they want that to look.

▶ Develop communication systems that identify and respect patient preferences along the continuum of care.

References

1. Joseph-Williams N, Elwyn G, Edwards A. Knowledge is not power for patients: a systematic review and thematic synthesis of patient-reported barriers and facilitators to shared decision-making. *Patient Educ Couns.* 2014;94(3):291-309. doi:10.1016/j.pec.2013.10.031. http://www.sciencedirect.com/science/article/pii/S0738399113004722. Accessed 5 November 2017.

2. Alston C, Berger Z, Brownlee S, et al. *Shared Decision-Making Strategies for Best Care.* National Academy of Sciences; 2014. https://nam.edu/wpcontent/uploads/2015/06/SDMforBestCare2.pdf. Accessed 21 December 2017.

3. Clayman M, Gulbrandsen P, Morris M. A patient in the clinic; a person in the world. Why shared decision making needs to center on the person rather than the medical encounter. *Patient Educ Couns.* 2017;100(3):600-604. doi:10.1016/j.pec.2016.10.016. https://www.ncbi.nlm.nih.gov/pubmed/27780646. Accessed 30 October 2017.

4. Gaasch WH. *Natural History, Epidemiology, and Prognosis of Aortic Stenosis.* 2017. https://www.uptodate.com/contents/natural-history-epidemiology-and-prognosis-of-aortic-stenosis. Accessed 27 November 2017.

5. Matthias MS, Salyers MP, Frankel RM. Re-thinking shared decision-making: Context matters. *Patient Educ Couns.* 2013;91(2):176-179. Available at http://www.sciencedirect.com/science/article/pii/S0738399113000347. Accessed 5 November 2017.

6. Committee on Quality Health Care in America, Institute of Medicine. *Crossing the Quality Chasm: A New Health System for the 21st Century.* Washington, DC: National Academy Press; 2001. Obtained 2 December 2017 at https://www.ncbi.nlm.nih.gov/books/NBK22857/.

7. Oshima E, Emanuel EJ. Shared decision making to improve care and reduce costs. *N Engl J Med.* 2013;368:6-8. Obtained online 5 November 2017. http://www.nejm.org/doi/full/10.1056/NEJMp1209500.

8. Pollard S, Bansback N, Bryan S. Physician attitudes toward shared decision making: a systematic review. *Patient Educ Couns.* 2015;98(9):1046-1057. Available at http://www.sciencedirect.com/science/article/pii/S0738399115002256. Accessed 5 November 2017.

9. *Strategy 6I: Shared Decision-Making.* Content last reviewed October 2017. Rockville, MD:Agency for Healthcare Research and Quality. Available at www.ahrq.gov/cahps/quality-improvement/improvement-guide/6-strategies-improving/communication/strategy6i-shared-decisionmaking.html. Accessed 10 November 2017.

10. Tulsky JA, Beach MC, Butow PN, et al. A research agenda for communication between health care professionals and patients living with serious illness. *JAMA Intern Med.* 2017;177(9):1361-1366. doi:10.1001/jamainternmed.2017.2015.
11. Ubel PA, Scherr KA, Fagerlin A. Empowerment failure: how shortcomings in physician communication unwittingly undermine patient autonomy. *Am J Bioeth.* 2017;17(11). Available at http://www.bioethics.net/articles/empowerment-failure-how-shortcomings-in-physician-communication-unwittingly-undermine-patient-autonomy/. Accessed 12 November 2017.
12. Coylewright M., Mack MJ, Holmes DR, O'Gara PT. A call for an evidence-based approach to the heart team for patients with severe aortic stenosis. *J Am Coll Cardiol.* 2015;65(14):1472-1480. Available at https://www.sciencedirect.com/science/article/pii/S0735109715006701?via%3Dihub. Accessed 5 November 2017.
13. Coylewright M, Palmer R, O'Neil E, et al. Patient-define goals for the treatment of severe aortic stenosis: a qualitative analysis. *Health Expect.* 2016;19(5):1036-1043.

CHAPTER 9

The Right Care in the Right Place: A United States Perspective on Procedure Planning

Janet Fredal Wyman, DNP, RN-CS, ACNS-BC

OBJECTIVES

▶ Discuss infrastructure requirements
▶ Present models of periprocedure staffing
▶ Discuss periprocedure approaches
▶ Highlight the importance of emergency intervention planning

Background

The first transcatheter aortic valve replacement (TAVR) was performed in France by Alain Cribier in 2002.[1] In the ensuing years, TAVR technology and the required supplies, resources, team, location, and infrastructure have evolved. Procedural care standards based on operator, institutional, local, regional, and national practice patterns, as well as regulatory requirements, are defined by the multidisciplinary team (MDT) and applied to the unique needs of each patient. The MDT determines before the procedure the appropriate equipment and specific procedural plan based on the patient's anatomy, physiology, and comorbidities. Each institution establishes site-specific standards and processes to ensure quality and consistency. In this chapter, the TAVR procedure has been described from the perspective of a high-volume, urban program in the United States.

Procedural Infrastructure

Procedure Room

The procedural setting for TAVR may be an operating room (OR), a hybrid OR, a hybrid cardiac catheterization laboratory (CCL), or a traditional CCL. In 2016, the Society of Thoracic Surgeons (STS)/American College of Cardiology (ACC) Transcatheter Valve Therapies (TVT) Registry found that in the United States, the vast majority of TAVRs were performed in a hybrid room located in either the OR suite (>60%) or CCL suites (>27%) and less than 13% of TAVR procedures were performed in a traditional CCL procedure room.[2] In 2017, Aufrett and colleagues reported the transcatheter aortic valve implant (TAVI) experience from the FRANCE 2 and FRANCE TAVI (2015) registry.[3] In 2015, the number of TAVRs performed in the traditional CCL had decreased from 72.2% to 54.8%. Hybrid room use increased from 15.8% to 35.7% in 2015. Procedures performed in the OR decreased from 11.0% to 4.9%. Taken together, the US and French TAVR registries describe practice through 2015 and 2016 that trend toward hybrid procedure rooms and away from standard (nonhybrid) OR or CCL rooms. Regardless of the procedural setting, international societal recommendations state the space must meet OR standards for sterility, air circulation, heating, and cooling.[4,5]

A critical cornerstone of the TAVR procedure is collaboration between interventional cardiology and cardiac surgery. Data regarding requirements for quality are emerging, allowing multiple professional societies to join together and define the criteria for performing these procedures. Societal recommendations[4,5] for hospitals were incorporated into the Center for Medicare and Medicaid Services (CMS) National Coverage Determination (NCD)[6] for TAVR and are summarized in Table 9.1.

In the United States on May 1, 2012, CMS issued the NCD for TAVR, which identified diagnosis and institutional and operator requirements for TAVR reimbursement.[6] First, TAVR is covered for the treatment of symptomatic aortic valve stenosis when provided according to a Food and Drug Administration–approved indication. Second, the procedure must be performed with a valve and delivery system that has received approval by the Food and Drug Administration and is used for its approved indication. Third, 2 cardiac surgeons have examined the patient face to face and evaluated the patient's suitability for open aortic valve replacement surgery and the rationale for their decision must be available to the Heart Team. Finally, the patient must continuously be under the care of an MDT of medical professionals (preprocedurally, intraprocedurally, and postprocedurally), or Heart Team, which may facilitate patient-centered care through the collaboration of medical specialties. The NCD specifies that Heart Team collaboration and decision making must be available for team members to review.

In addition to supporting the multisociety recommendations for procedure rooms, CMS defined institutional and operator requirements for TAVR procedures. The infrastructure recommendations included but were not limited to:

- On-site heart valve surgery program;
- Cardiac catheterization laboratory or hybrid OR/catheterization laboratory equipped with a fixed radiographic imaging system with flat-panel fluoroscopy, offering quality imaging;
- Noninvasive imaging, such as echocardiography, vascular ultrasound imaging, computed tomography (CT), and magnetic resonance imaging (MRI);
- Sufficient space, in a sterile environment, to accommodate the necessary equipment for cases with and without complications; and
- Postprocedural intensive care facility with personnel experienced in managing patients who have undergone open-heart valve procedures.[6]

TABLE 9.1. Qualification for TAVR Heart Teams and Hospital Programs[4]

Qualification	To Begin a TAVR Program for Heart Teams *Without* TAVR Experience	For Hospital Programs *With* TAVR Experience Must Maintain
Hospital criteria	• ≥50 total AVRs in the previous year before TAVR, including 10 high-risk patients, and • ≥2 physicians with cardiac surgery privileges, and • ≥1000 catheterizations per year, including 400 percutaneous coronary interventions (PCIs) per year	• ≥20 AVRs per year or ≥40 AVRs every 2 y; and • ≥2 physicians with cardiac surgery privileges; and • ≥1000 catheterizations per year, including ≥400 PCIs per year
Heart Team Criteria:		
a. Cardiovascular surgeon with	• ≥100 career AVRs, including 10 high-risk patients; or • ≥25 AVRs in 1 y; or • ≥50 AVRs in 2 y; and which include at least 20 AVRs in the last year before TAVR initiation	Cardiovascular surgeon and interventional cardiologist whose combined experience maintains the following: ≥ 20 TAVR procedures in the prior year, or
b. Interventional cardiologist with	• Professional experience with • 100 structural heart disease procedures lifetime; or • 30 left-sided structural procedures per year of which 60% should be balloon aortic valvuloplasty	≥ 40 TAVR procedures in the prior 2 y
c. Additional members of the Heart Team	Echocardiographers, imaging specialists, heart failure specialists, cardiac anesthesiologists, intensivists, nurses, and social workers	Echocardiographers, imaging specialists, heart failure specialists, cardiac anesthesiologists, intensivists, nurses, and social workers
Additional program criteria	Device-specific training as required by the manufacturer	

AVR, aortic valve replacement; TAVR, transcatheter aortic valve replacement.
Adapted from Centers for Medicare and Medicaid Services. *National Coverage Determination for Transcatheter Aortic Valve Replacement.* 2012. https://www.cms.gov/medicare-coverage-database/details/ ncd-details.aspx? NCDId=355&ncdver=1&NCAId=257&ver=4&NcaName=Transcath- eter+Aortic+Valve+Replacement+(TAVR)&bc= ACAAAAAACAAAAA%3D%3D&. Accessed September 24, 2012.

Procedural Team

In addition to defining the hospital infrastructure, CMS also defined criteria for the hospital program Heart Team implanting physicians. Two sets of qualifications were developed: one for Heart Teams and hospital programs without TAVR experience and one for those with TAVR experience. The 2 sets of criteria are provided in Table 9.1.

The Heart Team for valvular heart disease emerged from the interventional cardiologist (IC) and cardiothoracic surgeon (CTS) partnership applied in the Bypass Angioplasty Revascularization Investigation (BARI)[7] and Synergy Between Percutaneous Coronary Intervention with Taxus and Cardiac Surgery (SYNTAX)[8] trials. This collaborative model was adopted in the TAVR clinical trials.

Although international professional societies recommend a Heart Team involvement in the evaluation of the patient with valvular heart disease, there are differences in the recommended requirements for the TAVR procedural team.[5,9] In the United States, regulatory requirements for reimbursement mandate the inclusion of both a cardiac surgeon and an IC during the transcatheter valve replacement procedure and their joint performance of the intraoperative technical aspects of TAVR. Outside the United States, there are recommendations regarding procedural volumes and experience to perform a procedure; however, joint procedural participation is not required. No longer constrained by the historical context of the procedural specialty or location, transcatheter technology has prompted a sharing of skills and knowledge between interventional cardiology and cardiac surgery, including valve pathoanatomy and physiology; noninvasive multimodality imaging such as CT, echocardiography, and fluoroscopy; and tools and approaches for both catheter-based and surgical intervention.

Implanting Team

The contemporary TAVR team described in a 2017 multiprofessional society expert consensus document[9] is a comprehensive group that may include but is not limited to the cardiology valve (CV) expert, IC, CV imaging expert, CTS, CV anesthesiologist, and a valve coordinator or valve program clinician. The MDT extends into the TAVR procedural room. The implanting team (eg, IC, CTS, CV anesthesiologist, and CV imaging specialist) is a subgroup of the Heart Team, supported by a specialized procedural team trained in transcatheter heart valve (THV) procedures.

Focusing on the procedural roles of nursing and the allied health team, Table 9.2 identifies the roles and general responsibilities of the team members. Although key roles are necessary for all procedures, the case plan and procedural approach may require additional members.

Anesthesia Support

The anesthesia approach for the TAVR procedure may be provided by the CV anesthesiologist, an advanced practice nurse trained in anesthesiology (eg, certified registered nurse anesthetist), anesthesia technician, and/or registered nurses. The anesthesia team is responsible for managing sedation for the patient, as well as anticipating the significant hemodynamic transitions that may occur during a TAVR procedure. As TAVR technology has progressed, the level of sedation required has become less intense. TAVR procedures may be safely performed without general anesthesia (GA) (monitored anesthesia care, moderate and conscious sedation [CS]) regardless of patients' clinical presentation and complexity of comorbidities.[10,12]

The shift away from GA has many benefits. A meta-analysis performed by Villablanca et al reviewing 26 studies and over 10,000 patients concluded that the use of a minimalist approach with CS and local anesthesia (LA) was associated with a lower 30-day mortality rate, shorter procedural time, fluoroscopy time, length of stay and intensive care unit time, and reduced need for inotropic support.[13] There was no significant difference in the rates of procedural

TABLE 9.2. Example of TAVR Procedure Team Roles and Responsibilities

Key Roles	Training/ Credentialing	General Responsibilities
Proceduralists	Interventional Cardiologist and Cardiothoracic Surgeon	Implanting team Leads team Implants valve 1st and 2nd position (primary or secondary operator) predetermined
First assistant	2nd Proceduralist Interventional Fellow (Large Bore Training) Advanced Practice Provider w/ Interventional Training	Preprocedure physical assessment Verifies informed consent Physician: performs initial time-out Verifies transvenous pacemaker and power injector function Establishes initial line access Places preclosure devices Assists during procedure Follows with patient to postprocedure transfer Completes postprocedure report to team
CV imaging specialist	Advanced Cardiac Imaging Cardiologist Or CV Anesthesiologist	For procedures requiring TEE imaging: Assess annulus for valve sizing (before and during procedure) Assess valve post implantation: placement, leak, other valve disease Provides assistance on device placement
CV anesthesia	Anesthesiologist Or Nurse or CV Specialist	Determines method of anesthesia or sedation based on patient needs Administers and manages anesthesia, medications and fluids Oversees postprocedure recovery
Scrub tech	CV Technician	Prepare all tools and equipment before procedure Ensure all equipment is sterile Ensure patient is positioned and comfortable before and during procedure Manages sterile table during procedure Cleans equipment and tools following procedure
Nurse	Nurse	Documents patient care in chart Places orders (laboratory tests, treatments) in chart Administers medications (if conscious sedation) Provides equipment Manages pacemaker acer Manages power injector Runs activated clotting time Ensures patient remains comfortable during procedure
Circulator	Nurse or CV Technician	Provides equipment Manages pacemaker Manages power injector Runs activated clotting time Provides technical support during procedure

TABLE 9.2. Example of TAVR Procedure Team Roles and Responsibilities   (Continued)

Key Roles	Training/ Credentialing	General Responsibilities
Device specialist	CV Technician or Nurse with device training	Device/valve preparation
Case monitor	CV Technician	Documents each step of procedure (wires, devices, personnel transitions, etc.; Manage imaging; Monitor hemodynamics and ECG Assist with imaging transitions on monitor screens; Call for additional procedural support and resources as needed
Additional Team Members		
Surgical scrub (for procedures with cutdown access)	Surgical Assist	Prepare all surgical tools and equipment before procedure Ensure all surgical equipment is sterile Ensure patient is positioned and comfortable before and during procedure Manages sterile table during procedure Cleans surgical equipment and tools following procedure
Surgical circulating nurse		Provides surgical equipment Provides technical surgical support during procedure Ensures patient remains comfortable during procedure
Electrophysiologist		Implantation of permanent pacemaker
Vascular specialist		Establishes vascular access for alternate access cases as preferred: transcarotid, subclavian, etc.
Perfusionists		Available for emergent procedures

CV, cardiovascular; ECG, electrocardiogram; TAVR, transcatheter aortic valve replacement; TEE, transesophageal echocardiography.

success, annular rupture, or paravalvular leak. These studies suggest that conscious or moderate sedation may be associated with improvements in both outcome and process.

The transition to a less intensive anesthesia strategy may modify the intraprocedural role of anesthesiology; however, the potential for hemodynamic collapse and emergent intubation necessitates formal standards regarding the availability of cardiovascular anesthesia for emergencies. Practice varies in the United States and other countries, depending on institutional policies and regional scope of practice for nurses, anesthesiologists, and physicians in fellowship training.[14]

Nursing and Cardiovascular Technician Support

TAVR procedures require a specialized, trained procedural team. The composition of the team may vary based on practice regulations for the state or country in which the procedure is performed, the access site (eg, femoral or other) and approach (eg, percutaneous or surgical incision), and the type of anesthesia required. The procedural team must have competency and technical skills typical of the CCL and/or OR, as determined by the institution. For the purpose of this chapter, the aforementioned US high-volume urban center serves as the context.

The procedural staffing model for transfemoral TAVR may include 3 nurses and/or allied health professionals. One staff member functions as the sterile or "scrub" technician and is primarily responsible for maintaining the sterility of and equipment on the procedure table. Two staff function in "circulating" positions. Both provide equipment, test blood for activated clotting time (ACT), and are able to manage the power injector and transvenous pacemaker (TVP). At least one of these team members is a nurse, credentialed and licensed to perform and document the clinical assessment and care, specifically patient care orders (ie, laboratory tests, urinary catheter insertion) and medication administration. Cardiovascular technicians with the appropriate education, training, and certification (eg, registered cardiovascular invasive specialist or RCIS in the United States) may perform the roles of the scrub technician and one of the circulators.

Procedures that require a more invasive or alternate access may require additional team members. Transaortic, transapical (TA), transcarotid, or surgical vascular access may require team members with additional surgical training. In the United States, institutions may choose to add specialty technicians or surgical circulating nurses or alternately may cross-train staff in both CCL and OR team skills. The staffing model adopted for each institution varies and is influenced by numerous factors including team and resource availability, complexity of case, frequency of need, and operator preferences.

During the procedure, one team member may prepare the device for delivery. This is a timed and sterile procedure, which may be performed by a nurse or cardiovascular technician who has received additional device-specific training. Each device has a unique preparation process; the "Device Specialist" should have completed the device manufacturers' training for each device employed with repetitive proctored support. In some institutions, specialized device manufacturer staff may perform the device preparation.

The monitor role is responsible for documenting the time of all steps of the procedure, devices used, pacing runs, and entry and exit of personnel. The monitor may manage imaging screens, interpret hemodynamic and electrocardiographic data, as well as adjust the hemodynamic and imaging views based on procedural needs. This role may be performed by a cardiovascular technician or nurse trained in the procedure and early identification and prevention of adverse events.

Perfusion Support

The risk of conversion to emergent cardiac surgery during a TAVR procedure has been reported between 0.7%[15] and 1.3%.[2] Conversion to surgery was associated most frequently with LV perforation, annular rupture, and valve embolization or migration. Regardless of the cause, conversion requires emergent perfusion support. Carroll et al[16] found that there was a significant decrease in the frequency of conversion with increased TAVR procedural experience. With the highest rates during the first 30 cases at 1.3%, conversion rates decreased to 0.8% in the cohort of hospitals with a cumulative volume greater than 138 cases. Based on these results, the need for perfusion attendance during a procedure is low; however, the availability of perfusion support for emergent cases is indicated and determined by the institution.

Procedural Processes of Care

In 2009, the World Health Organization initiated the Safe Surgery Saves Lives program to reduce the number of surgical deaths occurring globally.[17] Checklists have been implemented in multiple settings for varied surgical types and show consistent improvement in quality and reduction in errors.[18] Templates, checklists, and order sets are key strategies for TAVR programs to standardize processes minimizing error and ensuring quality and consistency.

Preprocedural Planning

The 2017 ACC Expert Consensus Decision Pathway for TAVR provides a detailed process for preprocedural planning by the MDT.[9] Routine conferences are recommended, during which the MDT develops a procedural plan that provides full direction for the team regarding the procedure to be performed, addresses the unique risks of the patient, and provides guidance regarding special resources required. This case assessment and decision making should be readily available to the team before and during the procedure. An example of a case review with procedural plan is shown in Table 9.3.

During the MDT conference, anesthesiology may communicate specific concerns regarding the anesthesia approach and airway. Anesthesiology may perform a face-to-face assessment before TAVR, even on the day prior or day of the procedure; however, during the MDT conference anesthesiology may recognize anatomical or medical history issues that necessitate further exploration or may determine the mode of anesthesia.

Following the MDT decision, standardized procedural orders for TAVR may serve to schedule and communicate the procedural plans to the CCL or OR teams as well as the instructions communicated to the patient (Table 9.4.) The order should identify the specific valve type and size, access site, anesthesia approach, and vendor support to ensure that appropriate resources are available. Specific imaging needs for valve placement should be clarified: transesophageal echocardiogram assessment during the procedure or fluoroscopy-guided THV placement with transthoracic echocardiography post procedure.

Procedural Management of Coexisting Conditions

Poor renal function is associated with worse short- and long-term outcomes.[19] Given the prevalence of impaired renal function in this patient population, each institution must consider specific protocols to reduce nephrotoxicity, such as prehydration and preprocedural instructions for medications associated with drug-induced nephrotoxicity.

Contrast allergy must also be assessed and addressed for TAVR. For patients who have allergies to iodinated contrast requiring premedication, completion of pretreatment for the allergy should be verified with the patient and documented if complete. If an outpatient oral regimen for contrast allergy has not been completed before the procedure, a contrast allergy protocol including intravenous medications may be used.

Diabetes occurs in approximately 37% of patients undergoing TAVR.[2] The plan for management of diabetes medications should be defined and may include adjustments in insulin or medication dosing and timing of NPO status.

Over 40% of patients undergoing TAVR present with a prior history of atrial fibrillation.[2] Many of these patients will be given some form of anticoagulation for stroke risk reduction. The last dose of standard anticoagulation should be identified; if bridging therapy is required, the dosing plan with date and time of last bridging dose should also be included.

TABLE 9.3. Example Procedural Plan

- Last Name, First Name   MRN   DOB
- Procedure:
- Device:
  - Annulus/native valve and root anatomy/Calcium:
- Access:
- Anesthesia:
  - **Allergies:**
- Imaging:
- Complication management:
  - Airway concerns:
  - Coronary protection:
  - Pacer/Rhythm:
  - GFR: ; Max contrast load:
  - Vascular:
  - Hemodynamic support:
- **Pt Data:** Ht: cm; Wt: kg; BMI: --- (labs: date) Creat: GFR: Hb: Plts: Alb:
- **PMH:** (pertinent)
- **ECG:**
- **PFT** (date): FEV1: (%), FEV1/FVC: %, DLCO: (%);
- Carotid Doppler (date): Right: %, Left: %
- **Echo:** (date) EF: % PAP: mmHg

  ✓ Vmax: m/s Peak/Mean PG: mmHg, AV SVI: mL/m^2

  ✓ AVA: cm^2 AVA index: cm^2/m^2

  ✓ AI / MR / TR

- **Cath:** (date): LM: %, LAD: %, LCX: %, RCA: %

  ✓ Hemodynamics: RA: RV: PA: PCWP: LVEDP: CO (Fick): CI:

  ✓ Valve: BAV using mm balloon

  AV Peak/Mean Gradient: → mmHg AVA: → cm^2

- **CT: (date)** ------------------------------------ **Coplanar Angle:**

  ✓ Syst: Area: mm^2 Circ: mm; LVOT: mm^2; LCA Ht: mm; RCA Ht: mm;

  ✓ Sinus of Valsalva: mm; STJ Diam: mm; Root /_ °

  ✓ RtCIA: mm; RtEIA: mm; RtCFA: mm;

  ✓ LtCIA: mm; LtEIA: mm; LtCFA: mm;

AI, aortic insufficiency; Alb, albumin; AV SVI, aortic valve stroke volume index; AVA, aortic valve area; AVAI, aortic valve area index; BAV, balloon aortic valvuloplasty; BMI, body mass index; CFA, common femoral artery; CI, cardiac index; CIA, common iliac artery; CO, cardiac output; CT, computerized tomography; DLCO, diffusion lung carbon monoxide; DOB, date of birth; ECG, electrocardiogram; ECHO, echocardiogram; EF, ejection fraction; EIA, external iliac artery; FEV, forced expiratory volume; FVC, forced expiratory volume; GFR, glomerular filtration rate; Hb, hemoglobin; Ht, height; LAD, left anterior descending; LCA, left coronary artery; LCX, left circumflex; LM, left main; LVEDP, left ventricular end diastolic pressure; MG, mean gradient; MR, mitral regurgitation; MRN, medical record number; PA, pulmonary artery; PAP, pulmonary artery pressure; PCWP, pulmonary capillary wedge pressure; PFT, pulmonary function test; Plt, platelets; PMH, past medical history; Pt, patient; RA, right atrium; RCA, right coronary artery; Rt, right; RV, right ventricle; STJ, sinotubular junction; syst, systolic; TR, tricuspid regurgitation; Vmax, maximal velocity; Wt, weight.

TABLE 9.4. TAVR Procedure Orders

Planned Procedure Date:

Primary operator:

Referring physician:

Planned procedure: Approach:

Procedure type: (commercial vs. research)

Registry/clinical trial number:

     Research coordinator:

Equipment/devices:

Vendor support:

Imaging support: (3D-TEE/TTE/TEE)

Anesthesia: GA/MAC/conscious sedation

Renal function:

     For GFR <45, plan:

Allergies:

     Contrast allergy, plan:

Diabetes:

     DM medications, plan:

Anticoagulants: yes/no;

     Type:

     Last dose:

     Bridging plan: Yes/Not indicated

          Last bridging dose:

Interpreter services: Yes/Not indicated   Language:

3-D, three-dimensional; DM, diabetes mellitus; GA, general anesthesia; GFR, glomerular filtration rate; MAC, monitored anesthesia care; TAVR, transcatheter aortic valve replacement; TEE, transesophageal echocardiography; TTE, transthoracic echocardiography.

Procedural Safety Pause: The "Time-out"

In 2009, the World Health Organization published guidelines to reduce preventable surgical complications.[20] Recommendations for "time-outs" or "surgical pauses" are included that outline specific points before, during, and after the procedure when the members of the team verbally confirm the patient, the procedure, and protective steps or measures. It is a means to ensure clear communication and coordination of care among team members. There are 3 time-outs that occur during the TAVR procedure: (1) the preprocedure time-out is performed before sedation of the patient, (2) a critical time-out occurs before valve deployment, and (3) a postprocedure time-out occurs at the time of hand-off.

The preprocedure time-out is typically led by one of the implanting physicians and requires attendance of the team members providing the roles for sedation/anesthesia, circulation, and monitoring (eg, the anesthesiologist, a circulating nurse, and the cardiovascular technician). During this time-out, there is an oral review of the case plan with the team while the patient is alert, before administration of sedation. The patient should be involved to verify his/her identity and elements of their past medical history that affect the procedure, such as allergies and renal disease. During the preprocedure time-out, the team assignments are reviewed, all equipment needed for the procedure are verified as present and all emergent equipment tested, and appropriate functioning is confirmed. Table 9.5 provides an example of a preprocedure time-out template. Key elements of the plan should be posted and visible for the team to easily reference during the case.

The second time-out is a "critical stop" and takes place before deployment of the THV. The entire procedural team stops all activity, and the implanting physician deploying the valve leads the time-out. During the critical stop the case and expected procedural steps are reviewed. Anesthesia verifies administration of prophylactic antibiotics. The status of anticoagulation (eg, timing of and most recent ACT results) is reviewed. Appropriate function of the TVP is verified, and the appropriate imaging display is confirmed. This time-out actively assures that the patient and all members of the team are ready for valve deployment. Table 9.6 provides an example of a "Critical Time-out" checklist.

A third key time-out occurs at the time of hand-off to the managing care team. The procedure type, status of patient, lines placed, medications administered, hemodynamic status, and significant events are reviewed. A head-to-toe assessment helps ensure complete communication. Finally, the status of communication with family or patients support person should be identified. An example of the postprocedure hand-off is provided in Table 9.7.

The Procedure: Step by Step

Every TAVR procedure is unique based on the needs of the patient. To frame this section with a procedural overview, Table 9.8 reviews the key steps and documentation of a transfemoral TAVR procedure.

Anesthesia Approach

The mode of anesthesia used during a TAVR procedure is determined by the patient's clinical presentation, comorbidities, procedural approach/access site, and local practice. The approach to anesthesia spans GA, monitored anesthesia care or LA with CS, and CS administered by nursing.

In 2017, Villablanca et al performed a meta-analysis of 26 studies (N = 10,572 patients) reviewing the safety of TAVR under LA/CS as compared with GA.[13] Their findings for LA/CS supported a lower 30-day mortality rate, shorter procedure and fluoroscopy time, reduced

TABLE 9.5. Preprocedure Time-out (Performed Before Administration of Sedation)

Conducted by the Physician in Charge	
• Patient identity	• 2 identifiers: name, DOB, MRN • Patient verifies name and DOB
• Physician: planned primary operator	
• Consent signed	• Verify on chart

• Planned procedure	• Access route
	• Valve type and size
	• Type of anesthesia
	• Mallampati score
	• Unique aspects adjustments from MDT
	  • Depressed EF
	  • Pulmonary HTN
	  • Coronary protection
	  • Cerebral protection
	  • Other

• Allergies	• Contrast, antibiotics
• Investigations review	• Glomerular filtration rate • Hemoglobin • PT/INR • Verification type and screen complete
• Maximum contrast load	
• Planned antibiotic therapy available	
• Personnel and assigned roles	• Proceduralists: primary • First assist: Secondary/Fellow/APP • Anesthesiologist/CRNA • Scrub tech • Nurse or circulator • Pacer management, power injector • Back table staff: device specialist • Emergent equipment

APP, advanced practice provider; CRNA, certified registered nurse anesthetist; DOB, date of birth; EF, ejection fraction; HTN, hypertension; MDT, multidisciplinary team; MRN, medical record number; PT/INR, protime/international normalized ratio.

time in intensive care as well as hospital stay, and a reduced need for inotropic support. A study by Hyman et al using data from the STS/ACC TVT Registry described anesthesia use with patients undergoing TAVR from April 1, 2014, through June 30, 2015.[11] CS was used in 15.8% (1737 of 10,997) of the procedures. The use of CS was associated with lower procedural inotrope requirements, shorter intensive care unit and hospital lengths of stay, lower in-hospital and 30-day mortality rates, and lower combined 30-day death/stroke rates. Interestingly, after treatment-weighted adjustment, CS was associated with lower procedural success (97.9% vs 98.6%, $P < .001$).

TABLE 9.6. Critical Time-out (Performed Before Valve Implantation)

Conducted by the Proceduralist Placing Valve	
• Patient identification	• 2 identifiers: name, MRN, DOB
• Brief patient history	• Reason for implantation • Significant PMH/PSH
• Valve plan	• Device and size • Critical steps for sizing, deployment • Critical unexpected steps

• Review team members and assigned roles	• Proceduralists
	  • First operator: deploying valve
	  • Secondary operator/first assist
	• Anesthesia
	  • Status
	  • Confirms antibiotics administered ≤60 min before deployment
	• Cath lab staff
	  • Last ACT results
	  • Verify: pacer
	  • Verify: power injector
	  • Emergent equipment prepared

ACT, activated clotting time; DOB, date of birth; MRN, medical record number; PMH, past medical history; PSH, past social history.

TABLE 9.7. Postprocedural Hand-off to Management Team

Conducted by Anesthesiologist or First Assist	
• Patient identification	• 2 identifiers: name, MRN, DOB
• Preprocedure	• Diagnosis with brief HPI • Pertinent PMH
• Procedure performed	• Device, access

• Key concerns for recovery and management	• Type of anesthesia
	• Vital signs BP/HR/oximetry/ventilation support
	• ECG status: preprocedure and postprocedure
	• Arteriotomy access: location, sheath size, closure devices, time of closure, status
	• Lines: sites and status
	• Medications: preprocedure and intraprocedure
	• Blood products/fluid hydration
	• Last laboratory results
	• Postdeployment echo
	• Significant events
	  • Hemodynamic report
	  • Neurologic status
	  • Bleeding events

• Family member/support person communication	• Last communication

ACT, activated clotting time; BP, blood pressure; ECG, electrocardiogram; HPI, history of present illness; HR, heart rate; PMH, past medical history; PSH, past social history.

TABLE 9.8. TAVR Procedure Transfemoral Approach

1. Preprocedure verification completed. "History and physical" and signed consents on chart
2. Patient setup: Positioned supine and comfortable on the procedure table
   a. Safety measures (arm board, procedure table locked, grounding pad (if indicated)
   b. Monitoring application: BP/O$_2$ saturation monitors applied, ECG leads applied
   c. Two radiolucent defibrillator pads placed connected to defibrillator
   d. Body warming blanket placed under/around patient
   e. Preoperative checklist reviewed and instructions provided to patient
3. Initial time-out performed (see Table 10.5)
4. Patient preparation
   a. Sedation initiated: per predetermined anesthesia protocol
   b. Foley inserted (if indicated)
   c. Bilateral groin prep: clipped and prepped with chloraprep
   d. Patient draped in sterile fashion
5. Procedure preparation
   a. Ultrasound- and flouro-guided femoral artery and vein access established
   b. Local infiltration with 2% lidocaine (LI2%) of RFA cannulated with 7F introducer sheath. Preclose RFA with perclose ×2.
   c. LI2% of LFV cannulated with 6F introducer sheath.
   d. 6F internal mammary catheter advanced to aortoiliac bifurcation.
   e. LFA angiogram performed via RFA.
   f. LI2% of LFA cannulated with 7F introducer sheath.
   g. LI2% of Rt radial artery cannulated with 6F introducer sheath.
   h. TVP via LFV advanced to RV. Tested at 10 mA and rate of 180 bpm.
   i. Activated clotting time (ACT) assessed. Results reported to procedural team.
   j. Contralateral angiogram performed
   k. 4F glidecather advanced down Lt leg
   l. 6F multipurpose A2 catheter, Lunderquist wire, and 14F/45 cm cook sheath handed off
   m. LFA: Pigtail catheter advanced to aortic root
   n. LFA: Short sheath exchanged for 14F/45-cm sheath
   o. AL1 catheter advanced to aortic root
   p. Ao angiogram performed with power injector
   q. Grand Slam wire and embolic protection device advanced via Rt radial artery
   r. ACT assessed. Results reported to procedural team.
   s. 035 J guidewire introduced under fluoroscopic guidance. 6F pigtail catheter advanced to left ventricle. LV and aortic pressures recorded.
6. Critical time-out performed (see Table 10.6)
7. Valve placement
   a. Pigtail catheters removed over Lunderquist wire. Lunderquist remains in LV
   b. 14F sheath removed
   c. Valve system advanced across Ao valve
   d. Pacer on, Ao gram, valve deployed, pacer off
   e. Valve delivery system removed
   f. Simultaneous pressures: LV and aortic recorded
   g. Final aortogram performed
   h. ACT assessed. Results reported to procedural team
8. Procedural completion
   a. RFA and LFA angiogram performed with DSA
   b. Sheath/catheters removed, RFA perclose sutures tightened
   c. TR band to Rt radial artery
   d. Manual pressure applied to LFA and LFV until hemostasis achieved
   e. Patient transferred to holding area
9. Postprocedural hand-off report provided to managing team

ACT, activated clotting time; Ao, aortic; BP, blood pressure; DSA, digital subtraction angiography; ECG, electrocardiogram; LFA, left femoral artery; LFV, left femoral vein; Lt, left; LV, left ventricle; RFA, right femoral artery; Rt, right; RV, right ventricle; TAVR, transcatheter aortic valve replacement; TR, Terumo band; TVP, transvenous pacemaker.

Collectively, the results of both the Villablanca and Hyman analyses support the safety of CS. Each institution must review the evidence against its team and resources to determine selection criteria for each anesthesia approach. Table 9.9 provides comparison and points of consideration for the various modes of anesthesia for TAVR.[12]

TABLE 9.9. Considerations for Mode of Anesthesia

Monitored Anesthesia Care (MAC) or Local Anesthesia/Conscious Sedation (LA/CS)	General Anesthesia
• Access: percutaneous approaches; femoral, transcaval • Able to follow commands • No Foley, TEE • Postprocedural valve placement with transthoracic echo	• Access: transapical, transcarotid, transaortic • Difficult airway or intubation • Vascular disease requiring cutdown • Severe OSA • Morbid obesity • Inability to follow commands • Inability to lie supine • Need for TEE assessment
Monitoring resources	Monitoring resources
• 5-lead ECG • Pulse oximetry • Invasive blood pressure monitoring • End-tidal CO_2 monitoring	• 5-lead electrocardiography • Pulse oximetry • End-tidal CO_2 detection • Fraction of inspired oxygen • Fraction of inhaled inspired volatile gases • Temperature • Invasive blood pressure monitoring • PA monitoring: low EF or severe Pulm HTN
Administration characteristics	Administration characteristics

MAC [10]
 	
• Face mask with oxygen supplementation
• Titrated midazolam for anxiety
• Sedative infusions and meds (one or combination): propofol, ketamine, remifentanil, dexmedetomidine
 	
LA/CS [36]:
 	
• Face mask or nasal cannula with oxygen supplementation
• Midazolam and piritramide (0.1-0.3 mg/kg) body weight-adjusted. Repetitive dosing for patient comfort
• 1% lidocaine bilateral groins
	• Airway: endotracheal intubation
	• IV anesthesia
	• Induction: IV anesthetic, morphine derivative, muscle relaxant
	• Maintenance
	  • Inhalation anesthetic or continuous infusion of IV anesthesia
	  • Continuous infusion of remifentanil

ECG, electrocardiogram; EF, ejection fraction; HTN, hypertension; IV, intravenous; OSA, obstructive sleep apnea; TEE, transesophageal echocardiography.

Procedural Monitoring

During the TAVR procedure, rapid ventricular pacing, typically via a temporary TVP wire in the right ventricle, is used to create a brief period of virtual cardiac standstill to allow placement of a new prosthetic valve in an existing diseased valve that has abnormal forward flow. Sudden onset and termination of the TVP overrides native electrical conduction and cardiac contractions to effectively cease for a short period and abruptly resume. These sudden transitions result in increased myocardial demand and rapid alterations of the patient's hemodynamic state that require continuous noninvasive and invasive monitoring. The various types of monitoring and procedural lines are reviewed.

Noninvasive Monitoring

Electrocardiogram Monitoring

Continuous electrocardiogram monitoring is generally initiated in the preprocedural area and maintained throughout hospitalization. During the procedure, monitoring patches are placed on the chest in positions that do not obstruct fluoroscopic imaging and the cardiac rhythm is continuously monitored.

Transcutaneous Defibrillation Pads

Transcutaneous defibrillation pads may be placed before the start of the procedure. Pads are positioned to minimize obstruction for fluoroscopic procedural imaging and planned access sites. The defibrillator machine is placed close to the procedure table and connected to the patient, ready for emergent use.

Continuous Pulse Oximetry

Pulse oximetry may be initiated before the procedure. It is monitored and documented throughout the procedure. Pulse oximetry is an important monitoring tool for TAVR procedures employing the least-invasive means for ongoing evaluation of oxygenation.

Invasive Hemodynamic Monitoring

Continuous Systemic Arterial Monitoring

Continuous systemic arterial monitoring may be performed through femoral access lines or through a radial arterial line placed before the procedure. Systemic arterial blood pressure is continuously monitored with appropriate fluid and medication changes as indicated. For TAVRs employing GA, an arterial line also allows for the evaluation of arterial blood gases in the rare event they are required.

Continuous Pulmonary Arterial Monitoring

Although used routinely in the early years of TAVR, a pulmonary artery (PA) catheter is no longer considered a standard of care. However, PA pressure monitoring may be indicated in the presence of pulmonary hypertension or left ventricular dysfunction.[21] The decision for PA pressure monitoring may be made during the MDT conference or preprocedural assessment.

Laboratory Blood Testing

At the beginning of the procedure, the most recent blood tests are reviewed, including renal function testing (creatinine and estimated glomerular filtration rate), hemoglobin, hematocrit, platelet count, and prothrombin time. ACTs are assessed during the procedure to monitor the patient's anticoagulation status after receiving intravenous (IV) heparin. Anticoagulation is administered following placement of central lines. An expert consensus statement published in 2017 recommended maintaining an ACT of 250 to 300 seconds.[9] During the critical time-out preceding valve deployment, the timing of the last anticoagulant dose and ACT results are reviewed to ensure that the risk of thrombus formation is minimized (Table 9.6).

Procedural Lines
Temporary Transvenous Pacemaker

The TVP wire is placed intraprocedurally. For patients with a narrow QRS at baseline, the wire is generally placed through a femoral vein and removed after the procedure if the patient had a pre-existing permanent pacemaker or did not develop conduction disturbances during the procedure. For patients at increased risk for potential heart block (ie, pre-existing right bundle branch block or left anterior fascicular block, small left ventricular outflow tract [LVOT], or high ratio of annulus-to-LVOT diameter), the TVP wire may be placed in the right internal jugular vein. For this patient group, either a screw-in lead may be used at the beginning of the procedure or the TVP wire changed at the end of the procedure to facilitate patient mobility after the procedure while determining if a permanent pacemaker is indicated.

Arterial Line

If used, an arterial line, most commonly in the radial artery, may be placed for continuous blood pressure monitoring. Discontinuation of the arterial line is determined based on the patient's clinical need and institutional policy.

Intravenous Lines

Peripheral IV lines are used for administration of fluids and medications. Typically, at least one peripheral IV line is placed preprocedurally and maintained postprocedurally. Central or large-bore intravenous lines may be placed for rapid fluid and medication administration.

Urinary Catheter

The use of a urinary (eg, Foley) catheter may be determined upon access, form of anesthesia, and patient clinical history. A urinary catheter should be avoided in patients with urological issues, including urinary strictures, ureteral stents, and prostate enlargement. Emerging evidence suggests that the use of a urinary catheter for TAVR may be associated with an increased risk of infection, bleeding, and prolonged length of stay.[22] With LA/CS, transfemoral access, and the use of closure devices to expedite hemostasis and reduce the duration of postprocedural bed rest, many institutions no longer include routine placement of urinary catheters. As the urinary catheter is associated with an increased risk of adverse events in the elderly, there is sufficient evidence to revisit the use of a urinary catheter in historical TAVR protocols.[23-25]

Vascular Approach

Evaluation of the arterial vasculature for atherosclerotic burden and location, arterial size and tortuosity, and presence of thrombus must be performed to determine the access site and approach for TAVR. Sheath delivery systems vary based on valve type and size.

Transfemoral access is the least invasive approach and the preferred delivery route for TAVR.[9] Table 9.11 describes the recommended iliofemoral artery minimal lumen diameters for the most commonly used THVs. Figure 9.1 provides an illustration of TAVR with trans-femoral access showing placement of femoral access lines, pacing wire in right ventricle, and valve delivery. As catheter sizes have decreased (Figure 9.1), the percentage of TAVR procedures performed through the femoral artery has increased from 75.9% in 2012 to 86.6% in 2015.[10]

When iliofemoral arteries are too small, calcified or tortuous for the available introducer sheaths, alternative access routes must be considered. Alternate nonfemoral routes available include TA, transaortic, and transsubclavian. For centers with advanced operators and programs with specialized training, transcaval, transcarotid, and antegrade-aortic are also employed.

Transapical Approach

Transapical (TA) TAVR is performed through a left anterolateral mini-thoracotomy under flu-oroscopic and transesophageal echocardiogram guidance and most commonly under GA. In the United States, this antegrade approach was the most widely used alternate access over all others combined until 2015 (6.1% vs 6.8%, respectively).[10]

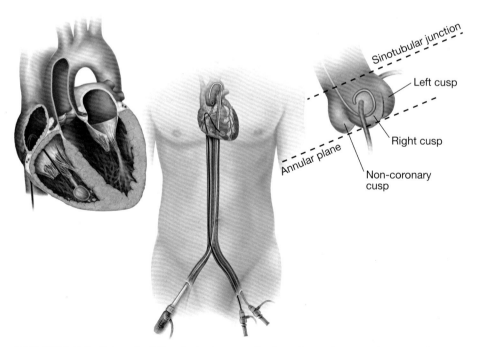

FIGURE 9.1. Setup depicting typical access for transfemoral transcatheter aortic valve replacement with delivery and nondelivery sides. Insets depict balloon-tipped pacing catheter in right ventricle and coplanar alignment of aortic cusps ("deployment angle") with an angled pigtail. (Reprinted with permission from Grover FL, Mack MJ, eds. *Cardiac Surgery*. Philadelphia, PA: Wolters Kluwer; 2017.)

The TA approach is used with the SAPIEN valve system (Edwards Lifesciences, Irvine, California). It involves implanting the THV directly through the left ventricle (LV) apex, antegrade through a small chest incision (approximately 1.5–3 cm) at approximately the sixth or fifth intercostal space. Hemostatic control of the LV is maintained during the procedure with 2 purse string sutures. Pacing during the procedure may be achieved with either transvenous or epicardial wires and is performed during balloon valvuloplasty and valve implantation, as well as sheath removal and suture-tying to decrease LV filling and pressure until the repair is complete. A postprocedural complication that is unique to the TA approach is the development of apical pseudoaneurysms.[26-28] The TA access should be performed only in a hybrid room with full OR and CCL capabilities. Figure 9.2 provides an illustration of TAVR via the TA approach.

Transaortic or Direct Aortic Approach

Transaortic or direct aortic access is an option for individuals with disease of the femoral vessels, descending or abdominal aorta, poor LV function, or atheroma or thrombus in the aortic arch or descending aorta. This approach involves performing a J-incision through the right second intercostal space. Double-purse string sutures are placed for bleeding management and closure at the end of the procedure. A needle is used to access the ascending aorta through a counter-incision placed in the right side of the neck. A guidewire is used to place a 7F sheath directly in the ascending aorta. The TAVR procedure is then performed retrograde through the ascending aorta, and balloon- and self-expanding THVs may be used.[29] As with the TA approach, trans- or direct aortic TAVR should be performed in a hybrid procedural room with both CCL and OR capabilities.

Transsubclavian Approach

The subclavian/axillary (SCA) access has been advocated as a preferred alternate access when the femoral route is not possible. Gleason et al advocate that the SCA route has the advantage of being in proximity of the access to the target site (aortic annulus) and the relatively straight course of the delivery system from the SCA to the annulus.[30] SCA access involves the use of cut down and general anesthesia, although percutaneous access has been reported.[31] Figure 9.3 shows the SCA access.

Transcaval Approach

Transcaval access is a percutaneous approach that involves advancing the introducer sheath into the femoral vein, traveling up the inferior vena cava to a predetermined site and crossing over into the adjacent infrarenal abdominal aorta.[32] The TAVR procedure is continued through the introducer sheath in this cross-over position. At the completion of the procedure, the caval-aortic access site is closed with a nitinol occluder device (see Figure 9.4).

The transcaval procedure can be performed in a hybrid room or CCL appropriately equipped for TAVR and peripheral interventional procedures. Key aspects of the procedure are detailed.

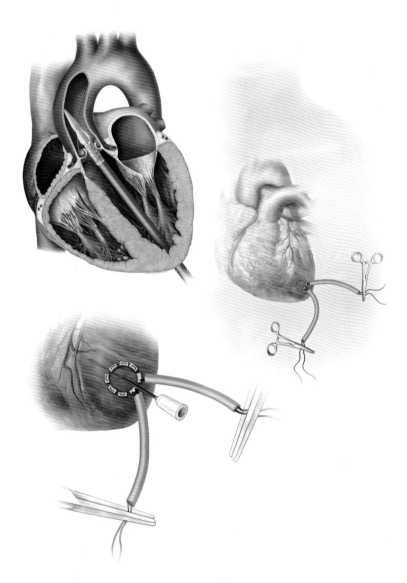

FIGURE 9.2. Transapical approach via anterior minithoracotomy. Insets depict location of apical purse string and puncture site as well as appropriate predeployment position for balloon-expanded transcatheter aortic valve replacement. (Reprinted with permission from Grover FL, Mack MJ, eds. *Cardiac Surgery*. Philadelphia, PA: Wolters Kluwer; 2017.)

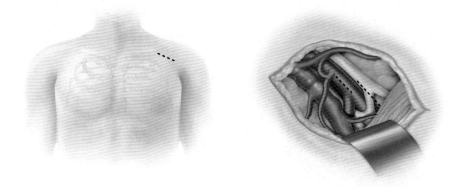

FIGURE 9.3. Axillary exposure for subclavian transcatheter aortic valve replacement delivery. (Reprinted with permission from Grover FL, Mack MJ, eds. *Cardiac Surgery*. Philadelphia, PA: Wolters Kluwer; 2017.)

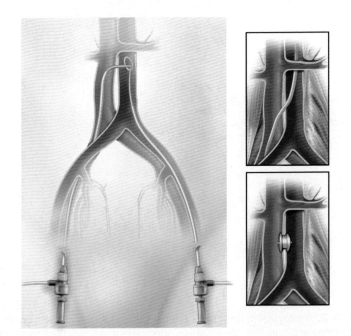

FIGURE 9.4. Transcaval transcatheter aortic valve replacement. Transcaval crossing with snare, device closure of arteriovenous communication. (Reprinted with permission from Grover FL, Mack MJ, eds. *Cardiac Surgery*. Philadelphia, PA: Wolters Kluwer; 2017.)

- Preprocedural planning with analysis of the contrast-enhanced, electrocardiogram-gated TAVR CT of chest, abdomen, and pelvis in less than 0.6-mm slices
- Identification of a calcium-free target in the aorta that is in close proximity to the inferior vena cava and safely away from the renal artery, renal vein, and aortoiliac bifurcation[32]
- Use of an electrified guidewire to burn through the vessels into the aorta, which is then captured and stabilized by a snare previously placed in the aorta
- Advancement of the introducer system over the guidewire to perform the TAVR procedure

Lederman, Babaliaros, and Greenbaum provide detailed instructions on how to perform the transcaval access and closure for TAVI.[32] This route was initially explored for candidates who were ineligible for femoral artery access and had a high or prohibitive risk of complications with all transthoracic routes.[33]

Transcarotid Approach

The transcarotid approach for TAVR is employed for individuals ineligible for other access routes. It is an extrathoracic approach that does not require manipulation of major neurovascular structures or the apex. As described by Thourani et al,[29] the right common carotid is exposed and after cross-clamping of the common carotid it is opened longitudinally for 2.5 cm. Cerebral perfusion may be maintained with a bypass shunt in the distal carotid. The J-tipped wire and 7F introducer sheath are placed in the ascending aorta, and the procedure is continued using a protocol similar to the transaortic approach. The procedure is also performed without bypass shunt using vascular clamps to achieve proximal and distal control of the carotid artery.[34] Figure 9.5 demonstrates the transcarotid setup with distal carotid bypass.

Procedural Complications

Preprocedural planning and anticipating complications are the most important steps in reducing risk, optimizing outcomes, and managing periprocedural complications and emergency interventions. Anticipating the worst is a key aspect of the MDT procedural planning. The preprocedural plan should include unique patient risks, the planned THV device and access, anticipated emergency intervention planning, as well as the resources needed. This procedural plan should be available to all members of the Heart Team, documented as appropriate in the patient medical record, and reviewed during the procedural time-outs. Table 9.10 reviews complications, associated variables, and options for emergent intervention. The 2 most frequent complications, stroke and conduction abnormalities, will be considered in detail.

Stroke

Stroke is one of the most concerning complications following TAVR. A study by Szeto et al[35] showed that arch calcification appeared to be associated with an increased risk of an embolic event and likely occurred during wire manipulation in the aortic arch and valve insertion. The 2016 Annual Report of the STS/ACC TVT Registry identified an in-hospital stroke incidence of 2.0% and a 30-day stroke rate of 1.9%.[10] Stroke following TAVR reaches across a spectrum of manifestations: major cerebrovascular accidents (CVAs) resulting in severe neurological deficits, CVA with mild cognitive or motor impairments, and subclinical cerebral infarcts with no

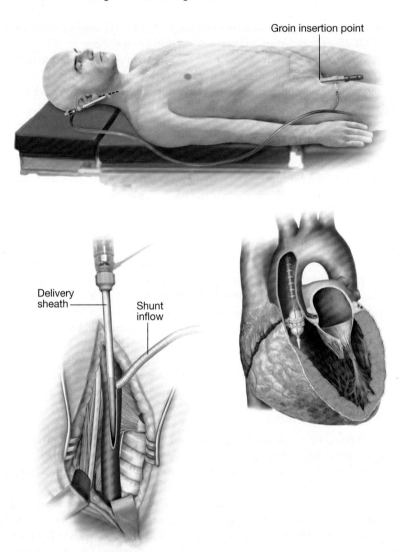

FIGURE 9.5. Setup for transcarotid transcatheter aortic valve replacement with depiction of common femoral to distal carotid shunt for cerebral protection. Inset shows longitudinal arteriotomy with proximal delivery sheath placement and distal carotid shunt in place. (Reprinted with permission from Grover FL, Mack MJ, eds. *Cardiac Surgery.* Philadelphia, PA: Wolters Kluwer; 2017.)

apparent deficits. The 2016 Neuro-TAVI trial reported that 32 of 34 patients who underwent TAVR and postprocedural diffusion-weighted MRI demonstrated cerebral emboli.[36] Systematic neurologic and cognitive evaluations were performed on these patients and showed that 1 in 5 of the patients had new, clinically evident neurologic impairment accompanied by imaging evidence of cerebral ischemia. The neurologic impairments continued to be evident in 15% of the

TABLE 9.10. Periprocedural Emergencies, Risk, and Treatment Plans

Complication	Anticipating Risk	Treatment Plans
Hemodynamic instability	• LV dysfunction • Prolonged pacing runs	• Identify and treat cause • Inotropic and fluid support • Mechanical ventricular support • Cardiopulmonary bypass
Coronary obstruction	• Coronary height measurements	• Prewire at-risk coronary artery • PCI • Cardiac support • Intentional laceration of obstructing leaflet
Complete heart block	• Pre-existing conduction defects (prolonged QRS, fascicular and first-degree block) • Overexpansion of native aortic annulus • Depth of valve within LVOT	• Transvenous pacing • Placement of PPM • Anticipated block: screw-in leads during procedure
Stroke	• Calcification in aortic arch[30]	• Embolic protection with filter device • Large emboli: catheter, mechanical retrieval
Aortic insufficiency • Central • Paravalvular	• Undersizing of valve • Uneven calcium distribution	• Balloon inflations of prosthetic valve • Valve in valve
Annular rupture	• Calcification of annulus • Calcification of LVOT • Oversizing of valve	• Reverse anticoagulation • Surgical repair • Pericardial drainage
Ventricular perforation	• Unanticipated with hemodynamic compromise • Delayed presentation	• Reverse anticoagulation • Surgical repair • Pericardial drainage • Percutaneous repair[38]
Valve embolization	• Undersizing of valve	• Conversion to surgical AVR • Wire stabilization of valve with percutaneous cardiac support
Aortic dissection	• Uncommon complication • Aortic disease	• Site dependent • Blood pressure control SBP<110 mm Hg • Stent graft from contralateral groin • Open surgical repair
Aortic rupture	• Device catheter trauma • Tortuous vessels • Steep angulation	• Emergent surgical or endovascular treatment

198 CHAPTER 9 The Right Care in the Right Place

TABLE 9.10. Periprocedural Emergencies, Risk, and Treatment Plans   (Continued)

Complication	Anticipating Risk	Treatment Plans
Vascular access complications: Iliofemoral dissection	• Preprocedural assessment of vessel size and calcification • Peripheral disease • Female gender • Renal failure	• Review of vessel with DSA • CTA w/distal run-off to id focus of dissection • Balloon procedure w/stent • Surgical repair
Vascular access complications: Iliofemoral rupture	• Preprocedural assessment of vessel size and calcification • Fragile vessels	• Rapid sheath reintroduction • Contralateral balloon delivery and inflation • Fluid repletion, quick anticoagulation reversal • Covered stent placement • Surgical intervention

AVR, aortic valve replacement; CTA, computed tomography angiography; DSA, digital subtraction angiography LV, left ventricle; LVOT, left ventricular outflow tract; PCI, percutaneous coronary intervention; PPM, permanent pacemaker; SBP, systolic blood pressure.
Adapted from Otto CM, Kumbhani DJ, Alexander KP, et al. 2017 ACC expert consensus decision pathway for transcatheter aortic valve replacement in the management of adults with aortic stenosis: a report of the American College of Cardiology Task Force on Clinical Expert Consensus Documents. *J Am Coll Cardiol.* 2017;69(10):1313-1346.

patients at 30 days.[36] These results suggest that stroke incidence may be higher than reported by current registries, as postprocedural neurologic imaging is not routinely performed. Recent trials and analyses have shown that the use of cerebral embolic protection during TAVR reduced the periprocedural silent ischemic brain lesions as demonstrated on MRI post-TAVR.[37-39]

In the 2016 CLaret Embolic Protection ANd TAVI Trial (CLEAN-TAVI) trial, 100 patients with severe symptomatic stenosis were randomly assigned to TAVI with a cerebral protection device or without. Postprocedural MRI was performed 2 days after the procedure. The number of new lesions was lower in the filter group, 4.00 versus 10.00 in the nonfilter group.[40] Although larger trials are indicated to assess the value of embolic protection during TAVR procedures, there is a clear need for strategies to reduce stroke incidence.

Conduction Defects

Development of conduction defects requiring permanent pacemaker (PPM) placement is one of the most common complications with TAVR. In the 2016 report from the STS/ACC TVT Registry, the 30-day new pacemaker implantation increased to 12%, previously reported as 8.8% in 2013.[10] Published in 2012, the PARTNER-2 trial showed that 30-day rates of PPM implantations in the balloon-expandable valve was 8.5%.[41] Historically, the incidence of PPM implantation with TAVR has been significant; estimated at 3.2% with surgical aortic valve replacement, this compares with as high as 25% with TAVR using the self-expanding CoreValve (Medtronic, Minneapolis, Minnesota). A meta-analysis published in 2013 showed that heart block requiring PPM implantation was the most common adverse outcome (13.1%) and was 5 times more common with the CoreValve than with the SAPIEN valve implanted using the transarterial route (25.2% vs 5.0%, respectively).[42]

The patient and procedural factors associated with the development of new left bundle branch block (LBBB) include pre-existing conduction abnormalities, female sex, previous coronary artery bypass graft surgery, diabetes, and the amount of calcification of the aortic valve.[43] The most common procedural characteristic associated with new LBBB is the depth of valve implantation into the LVOT and implantation of a self-expanding THV (eg, CoreValve involves progressive deployment from the ventricular side exerting force on the LVOT). The CoreValve is more often associated with the need for new pacemaker implantation.[43] The presence or development of any of these characteristics predictive of new-onset LBBB should alert the procedural team to an increased risk for continued pacemaker support following the procedure. Temporary pacemaker leads with screw-in tips or another form of stabilization should be considered at the outset of the procedure or on standby for internal jugular placement at the end of the procedure.

Emergency Intervention

One of the most difficult challenges in TAVR is overcoming emergency complications. Successful management begins during preprocedural planning with recognition of potential risk and planning for complications. Despite preprocedural plans, unexpected events occur; they are best managed with predefined protocols that verify that emergent equipment is available and functional at the outset of each procedure, clearly define resuscitative roles, and establish that emergency contacts are readily available. Emergency intervention planning should include protocols and resources for (1) emergent vascular repair, (2) management of severe hemodynamic instability, and (3) conversion to open heart surgery (OHS).

The 2016 annual report of the STS/ACC TVT registry reported the major vascular access site complication (VARC) rate as 1.3%.[10] Increased risks for vascular complications requiring emergent vascular repair have been identified as female gender, renal failure, peripheral vascular disease with significant calcification, and concomitant peripheral vascular disease.[44] Steps for managing are based on the type of complication occurring. Steps for managing ileofemoral rupture and dissection are reviewed in Table 9.11.

Aortic dissection is an uncommon but potentially fatal vascular complication of TAVR. The France TAVI data showed an aortic dissection rate between 0.2 and 0.4%.[3] The clinical signs of aortic dissection may manifest at any time during or after the procedure. Symptoms

TABLE 9.11. Access Vessel Dimension Based on Valve Type and Size

Valve Size (mm)	Edwards SAPIEN-XT (mm)	Edwards SAPIEN-3 (mm)	CoreValve Evolut-PRO (mm)	CoreValve Evolut-R (mm)
20		5.0		
23	6.0	5.5	5.0	5.0
26	6.5	5.5	5.0	5.0
29	7.0	6.0	5.0	5.0
31/34				5.5

of chest and abdominal pain, hypotension, and pressure difference greater than 20 mm Hg between the arms are all suggestive of dissection. Management is determined by the site and extent of vascular compromise. Strict blood pressure control is essential, maintaining a systolic <110 mm Hg using beta-blocker therapy or nondihydropyridine calcium channel blockers. Hypotension is managed with fluid volume administration.[44] Type A dissections, located in the ascending aorta, are indication for prompt surgical treatment, whereas type B dissections, located in the descending aorta, may be treated medically with endovascular repair a consideration.[44]

Severe hemodynamic instability, should it occur during TAVR, requires mechanical cardiac support (MCS), and a team well trained in its use should be available for every procedure. Emergency indications for MCS include cardiac arrest (ventricular tachycardia or fibrillation), refractory hypotension, cardiac tamponade, severe aortic insufficiency, postprocedural myocardial contracture (stone heart) or LV failure, valve embolization, and left main obstruction with percutaneous coronary intervention.[44] A 2016 single-center report regarding MCS use during TAVR found that the intra-aortic balloon pump was the most common MCS employed followed by temporary ventricular assist (eg, Impella), cardiopulmonary bypass, and extracorporeal membranous oxygenation.[45]

When life-threatening complications occur during TAVR, conversion to open OHS may be necessary; these complications may include valve embolization into the LV, paravalvular or central aortic regurgitation, coronary occlusion, annular rupture, or ventricular perforation. Conversion to OHS occurred in 0.4% of the patients followed in the France TAVI Registry[44] and in 1.3% in the STS/ACC TVT Registry.[16] Carroll et al[16] performed an assessment of procedural outcomes based on program experience and found that as program experience increased, conversion rate to OHS decreased. An emergency OHS protocol that delineates specific roles and responsibilities is essential for every new program. Table 9.12 provides an example of key concepts for an emergency OHS protocol.[46] Similar protocols should be developed for situations in which unexpected cardiopulmonary resuscitation is indicated or conversion from LA/CS to GA is required.

TABLE 9.12. Concepts for an Emergency Protocol for Conversion to Open Heart Surgery

Preprocedural Preparation	
Procedural team members defined with clear roles for procedure *and* during emergent transitions	Proceduralists: Interventional Cardiologist and Cardiac Surgeon Anesthesia/CRNA Scrub Nurse/First Assist Circulating Nurse Circulator#2: Nurse or CVT Monitor
Ventricular support	Cardiopulmonary bypass protocol defined Appropriate cannula and instruments available
Severe hemorrhage management	Cell saver set up Rapid fluid infusion device available Cross-match blood readily accessible

TABLE 9.12. Concepts for an Emergency Protocol for Conversion to Open Heart Surgery (Continued)

Intraoperative management	
Initiation of protocols	Protocol initiated by proceduralist in charge Circulator calls for additional nursing/CVT assistance
Room setup	CVT moves C-arm Circulator moves monitors and lines away from table Scrub assistant secures wires and moves to assistant side of table
Resuscitation	Proceduralist begins CPR Anesthesia calls for 2nd anesthesia team member Anesthesia secures airway if performed under sedation Anesthesia begins resuscitation with fluid and pharmacologic support as needed Rapid fluid infuser hooked up to patient
Perfusion	Perfusionist moves cell saver to surgical position Perfusionist moves pump to table Assistant takes lines up, clamps, and divides Circulator passes cannula and insertion tools to scrub nurse
Diagnosis and monitoring	Anesthesia continuously monitors hemodynamics and communicates vital signs to team Consider adjuncts of TEE for monitoring and diagnosis
Cannulation	Surgeon in charge exposes the heart, calls for heparin Anesthesia ensures appropriate heparin dose 2nd surgeon cannulates femorally, connects patient to CPB and initiates bypass

CPB, cardiopulmonary bypass; CPR, cardiopulmonary resuscitation; CRNA, certified registered nurse anesthetist; CVT, cardiovascular technician; TEE, transesophageal echocardiography.
Kapadia SR, Kodali S, Makkar R, et al. Protection against cerebral embolism during transcatheter aortic valve replacement. *J Am Coll Cardiol.* 2017;69(4):367-377.

Conclusions

Transcatheter treatment of the aortic valve has emerged as the preferred replacement strategy for severe symptomatic aortic stenosis; however, there is tremendous variation in how the procedure is performed. The primary objective of this chapter is to provide a framework for the procedural aspects of TAVR. There is no standard protocol; instead, each institution must develop its own processes that allow for operator and institutional preferences and the multidisciplinary Heart Team must plan each case according to unique patient needs. The general content of this chapter provides an in-depth description of the perspective of a high-volume large urban TAVR center in the United States. Examples of tools and checklists are provided. These examples may be applied in the context of the most recent professional society guidelines, and combined with local requirements and clinical practice, to assist with the development of a site-specific procedural pathway.

KEY TAKEAWAYS AND BEST PRACTICES

▶ Each institution must develop site-specific, patient-centric TAVR protocols that integrate evidence and best practices for patient-centered, procedural care.

▶ A multidisciplinary, multimodality approach to patient evaluation can be safely applied to a minimalist approach to the procedure: minimizing risks and exposure related to sedation/anesthesia, invasive lines, and invasive vascular access. Emerging evidence demonstrates that a minimalist approach with CS/LA and intraprocedural transthoracic echocardiography is associated with improved survival, procedural times, fluoroscopy times, intensive care unit times, and length of stay.

▶ Whenever safe and feasible for the patient and Heart Team, percutaneous transfemoral access is the preferred approach for TAVR. This is associated with the most favorable procedural and long-term outcomes when compared with alternative access. Emerging vascular access approaches, such as transcaval and transaxillary/subclavian, are also used and may also be performed percutaneously.

▶ Use of a urinary catheter at the time of TAVR, which has been associated with an increased risk of infection, bleeding, and prolonged length of stay, should be avoided except in select cases.

▶ The patient's goals, medical history, risk-benefit ratio, anatomy, and unique care requirements are key considerations to determine the right care and the right place for TAVR.

References

1. Cribier A, Eltchaninoff H, Bash A, et al. Percutaneous transcatheter implantation of an aortic valve prosthesis for calcific aortic stenosis: first human case description. *Circulation.* 2002;106(24):3006-3008.
2. Holmes DR, Nishimura RA, Grover FL, et al. Annual outcomes with transcatheter valve therapy: from the STS/ACC TVT registry. *Ann Thorac Surg.* 2016;101(2):789-800.
3. Auffret V, Lefevre T, Van Belle E, et al. Temporal trends in transcatheter aortic valve replacement in France: FRANCE 2 to FRANCE TAVI. *J Am Coll Cardiol.* 2017;70(1):42-55.
4. Tommaso CL, Bolman RM, Feldman T, et al. Multisociety (AATS, ACCF, SCAI, and STS) expert consensus statement: operator and institutional requirements for transcatheter valve repair and replacement, part 1: transcatheter aortic valve replacement. *J Am Coll Cardiol.* 2012;59(22):2028-2042.
5. Walters DL, Webster M, Pasupati S, et al. Position statement for the operator and institutional requirements for a transcatheter aortic valve implantation (TAVI) program. *Heart Lung Circ.* 2015;24(3):219-223.

6. Centers for Medicare and Medicaid Services. *National Coverage Determination for Transcatheter Aortic Valve Replacement*. 2012. https://www.cms.gov/medicare-coverage-database/details/ ncd-details. aspx?NCDId=355&ncdver=1&NCAId=257&ver=4&NcaName=Transcath- eter+Aortic+Valve+ Replacement+(TAVR)&bc=ACAAAAAACAAAAA%3D%3D&. Accessed September 24, 2012.

7. Bypass Angioplasty Revascularization Investigation I. Comparison of coronary bypass surgery with angioplasty in patients with multivessel disease. *N Engl J Med*. 1996;335(4):217-225.

8. Serruys PW, Morice MC, Kappetein AP, et al. Percutaneous coronary intervention versus coronary-artery bypass grafting for severe coronary artery disease. *N Engl J Med*. 2009;360(10):961-972.

9. Otto CM, Kumbhani DJ, Alexander KP, et al. 2017 ACC expert consensus decision pathway for transcatheter aortic valve replacement in the management of adults with aortic stenosis: a report of the American College of Cardiology Task Force on Clinical Expert Consensus Documents. *J Am Coll Cardiol*. 2017;69(10):1313-1346.

10. Grover FL, Vemulapalli S, Carroll JD, et al. 2016 annual report of The Society of Thoracic Surgeons/American College of Cardiology Transcatheter Valve Therapy Registry. *J Am Coll Cardiol*. 2017;69(10):1215-1230.

11. Hyman MC, Vemulapalli S, Szeto WY, et al. Conscious sedation versus general anesthesia for transcatheter aortic valve replacement: insights from the National Cardiovascular Data Registry Society of Thoracic Surgeons/American College of Cardiology Transcatheter Valve Therapy Registry. *Circulation*. 2017;136(22):2132-2140.

12. Pani S, Cagino J, Feustel P, et al. Patient selection and outcomes of transfemoral transcatheter aortic valve replacement performed with monitored anesthesia care versus general anesthesia. *J Cardiothorac Vasc Anesth*. 2017;31(6):2049-2054.

13. Villablanca PA, Mohananey D, Nikolic K, et al. Comparison of local versus general anesthesia in patients undergoing transcatheter aortic valve replacement: a meta-analysis. *Catheter Cardiovasc Interv*. 2017.

14. Krishnaswamy A, Latib A, Malik A, et al. Resource utilization for transfemoral transcatheter aortic valve replacement: an international comparison. *Catheter Cardiovasc Interv*. 2016;87(1):145-151.

15. Eggebrecht H, Vaquerizo B, Moris C, et al. Incidence and outcomes of emergent cardiac surgery during transfemoral transcatheter aortic valve implantation (TAVI): insights from the European Registry on Emergent Cardiac Surgery during TAVI (EuRECS-TAVI). *Eur Heart J*. 2017.

16. Carroll JD, Vemulapalli S, Dai D, et al. Procedural experience for transcatheter aortic valve replacement and relation to outcomes: the STS/ACC TVT registry. *J Am Coll Cardiol*. 2017;70(1):29-41.

17. *WHO Guidelines for Safe Surgery 2009: Safe Surgery Saves Lives*. Geneva 2009.

18. Haynes AB, Weiser TG, Berry WR, et al. A surgical safety checklist to reduce morbidity and mortality in a global population. *N Engl J Med*. 2009;360(5):491-499.

19. Ifedili IA, Bolorunduro O, Bob-Manuel T, et al. Impact of pre-existing kidney dysfunction on outcomes following transcatheter aortic valve replacement. *Curr Cardiol Rev*. 2017;13(4):283-292.

20. Vijayasekar C, Steele RJ. The World Health Organization's surgical safety checklist. *Surgeon*. 2009;7(5):260-262.

21. Afshar AH, Pourafkari L, Nader ND. Periprocedural considerations of transcatheter aortic valve implantation for anesthesiologists. *J Cardiovasc Thorac Res*. 2016;8(2):49-55.

22. Lauck SB, Kwon JY, Wood DA, et al. Avoidance of urinary catheterization to minimize in-hospital complications after transcatheter aortic valve implantation: an observational study. *Eur J Cardiovasc Nurs*. 2018;17(1):66-74.

23. Hooton TM, Bradley SF, Cardenas DD, et al. Diagnosis, prevention, and treatment of catheter-associated urinary tract infection in adults: 2009 International Clinical Practice Guidelines from the Infectious Diseases Society of America. *Clin Infect Dis*. 2010;50(5):625-663.

24. Chant C, Smith OM, Marshall JC, Friedrich JO. Relationship of catheter-associated urinary tract infection to mortality and length of stay in critically ill patients: a systematic review and meta-analysis of observational studies. *Crit Care Med*. 2011;39(5):1167-1173.

25. Eide LS, Ranhoff AH, Fridlund B, et al. Comparison of frequency, risk factors, and time course of postoperative delirium in octogenarians after transcatheter aortic valve implantation versus surgical aortic valve replacement. *Am J Cardiol*. 2015;115(6):802-809.

26. Manning MW, Diaz L, Jr., Weigner MB, Donnelly CL, Greenberg MR. Post transapical aortic valve replacement (TAVR) pseudoaneurysm. *West J Emerg Med*. 2014;15(7):895-896.

27. Al-Attar N, Raffoul R, Himbert D, Brochet E, Vahanian A, Nataf P. False aneurysm after transapical aortic valve implantation. *J Thorac Cardiovasc Surg*. 2009;137(1):e21-22.

28. Muraru D, Napodano M, Beltrame V, Badano LP. Left ventricular pseudoaneurysm after transapical aortic valve-in-valve implantation: use of transthoracic 3D echocardiography for guiding therapeutic approach. *Eur Heart J*. 2016;37(15):1255.

29. Thourani VH, Li C, Devireddy C, et al. High-risk patients with inoperative aortic stenosis: use of transapical, transaortic, and transcarotid techniques. *Ann Thorac Surg*. 2015;99(3):817-823; discussion 823-815.

30. Gleason TG, Schindler JT, Hagberg RC, et al. Subclavian/axillary access for self-expanding transcatheter aortic valve replacement renders equivalent outcomes as transfemoral. *Ann Thorac Surg*. 2017.

31. Schofer N, Deuschl F, Conradi L, et al. Preferential short cut or alternative route: the transaxillary access for transcatheter aortic valve implantation. *J Thorac Dis*. 2015;7(9):1543-1547.

32. Lederman RJ, Babaliaros VC, Greenbaum AB. How to perform transcaval access and closure for transcatheter aortic valve implantation. *Catheter Cardiovasc Interv*. 2015;86(7):1242-1254.

33. Greenbaum AB, O'Neill WW, Paone G, et al. Caval-aortic access to allow transcatheter aortic valve replacement in otherwise ineligible patients: initial human experience. *J Am Coll Cardiol*. 2014;63(25 Pt A):2795-2804.

34. Mylotte D, Sudre A, Teiger E, et al. Transcarotid transcatheter aortic valve replacement: feasibility and safety. *JACC Cardiovasc Interv*. 2016;9(5):472-480.

35. Szeto WY, Augoustides JG, Desai ND, et al. Cerebral embolic exposure during transfemoral and transapical transcatheter aortic valve replacement. *J Card Surg*. 2011;26(4):348-354.

36. Lansky AJ, Brown D, Pena C, et al. Neurologic complications of unprotected transcatheter aortic valve implantation (from the Neuro-TAVI trial). *Am J Cardiol*. 2016;118(10):1519-1526.

37. Kapadia SR, Kodali S, Makkar R, et al. Protection against cerebral embolism during transcatheter aortic valve replacement. *J Am Coll Cardiol*. 2017;69(4):367-377.

38. Seeger J, Gonska B, Otto M, Rottbauer W, Wohrle J. Cerebral embolic protection during transcatheter aortic valve replacement significantly reduces death and stroke compared with unprotected procedures. *JACC Cardiovasc interventions*. 2017;10(22):2297-2303.

39. Gallo M, Putzu A, Conti M, Pedrazzini G, Demertzis S, Ferrari E. Embolic protection devices for transcatheter aortic valve replacement. *Eur J Cardiothorac Surg*. 2017.

40. Haussig S, Mangner N, Dwyer MG, et al. Effect of a cerebral protection device on brain lesions following transcatheter aortic valve implantation in patients with severe aortic stenosis: The CLEAN-TAVI randomized clinical trial. *JAMA*. 2016;316(6):592-601.

41. Erkapic D, De Rosa S, Kelava A, Lehmann R, Fichtlscherer S, Hohnloser SH. Risk for permanent pacemaker after transcatheter aortic valve implantation: a comprehensive analysis of the literature. *J Cardiovasc Electrophysiol*. 2012;23(4):391-397.

42. Khatri PJ, Webb JG, Rodes-Cabau J, et al. Adverse effects associated with transcatheter aortic valve implantation: a meta-analysis of contemporary studies. *Ann Intern Med*. 2013;158(1):35-46.

43. Auffret V, Puri R, Urena M, et al. Conduction disturbances after transcatheter aortic valve replacement: current status and future perspectives. *Circulation*. 2017;136(11):1049-1069.

44. Chaudhry MA, Sardar MR. Vascular complications of transcatheter aortic valve replacement: a concise literature review. *World J Cardiol.* 2017;9(7):574-582.
45. Singh V, Damluji AA, Mendirichaga R, et al. Elective or emergency use of mechanical circulatory support devices during transcatheter aortic valve replacement. *J Interv Cardiol.* 2016;29(5):513-522.
46. Tam DY, Jones PM, Kiaii B, et al. Salvaging catastrophe in transcatheter aortic valve implantation: rehearsal, preassigned roles, and emergency preparedness. *Can J Anaesth.* 2015;62(8):918-926.

CHAPTER 10

Success Is When the Patient Goes Home: Postprocedure Care

Amanda Kirby, DNP, APNP, ACNP-BC

OBJECTIVES

▶ Outline recommendations for a comprehensive postprocedure care pathway

▶ Discuss strategies to mitigate risk of geriatric deconditioning

▶ Highlight the importance of discharge planning

Introduction

As discussed in prior chapters, a multidisciplinary Heart Team with well-developed pathways for evaluation, case selection, and procedural planning is essential for optimal postprocedure outcomes. The valve program clinician is well suited to manage the fundamental components of an individualized postprocedure patient care pathway. Clinical leadership is needed to balance vigilant monitoring of potential postprocedure complications and avoidance of prolonged hospitalization. For the multidisciplinary team involved from referral to discharge, program success is when the patient goes home. This chapter outlines the essential elements and priorities of the postprocedure period to achieve this goal.

Transcatheter aortic valve replacement (TAVR) programs have unique challenges to facilitate the goal of safe transition home. The patient population is largely geriatric with a varying burden of comorbidities and, in many cases, the potential for functional and/or cognitive decline. The familiarity that the Heart Team develops with individual patients during the comprehensive evaluation process, as described in chapter 4, supports the ability to identify risks for complications and adjust the care pathway accordingly. To this end, the priorities for care include vigilant monitoring of specified clinical targets, prevention of complications, and facilitation of return to baseline status.[1] These are dictated by procedural factors, common characteristics of the general patient population undergoing TAVR, and individual patient features. Procedural factors include the type of anesthesia, access site, occurrence of conduction disturbances or arrhythmias, and other postprocedure complications. Relevant patient characteristics include demographics, comorbid conditions, presence of frailty, functional or cognitive decline, and social support structure.

In 2017, the American College of Cardiology released an expert consensus document that included guidance for essential elements of postprocedure management.[2] These elements systematically focus on key milestones for recovery and risks for potential complications (Table 10.1). The development and utilization of standardized postprocedure order sets facilitate an organized approach to management of these clinical priorities and early detection of complications.

Infrastructure

Recovery Area

The postprocedure care plan should focus on relevant clinical factors and surveillance for potential complications. Individual patient features affect the recovery timeline, but discharge from the hospital should occur as soon as safe and feasible. The location for postprocedure recovery will vary from institution to institution. Many centers use recovery areas adjacent to the catheterization laboratory or operating room for the first several hours of monitoring

TABLE 10.1. Checklist for Post-TAVR Clinical Management

Key Steps	Essential Elements	Additional Details
Immediate Postprocedure Management		
Waking from sedation	☐ Early extubation (general anesthesia) ☐ Monitor mental status	
Postprocedure monitoring	☐ Telemetry and vital signs per hospital protocol for general or moderate sedation ☐ Monitor intake and output ☐ Laboratory results (complete blood count and metabolic panel) ☐ Monitor access (groin or thorax) site for bleeding, hematoma, pseudoaneurysm	☐ Ultrasound scan of groin site if concern for pseudoaneurysm ☐ Frequent neurological assessment
Pain management	☐ Provide appropriate pain management ☐ Monitor mental status	
Early mobilization	☐ Mobilize as soon as access site allows ☐ Manage comorbidities ☐ PT and OT assessment	☐ Encourage physical activity
Discharge planning	☐ Resume preoperative medications ☐ Plan discharge location ☐ Predischarge echocardiogram and ECG ☐ Schedule postdischarge clinic visits	☐ Family and social support ☐ Ability to perform ADLs ☐ Transportation ☐ Discharge medications ☐ Patient instructions and education

(Continued)

TABLE 10.1. Checklist for Post-TAVR Clinical Management (Continued)

Key Steps	Essential Elements	Additional Details
Long-Term Follow-up		
Timing	☐ TAVR team at 30 d ☐ Primary cardiologist at 6 mo and then annually ☐ Primary care MD or geriatrician at 3 mo and then as needed	☐ Hand-off from TAVR team to primary cardiologist at 30 d ☐ More frequent follow-up if needed for changes in symptoms, or transient conduction abnormalities ☐ Coordination of care among TAVR team, primary cardiologist, and primary care MD
Antithrombotic therapy	☐ ASA 75-100 mg daily lifelong ☐ Clopidogrel 75 mg daily for 3-6 mo ☐ Consider warfarin (INR 2.0-2.5) if at risk of AF or VTE	☐ Management when warfarin or NOAC needed for other indications
Concurrent cardiac disease	☐ Coronary disease ☐ Hypertension ☐ Heart failure ☐ Arrhythmias (especially AF) ☐ Manage cardiac risk factors (including diet and physical activity)	☐ Monitor laboratory results for blood counts, metabolic panel, renal function ☐ Assess pulmonary, renal, GI, and neurological function by primary care MD annually or as needed
Monitor for post-TAVR complications	☐ Echocardiography at 30 d then annually (if needed) ☐ ECG at 30 d and annually ☐ Consider 24 h ECG if bradycardia	☐ Paravalvular AR ☐ New heart block ☐ LV function ☐ PA systolic pressure
Dental hygiene and antibiotic prophylaxis	☐ Encourage optimal dental care ☐ Antibiotic prophylaxis per AHA/ACC guidelines	

ACC, American College of Cardiology; ADLs, activities of daily living; AF, atrial fibrillation; AHA, American Heart Association; AR, aortic regurgitation; ASA, aspirin; ECG, electrocardiogram; GI, gastrointestinal; INR, international normalized ratio; LV, left ventricular; MD, medical doctor; NOAC, new oral anticoagulant; OT, occupational therapy; PA, pulmonary artery; PT, physical therapy; TAVR, transcatheter aortic valve replacement; VTE, venous thromboembolism.

Reprinted with permission from Otto CM, Kumbhani DJ, Alexander KP, et al. 2017 ACC expert consensus decision pathway for transcatheter aortic valve replacement in the management of adults with aortic stenosis: a report of the American College of Cardiology Task Force on Clinical Expert Consensus Documents. *J Am Coll Cardiol.* 2017;69:1313-1346.

postprocedure, followed by transfer to a step-down telemetry unit for 1 to 2 days before discharge. Postprocedure recovery in a critical care unit is less common, especially in the case of an uncomplicated, femoral access TAVR. There may be circumstances associated with the use of alternative access or clinical instability when such a setting is necessary.

TABLE 10.2. Care Management Models

Primary Physician Care Model	Valve Service Care Model
• Primary physician follows patient throughout hospitalization • Oversight of all aspects of postprocedure care • May be assisted by residents/fellows and/or advanced practice providers • Supports continuity of care • May work best for new or growing programs as time for rounding on patients may be a factor	• Valve service coverage throughout hospitalization • Rotating assignment of Heart Team members • Service staffed by attending physicians, residents/fellows, and/or advanced practice providers • Oversight of all aspects of postprocedure care • Supports continuity of care • Requires adequate staffing resources • May work best for established, high-volume programs

Management Models

The implementation of a Heart Team care model for postprocedure patient management promotes consistency of care. Two examples are described in Table 10.2. It should be noted that these models are representative of collective experience and can be revised to suit the needs of individual programs based on program size, Heart Team preferences, and resources. The selection of a care model is a dynamic process that requires adjustment as a program evolves.

Priorities of Care

The valve program clinician plays a significant role in the postprocedure care pathway and leverages the familiarity acquired during the evaluation process to contribute to an individualized approach to care. The following section outlines the priorities and procedures for postprocedure monitoring by reviewing the goals of care, anticipated outcomes, and associated interventions. Importantly, institutional standards and protocols vary across programs and remain the primary resource for valve program clinicians and other team members to guide postprocedure care.

Recovery From Sedation/Anesthesia

Although general anesthesia remains the strategy of choice for many TAVR procedures, moderate sedation and local anesthesia are increasingly used.[2]

- Goal of care: Safe return to preprocedure level of function without residual effect of anesthesia/sedation
- Anticipated outcomes:
  - Extubation in the procedure room; stable ventilation and oxygenation
  - Intact neurological status
  - Hemodynamic stability
  - Ability to take oral fluids with advancement of diet according to institutional standards
  - Absence of pain
- Interventions:
  - Monitor vital signs and neurological status according to institutional standards
  - Monitor pain and discomfort

Hemostasis

Proficiency in vascular access monitoring is a core competency of nurses and allied health professionals who care for patients undergoing TAVR. Although there are variations in procedural approach to vascular access such as surgical cut down versus percutaneous access, the principles of postprocedure vascular access assessment remain the same. Staff members must be aware of institutional protocols regarding frequency of access assessment, bed rest parameters, and early warning signs of possible complications.

- Goal of care: Successful hemostasis
  - Successful deployment of vascular closure devices, if applicable
  - Safe and timely removal of vascular access sheaths
  - Access site hemostasis before transfer from procedure room
  - Maintenance of distal perfusion
- Anticipated outcomes:
  - Absence of vascular access injury and bleeding
  - Ability to mobilize according to institutional standards
  - Patient comfort
- Interventions:
  - Monitor access site(s) according to institutional standards with attention to the presence of bleeding, hematoma, pain, and swelling
  - Monitor distal perfusion according to institutional standards (eg, color, warmth, movement, sensation)
  - Monitor hemoglobin and hematocrit according to institutional standards

Cardiac Rhythm Monitoring

Atrioventricular (AV) block is the most common conduction disturbance following TAVR with both balloon-expandable and self-expanding TAVR platforms.[3] The risk for AV block is related to the anatomical proximity of the conduction system to the aortic valve; the need for a new permanent pacemaker varies with current-generation TAVR devices. The preexistence of right bundle branch block or left anterior fascicular block, small left ventricular outflow tract, and valve deployment depth are known predictors of increased risk of postimplantation conduction delays. The European Society of Cardiology has recommended monitoring of complete heart block and/or high-grade AV block for 7 days.[4] As evidence is still evolving, the uptake of this recommendation is not uniform across regions, including in the United States.

- Goal of care: Stable cardiac conduction and hemodynamic stability
- Anticipated outcomes:
  - Removal of transvenous pacemaker at end of procedure prior unless contraindicated
  - Maintenance of baseline rhythm
  - Early awareness of any changes (eg, lengthening PR interval)
  - Early intervention for new or worsening conduction disturbances or arrhythmias
- Interventions:
  - Obtain preprocedure electrocardiogram (ECG) for physicians or delegates to conduct screening of high-risk features and use for comparison

- Conduct telemetry and ECG monitoring and documentation of cardiac rhythm according to institutional standards
- Consider the avoidance of nodal blocking agents according to institutional standards
- If applicable, facilitate the removal of the temporary transvenous pacemaker as soon as clinically feasible to promote mobilization

Neurological Status

The incidence of both major and minor neurological events post TAVR continues to decrease; yet, stroke remains a devastating complication for some patients.[5] This is of particular concern as improved quality of life and the avoidance of disabling complications are priorities for patients and their families. The period of immediate postprocedure recovery requires close scrutiny of impaired neurological function to ensure early identification and treatment. Careful monitoring of the level of consciousness remains an essential standard of care. Abnormal findings must trigger communication with physicians or delegates, a more extensive neurological examination, diagnostic imaging, and/or emergency intervention if indicated.

- Goal of care: Stable neurological status
- Anticipated outcomes:
  - Preservation of baseline neurological status
  - Accurate monitoring
  - Early detection of alteration in the level of consciousness
  - Timely intervention to treat neurological complication
- Interventions:
  - Monitor neurological status according to institutional standards (eg, Glasgow Coma Scale, pupil size and reactivity)
  - Document and communicate altered level of consciousness
  - Facilitate diagnostic imaging (eg, computed tomography and/or magnetic resonance imaging) as indicated

Mobilization

Early mobilization is the most important strategy to avoid the rapid onset of muscle wasting and deconditioning associated with hospitalization and bedrest.[6] Expectations about anticipated time to mobilization should be clearly outlined in preprocedure patient education resources and consistently reinforced by all members of the health care team. Postprocedure bedrest is usually maintained for 4 to 6 hours to facilitate hemostasis.[6] Thereafter, a progressive mobilization pathway should include ambulation to the bathroom to assist with return to normal elimination patterns and transfer to a chair for meals to promote resumption of activities of daily living. For most patients, a nurse-led activity protocol is the most effective approach, whereas patients with more complex conditions may benefit from a physical therapy consultation. Families can play an essential role in emphasizing the importance of activity and self-care behavior.

- Goal of care: Rapid return to baseline mobilization and activities of daily living
- Anticipated outcomes:
  - Standardized strategy to achieve consistent early mobilization targets
  - Promotion of nursing role and competencies to lead post-TAVR mobilization protocol for most patients

- Early identification of inability to meet mobilization target and need for modified intervention and discharge plan
- Interventions:
  - Determine safety for early mobilization
  - Assist with ambulation to the bathroom
  - Facilitate transfer to chair for meals
  - Promote small, frequent periods of activity (including self-care)
  - Engage family to promote mobilization
  - Ensure availability of mobility aids, if used at baseline
  - Physical therapy consult for patients with new mobility deficits

Renal Function

Impaired renal function is a significant challenge for many patients undergoing TAVR and can be further compounded by the risk of acute kidney injury (AKI) in the postprocedure phase. AKI has been documented in as many as 8.3% to 58% of patients and has been shown to be associated with a 2- to 6-fold increase in post-TAVR mortality rates.[7-9] Consequently, identifying patients at increased risk for developing AKI following TAVR and close monitoring of renal function have substantial implications for the management of these higher-risk patients in the postoperative period. Risk factors for contrast-induced nephropathy include chronic kidney disease and diabetes, whereas the volume of periprocedure contrast administration can further worsen patients' renal vulnerabilities.

- Goal of care: Stable renal function and early awareness of postprocedure alterations in renal function
- Anticipated outcome:
  - Preservation of baseline renal status
- Interventions:
  - Record patients' renal baseline function and volume of contrast administration
  - Monitor renal function parameters (estimated glomerular filtration rate, creatinine, blood urea nitrogen) according to institutional standards
  - Promote adequate fluid intake; if not on fluid restrictions, encourage fluids
  - Monitor intake and output
  - Communicate signs and symptoms of worsening renal function; anticipate need for nephrology consultation as required

Mental Status

Delirium refers to the acute onset and fluctuating course of symptoms related to cognitive dysfunction, including decreased consciousness, inattention, disorientation, and impaired memory.[10] Predisposing factors include advanced age, preexisting cognitive impairment, and previous stroke, whereas surgery, medication changes, and hospitalization can be precipitating factors.[11] Delirium is potentially preventable and often unrecognized. This complication is common in over 30% of patients older than 70 years undergoing cardiac surgery and has a high morbidity and mortality rate. Data about incidence after TAVR are scarcer,[12] but careful vigilance and early intervention are essential to mitigate risks. General anesthesia and extended ventilation, use of opioids, and extended hospitalization increase patients' risk of developing delirium and warrant careful consideration.[13]

- Goals of care: Stable mental status
- Anticipated outcome:
  - Maintenance of baseline mental status without episodes of confusion or delirium
- Interventions:
  - Monitor mental status according to institutional standards
  - Avoid opioids and other medications that may contribute to confusion and/or delirium
  - Facilitate maintenance of normal sleep and wake cycle
  - Facilitate rapid recovery and discharge, if clinically feasible

Infection

Although the incidence of access and device-related infection is low,[14] the risks of other iatrogenic complications require heightened vigilance and prevention strategies. In particular, patients undergoing TAVR can be vulnerable to urinary tract infections secondary to catheterization, upper respiratory infections, or other hospital-acquired infections because of their age, frailty, impaired immunity, and overall health status.

- Goals of care: Prevention of infection
- Anticipated outcomes:
  - Freedom from infection
  - Early detection and treatment as required
- Interventions:
  - Avoidance of invasive lines; if clinically necessary, removal as soon as feasible
  - Avoidance of urinary catheter
  - Early mobilization
  - Laboratory specimen collection for infection surveillance according to institutional standards

Putting It All Together

The use of standardized protocols and prescribers' order sets are effective institutional strategies to promote best practices and ensure consistency of care across the program. For the purpose of providing an example, content for a nursing protocol or nursing care standard is outlined in Table 10.3, whereas Table 10.4 presents potential content for prescribers' orders.

Potential Complications

The priorities of care relate to the avoidance of the complications associated with TAVR. The evaluation of outcomes center on the standardized reporting of the Valve Academic Research Consortium (VARC-2)[15] discussed in detail in chapter 13. A working understanding of these quality indicators and how they are measured is essential for the valve program clinician to provide leadership. The VARC-2 quality indicators are outlined in Table 10.5.

In addition, length of stay should be considered an important quality indicator of postprocedure care. The increased awareness of the negative impact of extended hospitalization after TAVR and the opportunities to facilitate safe early discharge home for most patients signal the importance of monitoring length of stay to promote quality improvement.

TABLE 10.3. Potential Content for Postprocedure Nursing Care Protocol

Postprocedure Assessment

• Vital signs

• Neurological status

• Cardiac rhythm, PR interval, ST segment

• Heart sounds

• Respiratory rate, breathing, and breath sounds

• If recent extubation: trachea auscultation and assessment of potential stridor or respiratory impairment

• Signs of bleeding (blood at vascular access sites, swelling or palpable hematoma, bruising)

• Limb perfusion: color, warmth, movement, sensation, peripheral pulses

• Pain (vascular access sites, back/postural pain)

Interventions

Consider/notify the responsible physician/care provider immediately if postprocedure assessment findings reveal:

• Diminishing level of consciousness, asymmetrical physical responses that are changes from baseline

• Hemodynamic instability

• New arrhythmias, including new AV block/lengthening PR interval

• Decreasing QRS amplitude

• Distant or muffled heart sounds

• Labored respiratory efforts, increasing supplemental oxygen requirements, and/or asymmetrical chest expansion

• Urine output <0.5 mL/kg/hr or urinary retention not responsive to nursing interventions

• Active bleeding or expanding hematoma at any percutaneous sheath insertion and/or puncture site(s)

• Signs of diminished peripheral circulation or limb ischemia (eg, diminished pulse strength, cool skin, pale/dusky skin pallor, new sensory changes such as numbness/tingling)

• Change in clinical status

Components of Clinical Pathway

• Monitoring protocol

• Timing of removal of invasive lines

• Activity protocol (including bedrest and progressive nurse-led activity protocol)

• Elimination, hydration, nutrition protocols

• Patient teaching and discharge planning

TABLE 10.4. Potential Content for Postprocedure Prescribers' Orders

Monitoring:

- Telemetry
- Vital signs
- Vascular access site assessment
- Neurological assessment
- Removal of invasive lines (sheath, central line, temporary pacemaker as indicated)
- Consider statement about avoidance of urinary catheterization

Diet and Hydration

Activity:

- Bedrest time
- Activity protocol

Laboratory:

- CBC, electrolytes, renal profile
- INR as required

Diagnostics:

- ECG
- Transthoracic echocardiogram

Medications

- Resumption of baseline medications
- VTE prophylaxis as required
- Antiplatelet
- Anticoagulation
- Analgesia (consider statement to avoid opioids)

Discharge Target

CBC, complete blood count; ECG, electrocardiogram; INR, international normalized ratio; VTE, venous thromboembolism

TABLE 10.5. VARC-2 Quality Indicators

Mortality
Myocardial infarction
Stroke
Bleeding
Acute kidney injury
Vascular access site complications
Conduction disturbances and arrhythmias
Device success
Quality of life

Preparation for Discharge and Patient Teaching

Predischarge Diagnostics

The surveillance of laboratory values (eg, complete blood count, electrolyte, renal profile) is done to confirm the return to baseline values. The completion of a predischarge 12-lead ECG and the comparison with previous reports is essential to rule out new conduction delays, new onset of atrial arrhythmias, or other complications. Lastly, a postprocedure transthoracic echocardiogram is standard practice in TAVR centers. The most salient elements include confirmation of valve position, measurement of transvalvular gradients, absence of pericardial effusion, and reporting of biventricular function.[2]

Discharge Medications

Preprocedure medications should be resumed unless contraindicated to enable the patient's responsible physician to coordinate regimen changes. The optimal antithrombotic therapy after TAVR remains controversial; evidence continues to evolve rapidly. Dual antiplatelet therapy (aspirin and clopidogrel) has been used in the pivotal trials and subsequently adopted in clinical practice given the lack of clinical trial data.[16] There is debate about the effectiveness of a strategy of aspirin only to reduce the incidence of major life-threatening bleeding without increasing the risk of ischemic events.[17] Similarly, the role of warfarin to mitigate the risks of valve leaflet thrombosis and other thromboembolic events is also under investigation.[18] In this relatively unstable clinical context, the valve program clinician can play an important role in the implementation of medical recommendations to develop local agreements.

Discharge Teaching

Effective discharge teaching is an essential component of patient safety and an important strategy to facilitate transition of care from the TAVR center to home. Discharge teaching should start at the time of the initial assessment, be reinforced throughout the patient's admission, and be confirmed at the time of discharge. Consistent communication on the part of all team members about the target length of stay is essential to ensure that details about transportation, social support requirements, and follow-up are carefully planned. The period of transition of care and the risks of postdischarge fragmentation of health services can jeopardize patient safety and contribute to adverse events.[19] Table 10.6 includes possible components of a comprehensive discharge teaching plan.

Some valve programs have a standardized communication process in place to facilitate postdischarge communication, initiated by the center or the patient/family to mitigate the risks of adverse events and hospital readmission. Postprocedure "coaching" can be an effective strategy to ensure successful transitions of care.[20]

Staff Education

Ongoing education of the nursing and allied health team responsible for postprocedure patient care is an essential component of a successful TAVR program. Professional development focused on the unique components of the TAVR procedure, patient population, and processes of care helps to ensure that the clinical staff is aware of evolving evidence; ongoing dialogue and engagement with the frontline team provides the opportunity for revisions to established practices, quality improvement projects, and increased programmatic capacity. Sharing the patient pathway, care model, and patient case studies with staff regularly and involving them in brainstorming for improvement of patient care will gain support and continue their engagement in providing high-quality care.

TABLE 10.6. Components of a Comprehensive Discharge Teaching Plan

Discharge Teaching Plan Components
• Patient discharge education information sheet/brochure
• Referral to cardiac rehabilitation and information about activity
• Written information about discharge medications
• Wound care and signs of access-related complications
• Information about the TAVR device
• Confirmation of transportation plan for return home and availability of social support as required
• Follow-up appointments (including 30-d transthoracic echocardiogram)
• Contact information/instructions for communicating need for readmission and management of postdischarge complications
• Instructions about resumption of driving
• Prophylactic antibiotic requirements for future invasive and dental procedure

TAVR, transcatheter aortic valve replacement.

Conclusion

A standardized and efficient postprocedure care pathway for patients undergoing TAVR is essential for achieving optimal clinical outcomes. The development and consistent implementation of processes of care require the engagement of the multidisciplinary Heart Team, as well as the nursing staff who deliver postprocedure care. The valve program clinician is well qualified to take a leading role in the development and oversight of a postprocedure pathway that attends to the priorities of care for patients post TAVR and facilitates return to an optimal level of function.

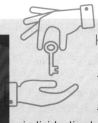

KEY TAKEAWAYS AND BEST PRACTICES

▶ The postprocedure care plan should focus on relevant clinical factors and surveillance for potential complications.

▶ The valve program clinician plays a significant role in the development of a postprocedure care pathway and an individualized approach to care.

▶ Careful attention needs to be paid to the vulnerabilities of the geriatric patient population undergoing TAVR to minimize postprocedure risk for complications.

▶ The collaboration of the multidisciplinary Heart Team is essential to achieve optimal outcomes.

References

1. Hawkey MC, Lauck SB, Perpetua EM, et al. Transcatheter aortic valve replacement program development: recommendations for best practice. *Catheter Cardiovasc Interv.* 2014;84:859-867.
2. Otto CM, Kumbhani DJ, Alexander KP, et al. 2017 ACC expert consensus decision pathway for transcatheter aortic valve replacement in the management of adults with aortic stenosis: a report of the American College of Cardiology Task Force on Clinical Expert Consensus Documents. *J Am Coll Cardiol.* 2017;69:1313-1346.
3. Bob-Manuel T, Nanda A, Latham S, et al. Permanent pacemaker insertion in patients with conduction abnormalities post transcatheter aortic valve replacement: a review and proposed guidelines. *Ann Transl Med.* 2017;6(1):11.
4. Brignole M, Auricchio A, Baron-Esquivias G, et al. 2013 ESC guidelines on cardiac pacing and cardiac resynchronization therapy: the task force on cardiac pacing and resynchronization therapy of the European Society of Cardiology (ESC). Developed in collaboration with the European Heart Rhythm Association (EHRA). *Europace.* 2013;15:1070-1118.
5. Kapadia SR, Kodali S, Makkar R, et al. Protection against cerebral embolism during transcatheter aortic valve replacement. *JACC.* 2017;69(4):367-377.
6. Lauck SB, Wood DA, Baumbusch J, et al. Vancouver transcatheter aortic valve replacement clinical pathway: minimalist approach, standardized care, and discharge criteria to reduce length of stay. *Circ Cardiovasc Qual Outcomes.* 2016;9(3):312-321.

7. Elhmidi Y, Bleiziffer S, Deutsch M-A, et al. Acute kidney injury after transcatheter aortic valve implantation: incidence, predictors and impact on mortality. *Arch Cardiovasc Dis*. 2014;107(2):133-139. doi:10.1016/j.acvd.2014.01.002.

8. Liao Y-B, Deng X-X, Meng Y, et al. Predictors and outcome of acute kidney injury after transcatheter aortic valve implantation – a systematic review and meta-analysis. *EuroIntervention*. 2016. doi:10.4244/EIJ-D-15-00254.

9. Gargiulo G, Capodanno D, Sannino A, et al. Moderate and severe pre-operative chronic kidney disease worsen clinical outcomes after transcatheter aortic valve implantation: meta-analysis of 4992 patients. *Circ Cardiovasc Interv*. 2015;8:e002220.

10. Inouye SK, Westendorp RGJ, Saczynski JS. Delirium in elderly people. *Lancet*. 2015;383:911-922.

11. Abawi M, Nijhoff F, Agostoni P, et al. Incidence, predictive factors, and effect of delirium after transcatheter aortic valve replacement. *JACC Cardiovasc Interv*. 2016;9(2):160-168. doi:10.1016/j.jcin.2015.09.037.

12. Soundhar A, Udesh R, Mehta A, et al. Delirium following transcatheter aortic valve replacement: national inpatient sample analysis. *J Cardiothorac Vasc Anesth*. 2017;31(6):1977-1984. doi:10.1053/j.jvca.2017.03.016.

13. Stachon P, Kaier K, Zirlik A, et al. Risk factors and outcome of postoperative delirium after transcatheter aortic valve replacement. *Clin Res Cardiol*. 2018. doi:10.1007/s00392-018-1241-3.

14. Amat-Santos IJ, Ribeiro HB, Urena M, et al. Prosthetic valve endocarditis after transcatheter valve replacement: a systematic review. *JACC Cardiovasc Interv*. 2015;8(2):334-346. doi:10.1016/j.jcin.2014.09.013.

15. Kappetein AP, Head SJ, Genereux P, et al. Updated standardized endpoint definitions for transcatheter aortic valve implantation: The Valve Academic Research Consortium-2 consensus document. *J Thorac Cardiovasc Surg*. 2013;145(1):6-23.

16. Nijenhuis VJ, Bennaghmouch N, van Kuijk JP, et al. Antithrombotic treatment in patients undergoing transcatheter aortic valve implantation (TAVI). *Thromb Haemost*. 2015;113(4):674-685.

17. Rodes-Cabau J, Masson JB, Welsh RC, et al. Aspirin versus aspirin plus Clopidogrel as antithrombotic treatment following transcatheter aortic valve replacement with a balloon-expandable valve: the ARTE (aspirin versus aspirin + clopidogrel following transcatheter aortic valve implantation) randomized clinical trial. *JACC Cardiovasc Interv*. 2017;10(13):1357-1365.

18. Gurevich S, Oestreich B, Kelly RF, et al. Routine use of anticoagulation after transcatheter aortic valve replacement: initial safety outcomes from a single-center experience. *Cardiovasc Revasc Med*. 2017. doi:10.1016/j.carrev.2017.12.001. pii:S1553-8389(17)30451-7.

19. Kothari AN, Loy VM, Brownlee SA, et al. Adverse effect of post-discharge care fragmentation on outcomes after readmissions after liver transplantation. *J Am Coll Surg*. 2017;225(1):62-67. doi:10.1016/j.jamcollsurg.2017.03.017.

20. Vora AN, Peterson ED, Hellkamp AS, et al. Care transitions after acute myocardial infarction for transferred-in versus direct-arrival patients. *Circ Cardiovasc Qual Outcomes*. 2016;9(2):109-116.

CHAPTER 11

Program Development and Optimization of Health Services

Elizabeth M. Perpetua, DNP, ACNP-BC, AACC

OBJECTIVES

▶ Describe the historical and current landscape of TAVR program development

▶ Apply a conceptual framework for program development, which incorporates a logic model of inputs, processes, outputs, and outcomes using the 5 Ws (why, who, what, where, when) and 3 Hs (how, how many, and how well)

▶ Provide specific examples and tools that may be used for TAVR program assessment and optimization

Introduction

Transcatheter aortic valve replacement (TAVR) and the programs that offer this therapy have evolved on pace with innovation, evidence, and guidelines. The international experience commenced in 2002 with Alain Cribier and colleagues, who performed the first TAVR in a patient with symptomatic severe aortic stenosis (AS) deemed ineligible for surgical aortic valve replacement (SAVR). Current indications for TAVR encompass patients at intermediate, high, and excessive surgical risk. Options for therapy include a full cadre of transcatheter valves and approaches for the treatment of aortic valve disease and failed aortic surgical prosthetic valves. Technological advances and emerging evidence have catalyzed major changes in cardiovascular care over a short period of time and have necessitated dynamic development and real-time optimization of the programs offering transcatheter valve therapy.

The purpose of this chapter is to review TAVR program development and optimization. The aims are to provide for program development: (1) a historical perspective; (2) a conceptual framework including the inputs, processes, and outputs for TAVR; and (3) specific examples and tools, which may facilitate site-specific translation and implementation of best practices.

Historical Perspective

Clinical trial constructs were incorporated into TAVR programs globally. A multidisciplinary Heart Team retained responsibility for diagnosis of symptomatic severe valvular heart disease (VHD) and objective evaluation of surgical risk and likelihood to benefit. Coordination of care across the continuum was emphasized and performed in some countries (eg, Canada[1] and the United States[2]) by a designated clinical coordinator instead of a research coordinator. Procedural standards included a room with fixed fluoroscopic imaging and a team of physicians and staff with hybrid cardiac catheterization laboratory and operating room competencies. Enrollment into postmarket registries was mandated to monitor safety and outcomes, later defined by the Valve Academic Research Consortium.[3-5]

Following *Conformité Européenne* mark of the Edwards Lifesciences SAPIEN and Medtronic CoreValve transcatheter heart valves,[6] Europe's transcatheter aortic valve implantation programs expanded from 37 in 2007 to nearly 350 in 2011.[7] During this time frame, over 34,000 patients underwent TAVR in 11 European countries, predominantly in Germany, Italy, and France.[7,8] The European experience was well underway before TAVR approval by the US Food and Drug Administration (FDA) in November 2011.

In the United States, much of the clinical trial requirements were mirrored in multisociety recommendations of the American Association of Thoracic Surgeons (AATS), American College of Cardiology (ACC), American Heart Association (AHA), American Society of Echocardiography (ASE), Society of Coronary Angiography and Intervention (SCAI), and Society of Thoracic Surgeons (STS).[9] Following FDA approval, Medicare's National Coverage Determination (NCD) for TAVR (May 2012) detailed qualifying criteria to begin a TAVR program. This unprecedented alignment of governmental agencies, payers, and professional societies propelled a shift to care that was not only clinically driven but also regulatory driven. As per the multisociety recommendations for TAVR operator and institutional requirements, the NCD detailed hospital infrastructure, Heart Team membership and roles, physician and hospital procedural volume prerequisites (eg, 1000 catheterizations, 400 percutaneous coronary interventions [PCIs], 30 left-sided structural interventional procedures, and 50 aortic valve replacements in the past year), and ongoing minimum TAVR volumes (20 cases per year or 40 over 2 years).[10] Although some countries, including Australia and New Zealand,[11] adopted many of these same recommendations for procedural volume, others identified minimum volume thresholds only for TAVR (eg, 25-50 TAVRs per year in Canada[12]).

Mandates from the Centers for Medicare and Medicaid Services (CMS) for reimbursement were rigid: 2 face-to-face surgical consultations; a cardiothoracic surgeon (CTS) and interventional cardiologist (IC) who met procedural volume thresholds; and joint performance of "the intraoperative technical aspects of TAVR" by the CTS and IC.[10] This diverged from the European Society of Cardiology (ESC)/European Association for Cardiothoracic Surgery (EACTS) 2012 guidelines, which did not require an intraprocedural dyad of a CTS and IC. Outside of the United States, the procedure generally uses 2 implanting physicians, including a CTS or IC, but does not by mandate require one implanter from each specialty (eg, Canada, Italy, United Kingdom). TAVR was also provided in hospitals without cardiac surgery, a practice found to be safe in a single prospective registry[13] and continued in Germany until 2016. On the other hand, US societal guidelines and reimbursement criteria appeared to prevent against overuse of this novel therapy. Appropriate use criteria for AS and TAVR would eventually be established in 2017.[14]

For many US hospitals, adherence to reimbursement eligibility criteria drove program development. In the United States, this led to a presumption that, to be reimbursed for the procedure, programs must collect all STS/ACC Transcatheter Valve Therapy (TVT) Registry data (eg, percent of carotid artery stenosis, forced expiratory volume) for all enrolled patients.[15] Clinical pathways therefore incorporated the tests required to acquire these registry data. As evidence and indications expanded, the clinical need, costs, and patient hardship posed by potentially unwarranted studies (eg, carotid artery ultrasound scan[16,17]) were growing concerns. However, the linkage of the NCD criteria and national registry implied that programs must obtain and submit all STS/ACC TVT Registry data to meet the requirements to offer TAVR.

Although regulatory requirements may influence and at times constrain best practices, the emphasis in program development internationally has been the "right care for the right patient." This textbook aims to describe care that is (1) clinically indicated; (2) evidence based; (3) provided by a multidisciplinary team (MDT) that objectively and judiciously evaluates, communicates, and assists patients to access the options for treatment; and (4) patient centered and personalized such that patient wishes are integral to care planning and risks are weighed against objective and subjective benefits, including not only quantity but also quality of life. These patient care aims have been described throughout this reference.

Dispersion and Adoption

The up-front investment and prescriptive requirements to establish a TAVR program may have been perceived as a barrier to entry. This fundamental level of standardization, however, especially when matched with TAVR-specific reimbursement criteria, may have also contributed to TAVR's rapid adoption in the United States and globally.[8] As of January 2018, there are nearly 570 TAVR programs in the United States,[18] more than 25 centers in Canada,[19] and over 100 in Germany.[20] If the innovators were clinical trial centers, early adopters were generally tertiary and other quaternary hospitals with responsibility for a large catchment of patients. The life cycle of technology adoption for TAVR has been expeditious: programs comprising the early and even the late majority of hospitals are providing TAVR in 2018.

This rapid adoption may also reflect the level of surveillance of TAVR program compliance with eligibility criteria. Eligibility is based on hospital self-report of volumes and outcomes, which has not generally been monitored or verified before payment, withholding, or audit. In 2012, it was estimated that only 400 US programs (approximately 1 TAVR program for every 3 open heart surgery programs) met all volume requirements set forth in the CMS NCD.[21] By 2015, the total number of TAVR programs in the United States exceeded the number of estimated eligible programs.

The issue of program eligibility may detract from perhaps a more important question: How many TAVR programs are needed to serve the population of patients with severe AS? The global incidence of AS is estimated to be as low as 4% to as high as 10% in those older than 65 years,[22-24] compounded by the aging of the world population: persons older than 65 years are expected to double by the year 2050.[25]

Several approaches are used at the local, regional, and national levels by hospitals, governments, and industry vendors to estimate the number of patients who may warrant treatment. Data may be obtained via various methodologies including software algorithms to analyze data ranging from website searches for AS to echocardiographic parameters, medical diagnosis, and procedural codes in electronic medical records and imaging systems; retrospective review of utilization and adoption; and epidemiological modeling. Using various strategies to anticipate the therapy demand may be useful for health system program development.

A deceptively simple method to determine TAVR need and access includes retrospective review of utilization and adoption. In the United States, nearly 95,000 commercial TAVRs were entered into the STS/ACC TVT Registry from 2012 to 2016.[18] Of these cases, nearly 40,000 were performed in 2016 across approximately 485 centers, which corresponds to an average of nearly 80 cases per program. As new sites continue to launch (85 US sites in 2016), the mean case volume has limited applicability; case volumes range considerably across US sites. At the site level, annualizing the number of cases based on a defined period (eg, rolling 6 months, previous calendar or fiscal year) can assist in understanding trends and growth. That being said, projecting the number of patients who need treatment based solely on the case volumes of the previous year may be misleading.

The German example has been studied to better understand TAVR adoption and program demand. In 2014, Germany reported over 13,000 TAVRs, for a population of 81 million (164 TAVR procedures per million inhabitants, a penetration rate exceeding 50%-60%).[26] This translates to 132 cases per year across the 100 TAVR centers in Germany, with 25% of centers performing fewer than 100 cases per year and 21% of centers performing more than 500 TAVR per year. When the number of TAVR centers in Germany decreased in 2016 following a ban in hospitals without cardiac surgery, it was approximated that there was 1 center for every 1 million people in Germany.[20] This is in contrast to the United States, where over 16,000 TAVR procedures were reported in 2014 to the STS/ACC TVT Registry,[18] for a population of over 315 million,[27] or approximately 50 TAVR per 1 million inhabitants.[20] Concerns were raised by US professional societies that the number of TAVR programs exceeds the need.

Rapid dispersion of TAVR has been scrutinized in Germany and the United States. Using the German experience as a comparator, the need in the United States has been hypothesized at 26,240 TAVR procedures per year.[28] Across the 560 US TAVR centers in 2018,[18] this corresponds to a mean case volume of less than 50 per site per year. Limiting the number of US sites (eg, 350 centers, akin to the German experience and "ample for satisfactory geographical access"[28]) has been proposed by professional societies[29] in the spirit of centralizing systems of care and assuring quality at a macro level. At the micro level, however, it is the patient and family that must sustain the burden of accessing these sites. An important consideration for limiting the number of TAVR centers is whether this in turn limits patient access.

Epidemiological models for current estimates and future projections of patients with AS may also be performed. Applying an epidemiological model to systematic reviews and meta-analyses, Durko and colleagues estimated that, among the United States, Canada, and 27 European countries, there are currently 180,000 patients who are potential candidates for TAVR. Should the indication expand to patients at low surgical risk, the number of candidates increases to 270,000.[30] Specifically for the United States, Durko et al projected that there are approximately 50,000 annual candidates for TAVR with current indications (symptomatic severe AS and intermediate or greater surgical risk). This projection increases to over 80,000 patients if TAVR becomes indicated in low-risk patients, as is expected in 2019.[30] The estimates may be distilled to the state, county, and city level based on census data.

Despite the challenges of geographical access and health system heterogeneity, regional systems of care for VHD have been developed or considered by other countries.[29] Stub and colleagues[31] described a Canadian provincial model of a centrally funded and coordinated TAVR program with multidisciplinary oversight of access, quality, planning, and evaluation in 4 provincial sites. Local Heart Teams made treatment decisions and performed TAVR. Complicated or low-volume procedures (ie, nontransfemoral TAVR) were centralized to a single site. Observed outcomes (2012-2014; $N = 583$) were equal to or better than US benchmarks[32] for a similar time period: all-cause in-hospital mortality rate of 3.1% and disability stroke of 1.9%; median length of stay of 3 days with 92.8% of patients discharged to home; and all-cause 30-day mortality of 3.5%.[31] Processes of care and coordination supported referral to the central site. Inspired by this work, US professional societies have explored the establishment of systems of care to optimize the management of VHD. The development of a regional system of care must consider the differences between health systems (ie, single-payer health system vs nonuniform health system) and hospital-level variation (ie, academic, not for profit, private).[31,33]

Program Volumes and Outcomes

Central to health care program development is the establishment of standards for safety and quality, which are presently measured by the markers of procedural volume and primary outcomes (eg, mortality and adverse event rates). Volume is frequently used as a surrogate indicator for expertise and quality, which are subsequently inferred by outcome. Volume-outcome relationships have been studied for other procedures (eg, aortic valve surgery,[34] PCI[35]) and suggest an inverse relationship between mortality and hospital procedural volume, largely depending on the implanting physician (eg, operator) volume. These data are emerging for TAVR.

Retrospective reviews of several international registries demonstrate a decrease in the average observed and risk-adjusted mortality associated with an increase in procedural volume.[36-39] In a US study of relationship of procedural volume and outcome (42,988 commercial TAVR cases; 395 hospitals), Carroll et al[38] found that an increased site volume was significantly associated with lower in-hospital risk-adjusted mortality ($P < .02$), vascular complications ($P < .003$), and bleeding ($P < .001$). Applying a volume-outcome model, risk-adjusted adverse outcomes decreased over the first 400 cases, including mortality (3.6%-2.2%), bleeding (9.6%-5.1%), vascular complications (6.1%-4.2%), and stroke (2.1%-1.7%).

The volume-outcomes relationship described by Carroll and colleagues is criticized on 2 aspects. First, volumes are not direct measures of quality. Second, although the study period was from 2012 to 2015, the devices and vascular access approaches used during that time frame are already outdated. Transapical access, which has been shown to have poorer overall outcomes, was used in nearly 30% of these cases. Also, these cases were performed using transcatheter heart valves and delivery systems that are no longer used due to advances in technology. A current inquiry may better represent contemporary TAVR practice, as technology and clinical practice has changed considerably from 2015 to 2018. That said, although the nature of the relationship remains unclear, regulatory bodies and professional societies continue to use procedural volume and outcome measures as criteria for program eligibility and payment.

It is unclear whether these findings are indicative of the TAVR learning curve, which may be less steep as technology has advanced (ie, third-generation balloon- and self-expandable valves in 2018). It appeared that 50 cases signified an inflection point for improved outcomes.[40] Based on these data, an increase from 20 to 50 cases per year has been proposed as the minimum volume for TAVR programs in the United States.[29,40] However, volume is a component of but not a direct measure of quality. Thus, direct measures of quality are needed and have yet to be defined.

Prospective patient enrollment into national registries has allowed for postmarket surveillance of TAVR device use and outcomes. Outcomes have been historically reported in aggregate, and quality assurance has been the responsibility of the TAVR center. The 2018 multisociety document on TAVR operational and institutional requirements recommended public reporting of site-level performance.[40] The primary metrics to monitor include in-hospital risk-adjusted all-cause mortality, discharge to home, 30-day all-cause mortality, all-cause neurologic events including transient ischemic attacks, major vascular complications, major bleeding, and moderate or greater aortic insufficiency. A TAVR center's average values for the 4 most recent consecutive quarters would be compared against the 4 most recent consecutive quarters of national data. To maintain an active TAVR program in the US, a site must not be in the lowest (worst) 10% for national benchmarks of any primary outcome for 2 or more consecutive quarters.[40] These recommendations may represent the next level of quality and outcome surveillance by professional societies and possibly enforcement by regulatory bodies.

Current Perspectives

After nearly 20 years of TAVR, what does the quintessential program look like? What clinical practices remain intact in these programs? Multidisciplinary Heart Teams, including a CTS and IC, remain the standard globally. The gold standard to evaluate valve disease and severity is transthoracic echocardiography and consultation for symptoms and surgical risk, using multiple risk scores.[14,41] Procedural risks and approach are guided by the data derived from multimodality imaging (ie, cardiac catheterization, coronary angiography, and computed tomography angiography).[14,41]

Commensurate with the advances in technology, expanded indication to intermediate-risk patients, and implementation of risk-stratified clinical pathways, opportunities to further streamline the procedure and hospital course have been shown to be safe and effective.[42,43] The procedural approach is primarily transfemoral, with a growing number of procedures performed under moderate sedation.[32] Patients may be admitted after the procedure to a cardiac monitoring unit (eg, telemetry or step-down unit) instead of a critical care unit, depending on procedural complications and nursing care needs.[42,43] Next-day discharge protocols focus on minimizing and discontinuing invasive lines,[44] ambulating early, promoting nutrition and sleep, and ensuring adequate support at home as part of the initial evaluation.[42]

In July 2018, the new multisocietal recommendations for TAVR operator and institutional requirements[40] were published and CMS convened a Medicare Evidence Development and Coverage Advisory Committee meeting to review the TAVR NCD.[45] Changes to these important documents may drive clinical practice into the modern era. The quantity and intensity of needs and resources to support TAVR have changed over time. This continuous evolution warrants a dynamic strategy to TAVR program development.

Program Development

The framework for program development (Figure 11.1) described in this chapter is a modified logic model[46] comprising 4 components answering basic questions: (1) Inputs (Why? Who? What? Where? When?), (2) Processes (How?), (3) Outputs (How many?), and (4) Outcomes (How well?). Although expert consensus statements, societal guidelines, and regulatory compliance may comprise the fundamentals of TAVR program development, this holistic model incorporates aspects of organizational culture and strategic planning pillars (eg, people, service, quality, finance/growth/value, and innovation).

Inputs comprise the content for the processes. Processes occur along a time interval, which in this case represents the continuum of care from referral to follow-up surveillance. Outputs and Outcomes are the quantitative and qualitative results that are produced by these processes. Outputs and Outcomes may be evaluated for further program development and optimization and are described in detail elsewhere in this text.

Inputs

Inputs are the answers to these questions: "Why? Who? What? When? Where?" These underpinnings of program development are identified in Figure 11.1 and detailed further in Table 11.1. The Inputs for program development are not static; it must be expected that content will change over time based on evidence, guidelines, and needs. There will also be national, regional, local, and site-level variation of the underlying Inputs of TAVR programs.

Why: Foundational Underpinnings

The foundational underpinnings (the "why") for programmatic development include scientific evidence, societal guidelines, regulations, policy, and quality requirements (Table 11.1). These various sources of evidence propel approvals of TAVR device indications from regulatory

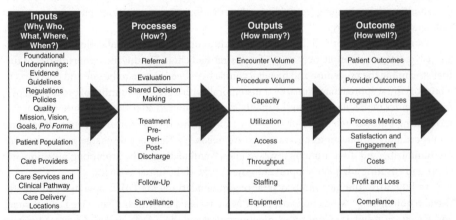

Inputs (Why, Who, What, Where, When?)	Processes (How?)	Outputs (How many?)	Outcome (How well?)
Foundational Underpinnings: Evidence Guidelines Regulations Policies Quality	Referral	Encounter Volume	Patient Outcomes
	Evaluation	Procedure Volume	Provider Outcomes
	Shared Decision Making	Capacity	Program Outcomes
Mission, Vision, Goals, *Pro Forma*	Treatment Pre- Peri- Post- Discharge	Utilization	Process Metrics
Patient Population		Access	Satisfaction and Engagement
Care Providers		Throughput	Costs
Care Services and Clinical Pathway	Follow-Up	Staffing	Profit and Loss
Care Delivery Locations	Surveillance	Equipment	Compliance

FIGURE 11.1. A logic model for transcatheter aortic valve replacement (TAVR) program development. Depicted here is a logic model of Inputs, Processes, Outputs, and Outcomes applied to TAVR program development. Framework variables and definitions may vary across programs. (©Perpetua Associates, used with permission.)

TABLE 11.1. Framework for Program Development: Examples of Inputs

Foundational Underpinnings (Why)	Patient Population and Care Providers (Who)	Patient Care Services and Clinical Pathway (What/When)	Care Delivery Locations (Where)

Science and guidelines
• Clinical trial evidence
• Registry data
• Societal guidelines
• VARC-2
 	
Regulations, policy, quality
• National
  • FDA
  • CE Mark
  • CMS
• Regional
• Hospital
 	
Program
• Mission
• Vision
• Goals/objectives
• Key results
	Patient population
	Diseased valve
	• Native AV disease
	• Prosthetic AV disease
	
	Valve disease
	• AS
	• AI
	• Mixed AS/AI
	
	Valve disease severity
	• Moderate
	• Moderate-severe
	• Severe
	
	Symptoms
	• Asymptomatic
	• Symptomatic
	
	Surgical risk
	• Inoperable
	• High
	• Intermediate
	• Low
	
	Care providers
	• Core team
	• Extended team
		Evaluation
		• Multidisciplinary team consultation
		• Echocardiography
		• Cardiac catheterization
		• CTA
		• Laboratory testing
		• ECG
		• Pulmonary laboratory
		
		Treatment
		• TAVR
		• SAVR
		• BAV
		• Medical therapy
		• Palliative care
		• Clinical trial
		
		Documentation
		• Electronic health record
		• Other tracking tools or databases
			Site characteristics
			• Hospital type and health system model
			• Hospital culture
			• Physician practice model
			• Payer model and payers
			• Administrative leadership model
			
			Care delivery sites
			• Referring center
			• Valve center
			• Inpatient units
			• Admitting unit
			• Procedural area
			• Recovery unit
			
			Departments
			• Cardiology
			• Cardiothoracic surgery
			• Anesthesiology
			• Echocardiography
			• Radiology
			• Ambulatory care
			• Inpatient care
			• Nursing
			• Research
			• Quality
			• Finance
			• Business development
			• Information technology discharge unit

AI, aortic insufficiency; AV, aortic valve; BAV, balloon aortic valvuloplasty; CE, *Conformité Européenne*; CMS, Centers for Medicare and Medicaid Services; CTA, computerized tomography with angiography; ECG, electrocardiography; FDA, Food and Drug Administration; SAVR, surgical aortic valve replacement; TAVR, transcatheter aortic valve replacement; VARC2, Valve Academic Research Consortium, second.

bodies internationally (eg, *Conformité Européenne* Mark in Europe and FDA approval in the United States) and adoption into societal guidelines (eg, ESC/EACTS,[4] Canadian Cardiovascular Society,[12] AATS/ACC/AHA/ASE/SCAI/STS[5,14,40]). Policies for TAVR span the local, regional, and national levels, as governmental and commercial insurers guide clinical practice and its payment. In the United States, the CMS NCD detailed the eligibility criteria for the establishment and reimbursement of TAVR programs, inclusive of staffing and infrastructure. In other countries, policy and payment are based on the health care system: national health service (eg, New Zealand, Spain, United Kingdom), single-payer national health insurance system (eg, Canada, Denmark, Sweden), or a multipayer universal health insurance fund (eg, France, Germany, Japan). Hospitals may be mandated at the local or national level to prospectively enroll patients into quality registries (eg, Canadian Quality Working Group Initiative,[47] STS/ACC TVT Registry[18]), which necessitate collection of patient and program data largely based on Valve Academic Research Consortium-2[3] definitions. Taken together, it is evidence, guidelines, regulations and policies, and quality requirements that provide the basis for TAVR program development.

In addition, a program may have a mission and vision statement with corresponding goals or objectives and key results. There are subtle differences between a mission and a vision, and they are frequently confused or conflated.

The mission is the guiding purpose of the program, given what it sets out to do currently. In the context of competing priorities, the mission frequently serves to direct decision making. Take, for example, the mission to provide safe and excellent patient-centered care for every patient, every time. Embedding this mission into decision making and process may provide clarity for the program and team. The team may ask themselves, "Is our care safe? Is our care excellent? Does our care put the patient at the center? Do we provide safe, excellent, patient-centered care for every patient? Do we do this every time? If not, why not?"

The vision is what the program wishes to be in the future. For instance, a TAVR program may have the vision of becoming a world-class comprehensive valve center that transforms cardiovascular care through the integration of clinical practice, education, and bench-to-bedside and clinical research and innovation. Selection of current and future initiatives may be based on alignment with this vision. Goals, or objectives, and key results may be derived from the mission and vision. The objective that all patients are evaluated and treated safely and expeditiously may be accompanied with the key results of all patients evaluated within 7 days and treated within 30 days. These results are binary and measurable. Patients are either evaluated within 7 days or they are not and treated within 30 days or they are not. The more clearly an organization and its teams can articulate and adhere to the mission, vision, goals/objectives, and key results, the greater the potential for growth and success.[48] From this, a *pro forma*, or business plan, may be formulated. Taken together, the integration of foundational underpinnings, mission and vision, objectives and key results, and a business plan ensures that programs "begin with the end in mind."

Who: Patient Population and Care Providers

Defining the patient population ("who") is key to program development, as patients must be at the center of care. Patients who have native or prosthetic aortic valve disease comprise the population who may undergo TAVR. Programs may estimate the number of patients based on the disease prevalence and incidence given their geographical catchment, health system affiliations, and payer contracts. A specific cohort of patients with native and aortic valve disease may be further refined at the program level. As seen in Table 11.1, the target cohort for the program may be as broad as all-comer patients with significant valve disease or progressively specified by the type of aortic valve disease, severity of disease, and surgical risk.

The program must define their patient population, referred to in Figure 11.2, as the valve patient cohort. Examples of referred subcohorts to consider are identified: (1) all patients referred with (significant) valve disease; (2) patients referred for definitive intervention; (3) query for patients with native valve disease or patients who have had previous valve surgery (ie, patients with a high likelihood of requiring repeat intervention given limited durability of most valve interventions).

Figure 11.2 depicts how the valve patient cohort targeted by the program determines the necessary services and care teams ("who"). The patient population characteristics determine the algorithm for evaluation by designated care providers: (1) referring or local primary care providers and cardiologists, (2) valve cardiology team (eg, cardiologists with specialty in VHD echocardiography), (3) interventional cardiology, (4) cardiothoracic surgery, or (5) Heart Team, including interventional cardiology and cardiothoracic surgery.

Figure 11.3 demonstrates the depth and breadth of required staffing considerations, as many departments are involved in patient care activities for valve/TAVR programs from referral to follow-up. The specific roles and responsibilities of core and extended MDT members are discussed elsewhere in this text.

What and When: Patient Care Services and Clinical Pathway

The foundational underpinnings ("why") and patient population and care providers ("who") determine the services provided, clinical pathway, and time targets for evaluation and treatment

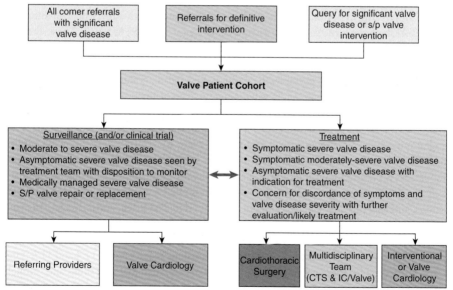

FIGURE 11.2. Inputs for program development: patient population and care providers. For the Inputs of "Patient Population and Care Providers" ("who"), an algorithm is proposed for programs to define their Valve Patient Cohort, which may comprise various types of patient referrals as seen in this figure. The characteristics of the Valve Patient Cohort warrant surveillance or treatment, which in turn determines the necessary care providers. Elements of this algorithm and their definitions may vary across programs. CTS, cardiothoracic surgery; IC, interventional cardiology; s/p, status post. (©Perpetua Associates, used with permission.)

HEART VALVE CENTER				
Evaluation	**Pre-Procedure**	**Peri-Procedure**	**Post-Procedure**	**Follow-Up**
Physician Team				
Core Clinical and Coordination Team				
Diagnostic Imaging Team (Echocardiography and Radiology)				
Clinic staff Diagnostics staff Referring staff Consult staff	Clinic staff Pre-procedure / inpatient staff	Cath lab staff OR staff Anesthesia staff Perfusion	Recovery unit staff Admit unit staff Discharge unit staff Ancillary services	Clinic staff Diagnostics staff Referring staff Consult staff
Researh and Quality Teams				
Administrative and Operations Teams				
Finance (Financial Clearance, Billing/Coding) Teams				

FIGURE 11.3. Inputs for program development: staffing the heart valve center. For the Input of "Care Providers" ("who"), this figure depicts the entire program footprint of core and extended multidisciplinary team members involved in patient care across the continuum. As programs grow, core team members (eg, physicians, core clinical ad coordination team members such as APPs, nurses, and schedulers) are often considered when staffing needs are evaluated. However, it is imperative that Extended Team members (eg, echosonographers, radiology technicians, cardiac catheterization laboratory staff, inpatient nursing staff) are also included in the staffing model of a heart valve center. Elements of this figure and their definitions may vary across programs. (©Perpetua Associates, used with permission.)

("what" and "when"). Components of the evaluation range from consultations to diagnostic studies, and treatment options, as indicated, may include medical therapy, which encompasses surveillance, balloon aortic valvuloplasty, and palliative care; TAVR; or SAVR. These elements of evaluation and treatment are listed in Table 11.1.

There is site-level variation for standardized referral and clinical processes, collectively referred to as pathways. For example, the pathway for referral, evaluation, and treatment may vary between a TAVR program and a valve program. The distinction is a shift of focus to the patient and the disease, rather than on the procedure or the device. A heart valve program (or center) may serve all patients (all-comer) with significant valve disease, whereas the TAVR program may receive patients with symptomatic severe AS referred only following surgical consultation and deemed at intermediate or greater surgical risk. The latter may be the eponymous TAVR program focusing only on patients already evaluated by a cardiac surgeon and likely for TAVR. The former may be the valve program that encompasses all VHD, treatment options, and care providers inclusive of but not limited to TAVR (eg, aortic, mitral, tricuspid, pulmonic valve disease, and all catheter-based and surgical therapies in commercial use and clinical trial). Examples of a referral and clinical pathway for a patient-centered, disease-based program, rather than a procedure-centric program, are depicted in Figures 11.4 and 11.5. Time targets are critical for these pathways and processes of care, such that wait times and throughput may be measured.

The disease-based program that offers not only commercially available treatment but also that in clinical trial may expand the program's patient population and therapeutic options. As of January 2018, for example, TAVR is being studied in asymptomatic patients with severe AS (Evaluation of Transcatheter Aortic Valve Replacement Compared to SurveilLance for Patients With AsYmptomatic Severe Aortic Stenosis [EARLY-TAVR][49]) and patients with moderate AS and left ventricular hypertrophy with heart failure (Transcatheter Aortic Valve Replacement

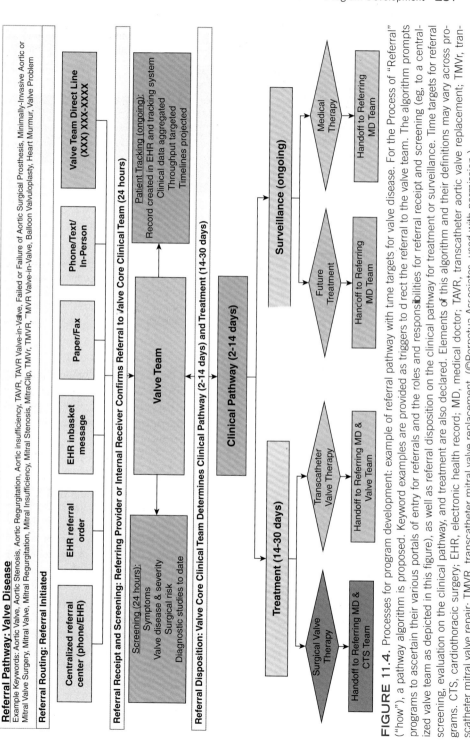

FIGURE 11.4. Processes for program development: example of referral pathway with time targets for valve disease. For the Process of "Referral" ("how"), a pathway algorithm is proposed. Keyword examples are provided as triggers to direct the referral to the valve team. The algorithm prompts programs to ascertain their various portals of entry for referrals and the roles and responsibilities for referral receipt and screening (eg, to a centralized valve team as depicted in this figure), as well as referral disposition on the clinical pathway for treatment or surveillance. Time targets for referral screening, evaluation on the clinical pathway, and treatment are also declared. Elements of this algorithm and their definitions may vary across programs. CTS, cardiothoracic surgery; EHR, electronic health record; MD, medical doctor; TAVR, transcatheter aortic valve replacement; TMVr, transcatheter mitral valve repair; TMVR, transcatheter mitral valve replacement. (©Perpetua Associates, used with permission.)

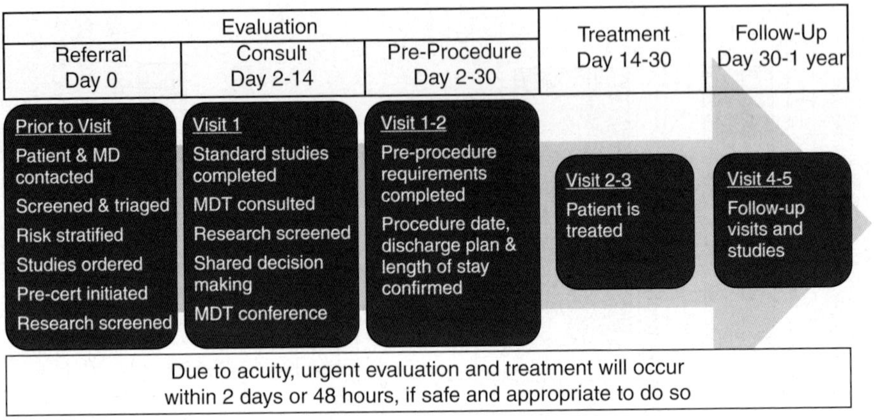

Evaluation			Treatment	Follow-Up
Referral Day 0	Consult Day 2-14	Pre-Procedure Day 2-30	Day 14-30	Day 30-1 year
Prior to Visit Patient & MD contacted Screened & triaged Risk stratified Studies ordered Pre-cert initiated Research screened	Visit 1 Standard studies completed MDT consulted Research screened Shared decision making MDT conference	Visit 1-2 Pre-procedure requirements completed Procedure date, discharge plan & length of stay confirmed	Visit 2-3 Patient is treated	Visit 4-5 Follow-up visits and studies

Due to acuity, urgent evaluation and treatment will occur
within 2 days or 48 hours, if safe and appropriate to do so

FIGURE 11.5. Processes for program development: example of clinical pathway overview with time targets. For the Processes from "Referral" to "Follow-up," this figure depicts a clinical pathway algorithm inclusive of elements and time targets for each patient visit. This pathway assumes and embeds the principles of safe, clinically indicated, expeditious, and risk-stratified care while minimizing the number of trips for the patient as consistent with patient and family preferences. Time targets include considerations for the urgent and the elective patient. Elements of this pathway and their definitions may vary across programs. MD, medical doctor; MDT, multidisciplinary team. (©Perpetua Associates, used with permission.)

to Unload the Left Ventricle in Patients with Advanced Heart Failure: A Randomized Trial [TAVR-UNLOAD][50]). It is anticipated that as early as 2019, TAVR may receive approval for use in patients with symptomatic severe AS at low surgical risk, which broadens the target population. Collectively, program development is based on the patient population and the subsequent evaluation components given current and future treatment options.

Where: Location

There are several considerations for program development (Table 11.1) pertaining to the locations (the "where") of the TAVR program: the culture, structure, and staff of the health system, hospitals, and departments; the center or program leadership and charter; and the specific areas of care delivery. A program's health system may include variation between hospital types (eg, academic, private, not for- profit); physician practice and compensation models (eg, hospital employed vs private practice); payers and models for payment/reimbursement (eg, TAVR-specific diagnosis-related groups; bundled payments). An academic tertiary medical center may have an increased number of patients referred from outside of the center, which may require more effort for communication and coordination than patients who are primarily managed within the center. A hospital with an increased number of internal patient referrals (eg, an integrated health system or single payer health system) may require less effort to acquire medical records or payment authorization. Schedule requirements, compensation packages, and medical records may be more transparent and similar within provider groups of the same model. Administrative leadership and service departments may also differ in their composition and degree of stakeholder buy-in across each location. The Inputs and the Processes of program development may increase with heterogeneity in the system and program.

Given the context, a TAVR program may have defined the leadership, mission, and vision, as well as the areas and resources of care delivery. Stub and colleagues[31] exemplify a regional system of care for TAVR, whereas Nishimura and colleagues[29] propose a hub-and-spoke model of care for VHD. Leadership may comprise a triad of a medical director, surgical director, and administrator.[51] Valve program staff may include a valve program clinician (VPC), clinical staff (nurses, nurse practitioners, or physician assistant), or administrative or clerical support staff. In addition to the MDT membership and meeting structure, the program at large may have a valve practice committee or council with champions from each care delivery area (eg, clinic, diagnostic laboratories, cardiac catheterization laboratory, operating room, pre-/peri-/post-TAVR inpatients units) focused on education and best practices. Some programs may have an informal leadership structure, or a virtual valve clinic, or no designated physical location or staff. Other programs may have a formal, brick-and-mortar space with a specific cost center and service line. Although there is bound to be differences across programs, it is critical that these characteristics are clearly delineated and communicated.

How: Processes

The Inputs (5 Ws: Why, Who, What, When, Where) are combined to inform the Processes (How). Along the timeline of care delivery there are many processes. Clinical pathways are processes that are standardized then further personalized to deliver care to the patient. Operational logistics and processes are also embedded to support the clinical pathway and program. The specific roles and responsibilities of core and extended MDT members may be determined by formal agreement and facilitated via job descriptions, TAVR-specific education and training, standardized order sets, and documentation templates inclusive of quality and process measures.

A cross-functional process map (eg, swim lanes) is a process flow diagram to depict processes and subprocesses. Columns may represent the departments or persons involved in the process, whereas the rows represent steps completed over time. This mapping allows for delineation of roles and responsibilities, as well as the identification of gaps and bottlenecks, in a specific process or subprocesses. Table 11.2 is an example of a swim lanes template that may be used to assist in defining and communicating team member roles along the continuum of care. The rows of Table 11.2 list roles or positions of core and extended MDT members. The columns in Table 11.2 list the points of patient encounter across the continuum of care: referral, evaluation, shared decision making, treatment (preprocedure, periprocedure, postprocedure), and follow-up. A specific example of a referral intake and screening cross-functional process map, with swim lanes for an advanced practice provider, nurse, and scheduler, is depicted in Figure 11.6.

How Many and How Well: Outputs and Outcomes

Again, program development must begin with the end in mind. The TAVR program may define the desired goals, objectives, and key results a priori in a business plan and on an ongoing basis, commensurate with national and local benchmarks. Outputs may be described as results that reveal "How many?" with a focus on quantity or volumes. Outcomes may be generalized as results that answer "How well?" with an emphasis on quality, performance, and experience. Understanding and bridging the gap between observed and expected Outputs and Outcomes (Figure 11.1) is critical to program assessment and optimization.

Examples of Outputs include volumes of encounters (new referrals, provider appointments, diagnostic testing appointments) and procedures (TAVR, SAVR, balloon

TABLE 11.2. Example of a Swim Lanes Template for Processes of Care

	Referral	Evaluation	Shared Decision Making	Treatment			Follow-up
				Pre	Intra	Post	
Core Multidisciplinary Team							
Valve program scheduler							
Valve program clinician (coordinator)							
Valve program nurse(s)							
Valve program advanced practice provider							
Interventional cardiologist							
Cardiothoracic surgeon							
Valve cardiologist							
Echocardiographer							
Echosonographer							
Anesthesiology							
Extended Multidisciplinary Team							
Referring provider							
Consultative specialists							
Radiologist							
Radiology technician							

Diagnostic testing staff	Research staff	Procedural staff	Circulator	Sterile "scrub"	Clinical monitor	Perfusion	Admit unit service and staff	Recovery unit service and staff	Inpatient unit service and staff

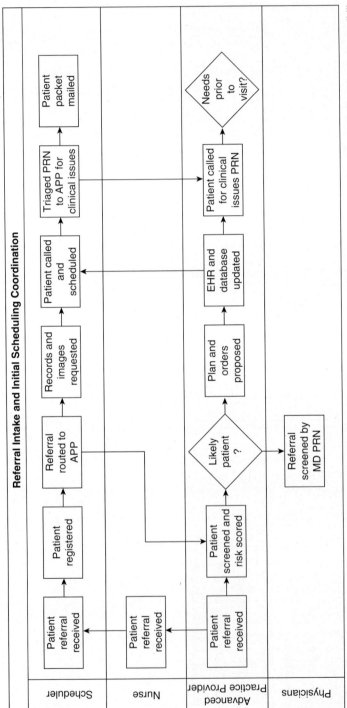

FIGURE 11.6. Example of cross-functional process map for referral intake and scheduling coordination. Depicted here are the broad responsibilities of key MDT members for this interval of the continuum of care.

aortic valvuloplasty, PCI, cardiac catheterization). Table 11.3 demonstrates encounter volumes, which are categorized as direct or indirect and generally measurable by an organization via the electronic health record. Direct encounters, or face-to-face visits with the patient, are typically billable and most conventionally measured by the health system (eg, relative value units). Indirect encounters are contacts with patients and their health information often through means that are not face-to-face interactions, yet are quantifiable, such as communication and action based on review of records or test results, phone calls, e-mails, or electronic health record messaging.

For the purposes of demonstration in Table 11.3, conservative assumptions were used, including (1) for patients referred to the TAVR program, 50% proceed to TAVR, 25% proceed to SAVR, and 25% proceed to medical therapy or monitoring; (2) evaluation includes interventional cardiology and cardiothoracic surgery consults for each patient; transthoracic echocardiogram, computed tomography angiogram, cardiac catheterization, and pulmonary function testing for each patient; second cardiothoracic surgical consultation for patients who proceed to TAVR; (3) preprocedure requirements include an electrocardiogram, chest radiograph, laboratory studies, and a history and physical visit or preprocedure clinic visit;

TABLE 11.3. Example of Encounter Volumes for a US TAVR Program

Encounters	Annual Volume of TAVR Procedures				
	1	20	50	100	200
Referrals	2	40	100	200	400
Direct Encounters					
Provider consultations	3	60	150	300	600
Initial diagnostic tests	4	80	200	400	800
Preprocedure tests and visits	4	80	200	400	800
Definitive procedure (TAVR/SAVR)	1	20	50	100	200
Follow-up tests and visits	5	100	250	500	1000
Indirect Encounters					
Order entry	6	120	300	600	1200
Results review	6	120	300	600	1200
Authorizations	6	120	300	600	1200
Encounter scheduling	13	260	650	1300	2600
Total Encounters	50	1000	2500	5000	10,000

SAVR, surgical aortic valve replacement; TAVR, transcatheter aortic valve replacement.

(4) follow-up includes a provider visit, echocardiogram, and electrocardiogram at 30 days and 1 year per the requirements of the TVT Registry. A TAVR program may model and evaluate its own Outputs based on the previous and projected volumes and the encounters included in the clinical pathway.

The exponential growth in encounter volumes is evident here and can be used to project program needs. For example, Table 11.3 lists 50 encounters for 1 TAVR procedure, 2500 encounters for 50 TAVR procedures, and 10,000 encounters for 200 TAVR procedures. These encounter volumes may be helpful to ascertain capacity; utilization, access, and throughput given the patient demand; and the efficiency and effectiveness of processes of the program itself and competing programs sharing the same resources. The Inputs of staffing and equipment are also observed as Outputs in terms of their adequacy in meeting demands and objectives.

Results also include Outcomes of the patient, provider, and program; process metrics such as length of stay and discharge disposition; patient satisfaction scores; employee engagement scores and metrics such as retention and turnover; costs, profits, and loss; and compliance with regulatory bodies and requirements. Some of these measures are described in detail elsewhere in this text.

Program development must account for the anticipated drivers of change in the immediate, short term, and long term. As described previously, program outcomes are typically reviewed at the site level. Specific patient outcomes are reported in aggregate by national/regional quality registries. Sites must consider the impact of the proposed shift to public reporting and minimum thresholds for quality and outcomes. Program evaluation and quality are further discussed in the following chapter.

Program Optimization

Now widely applied to health care, program optimization is rooted in mathematical modeling and operations research. Also termed the "science of better," data describing variables and processes are collected, analyzed, and transformed into insights to increase efficiency, increase effectiveness, decrease waste, and decrease costs.[52] The sciences of dissemination and implementation study the processes of meeting these aims and may evaluate operational processes in clinical care. In health care, program optimization may refer to the following objectives:

1. Improve safety, quality, outcomes, and process metrics;
2. Increase access;
3. Increase utilization at the highest-intended yet safest level;
4. Decrease wait times;
5. Increase satisfaction, retention, and engagement of patients, referring providers, and team members/staff;
6. Decrease costs and resources;
7. Eliminate waste.

Central to these objectives is the VPC, who serves as the hub for the many spokes of a TAVR program.

Valve Program Clinician

Managing and optimizing the dynamic Inputs, Processes, Outputs, and Outcomes integral to TAVR program development may be daunting to the MDT. Prominent challenges include the complexity of seemingly ever-evolving requirements, rapid growth of the therapy, and competing priorities of the hospital and MDT membership and resources. In the TAVR programs that use the position(s), the VPC, or valve program coordinator, frequently has patient-facing and program development responsibilities.[2,51]

These program linchpins may possess not only content expertise for this specialty but also deep and broad experience within their institutions and referring health systems and relationships that facilitate clinical and operational program success.[51] The VPC has, as a result, been identified as a champion for enhancing program value.[51] Specific strategies and tactics in which the VPC may play a pivotal role to optimize the TAVR program are listed in Table 11.4.

The VPC role has expanded with the growth of TAVR, compounded by postmarket approval in rapid succession for additional catheter-based structural heart and valve therapies (eg, transcatheter mitral valve repair, transcatheter mitral valve replacement in failed surgical mitral prosthetic rings or valves; transcatheter tricuspid therapies; transcatheter left atrial appendage occlusion), many of which have similar program requirements. The key role and the described phenotype, particularly of VPCs in the early era of TAVR, have culminated for some in a transition to administrative, director, or manager positions in their respective programs and centers.[51,53]

TABLE 11.4. Strategies and Tactics for TAVR Program Optimization

Build the Effective Multidisciplinary Team and Program

1. Effectively distribute team member responsibilities, particularly of the valve program coordinator/clinician, to ensure skill-task alignment and accommodate increasing volume

2. Engage ancillary providers in collaborative patient care

3. Implement clinical pathways that integrate evidence, guidelines, and regulations while reducing complexity

Ensure Appropriate Patient Identification and Referrals

4. Support referring physicians in timely patient identification

5. Leverage echocardiographic surveillance to identify at-risk patients

Optimize the Screening Clinic

6. Prescreen patients to maximize valve clinic capacity and reduce unnecessary testing

7. Develop a patient-centered screening schedule

8. Initiate patient and family screening and education before the valve clinic evaluation

9. Evaluate comprehensive clinical and nonclinical risk factors during screening

(Continued)

TABLE 11.4. Strategies and Tactics for TAVR Program Optimization (Continued)

Improve Procedural Efficiency

10. Optimize procedural scheduling based on data describing utilization, physician and laboratory availability, and need projections

11. Implement clinical protocols that reduce procedural complexity, including moderate sedation

Optimize Postprocedure Recovery

12. Streamline postprocedure recovery pathways that are specific to TAVR, and not adapted from SAVR

13. Educate and empower postprocedure staff to manage expedited recovery pathway

14. Develop rhythm management protocols for earlier identification and treatment of conduction disturbances that prolong length of stay and compromise outcomes

Coordinate Discharge and Long-Term Surveillance

15. Screen for discharge disposition at the time of referral and prioritize discharge to home whenever possible

16. Reinforce the importance of cardiac rehabilitation

17. Hardwire a coordinated long-term follow-up strategy

Leverage Data to Drive Value

18. Prioritize complete and timely registry submission

19. Ensure accurate documentation to capture acuity of patient and care provided, facilitating appropriate payment

20. Monitor program impact through comprehensive evaluation and value analysis

SAVR, surgical aortic valve replacement; TAVR, transcatheter aortic valve replacement.
Adapted from the Advisory Board Company. *Enhancing TAVR Program Value.* 2017.

For all programs, growth demands that responsibilities of the MDT, namely, the VPC, are skill-task aligned to allow for work at the top of licensure. For example, a registered nurse or advanced practice provider (APP) such as a nurse practitioner or physician assistant who spends 60% of his/her full time equivalent (FTE) performing scheduling or clerical tasks is not working at the top of his/her license. Poor skill-task alignment may result in decreased throughput, decreased job satisfaction, increased labor costs, and unrealized gains due to non–revenue producing or non–value added time.[54] As TAVR programs expand and VPCs advance in their roles, it is paramount to evaluate how best to allocate FTEs and optimize the staffing model for clinical coordination.

A model for skill-task alignment is depicted in Figure 11.7. Although this model has its limitations and use of the cognitive domains[55] is not exclusive to a particular position or role, this model is intended as a visual tool to guide skill-task alignment.

Various tools may be employed to assess staffing; however, this evaluation may prove challenging for TAVR program coordination given that responsibilities occur predominantly in the ambulatory care setting and do not often lend itself to tracking via the conventional metrics

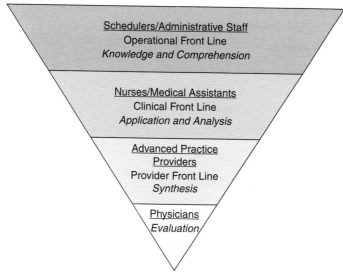

FIGURE 11.7. Skill task alignment for valve program staff. Based on Bloom's Taxonomy of the Cognitive Domain,[55] the blocks of this pyramid depict the level of data or knowledge usage most common to staff members as inferred by ascending levels. Staff members, however, may use all levels of the cognitive domain for the respective scope and licensure and are not limited to a single domain. The associated quantity and state of data from their raw to most synthesized state may be inferred by the block size and level. Skill-task alignment is promoted by distributing work according to the function of the designated role. For example, in this model, advanced practice providers (nurse practitioners and physicians assistants) function at the top of their licenses by serving as the provider front line and allowing nurses and medical assistants to serve as the clinical front line (eg, triaging patient calls, providing patient education). Nurses and medical assistants empower schedulers and administrative staff to serve as the operational front line (eg, scheduling appointments and obtaining medical records). Elements of this figure and its definitions may vary across programs. (©Perpetua Associates, used with permission.)

used in the inpatient setting. As described previously, the duties performed by the TAVR program staff (eg, VPC and/or core clinical and coordination team including program registered nurses, APPs, or administrative coordinators) may not occur in the context of revenue-generating patient visits or encounters that are readily tracked. Table 11.5 offers an example of a swim lane snapshot for the initial patient referral intake, with time trials to assess efficiency and effectiveness and enhance skill-task alignment.

The primary function of the VPC is to steward the patient journey from referral to follow-up. However, the VPC is frequently charged with improving processes, safety, and quality to care for patients. The VPC's knowledge and application of specific methodologies and tools to improve and optimize performance may be a powerful accelerator to enhance program growth and value.

Methodologies and Tools

Although the application of implementation science is outside of the scope of this text, an introduction to methodologies such as the Institute for Healthcare Improvement (IHI) Triple and Quadruple Aim, Toyota (Lean) Production System, and Six Sigma may be useful. Specific

TABLE 11.5. Referral Screening and Coordination Snapshot and Time Trial: Optimizing Skill-Task Alignment by Role, Responsibilities, and Scope

Without Skill-Task Alignment		
Role	**Referral, Screening, and Coordination**	**Minutes per Patient**
Valve program clinician/ coordinator	Initial record review/chart screen	20
	Ensure patient is registered and in electronic medical record	5
	Enter into patient database	5
	Forecast next likely dates for evaluation	10
	Notify referring provider of referral	10
	Initial patient call	30
	Update medical record, calculate initial risk scores, triage	20
	Propose orders, verify allergies, medications, recent laboratory tests	30
	Obtain additional records and images	30
	Obtain preauthorizations as needed	30
	Schedule for departments (clinics, echo laboratory, radiology, etc)	40
	Total time	**240**
With Skill-Task Alignment		
Valve program scheduler (nonclinical)	Initial record review/chart screen and provide to valve program clinician	10
	Ensure patient is registered and in electronic medical record	5
	Enter into patient database	5
	Forecast next likely dates for evaluation	10
	Initial patient call and triage to clinician/coordinator	30
	Schedule w/departments (clinics, echo laboratory, radiology, etc)	40
	Obtain additional records and images	30
	Obtain preauthorizations as needed	30
	Follow-up on records, images, and preauthorizations	20
	Scheduler total time	**180**

TABLE 11.5. Referral Screening and Coordination Snapshot and Time Trial: Optimizing Skill-Task Alignment by Role, Responsibilities, and Scope   (Continued)

Role	Referral Screening and Coordination	Minutes Per Patient
Valve program clinician/ coordinator	Review and screen records, update medical record, calculate initial risk scores, triage, and call patient as needed	35
	Propose/sign orders, verify allergies, medications, recent laboratory tests	15
	Notify referring physician of referral receipt	10
	Clinician coordinator total time	**60**
	Before scheduler hired	240
	After scheduler hired	60
	Time gained after scheduler hired	**180**

tools used for gap analysis, including the aforementioned cross-functional process map, swim lanes the Plan-Do-Study-Act (PDSA) cycle,[56] and Situation, Background, Assessment, Recommendation (SBAR),[57] may also assist VPCs, TAVR program teams, and leadership in the process of optimization.

Triple and Quadruple Aim

In health care, the IHI Triple Aim may be used to describe the goals of program optimization: improving the patient experience of care (quality, satisfaction, and engagement); improving the health of populations; and reducing the per capita cost of health care.[58] Many tools are available from the IHI, including self-assessment tools, videos, and surveys for integrating the Triple Aim framework into an organization or program.

The guiding principles may be embedded into TAVR program development. Minneapolis Heart Institute in Minnesota, for example, has presented their efforts to meet the triple aim by managing the patients in their health care system from initial diagnosis of VHD by echocardiogram. Synthesizing data from the electronic medical record, echocardiographic monitoring, finance, and national registries, Minneapolis Heart Institute's cohort of patients with VHD is provided case management via best practice alerts and tracked for outcomes and costs.[59]

The Quadruple Aim is the addition of a fourth objective addressing an organization's most valuable resources: its people. Satisfaction, engagement, and retention are associated with productivity and success, and the opportunity to use one's strengths has been found to cultivate resilience and may prevent burnout.[60] The IHI has several resources for organizations that seek to apply a fourth aim, emphasizing opportunities for finding love and joy in one's work.

Toyota (Lean) Production System

Founded by Taiichi Ohno between 1948 and 1975, the Toyota Production System (TPS) or Toyota Lean Management System uses a variety of strategies to accomplish the elimination of 7 sources of waste: overproduction, time on hand, transportation, processing, inventory or stock at hand, movement, defects, and underutilized workers. Unique and fundamental to TPS is the principle that those who do the work possess knowledge of the problems and the best solutions. A variety of *Kaizen* (continuous improvement) strategies are employed, including process mapping along the production (value) stream using time trials and defined metrics; 3 Ps: Production, Preparation, Process; and 5 S: Sort, Set in Order, Shine, Standardize, and Sustain (described elsewhere in this text).[61]

Although many health systems use TPS methodologies for project management, in 2002, Virginia Mason Medical Center in Seattle, Washington, became the first in the United States to integrate TPS and its basic tenets into a system-wide structure known as the Virginia Mason Production System (VMPS). The reported benefits of the VMPS include increased value-added time for patients with their providers and increased safety with decreased delays due to timely results and treatments, skill-task alignment for staff, and the elimination of waste. For example, VMPS initiatives decreased the time required to report laboratory test results to the patient by more than 85% and decreased nurse walking distance in the hospital by 750 miles per day, reallocating to direct patient care the 250 hours spent walking.[62] At Virginia Mason, *Kaizen* for TAVR has taken the form of Rapid Process Improvement Workshops to apply a population health approach for VHD, as well as *Kaizen* events for discrete intervals of the clinical pathway (eg, day of procedure, discharge, follow-up with referring provider).

Six Sigma

Six Sigma is a data-driven quality program introduced by Bill Smith in 1985 at Motorola.[63] Named for its aim to drive toward 6 standard deviations between the mean and the near specification limit for a defect, it employs 2 main methodologies: DMAIC (define, measure, analyze, improve, control) and DMADV (define, measure, analyze, design, verify). The former method, DMAIC, is to improve existing processes that fall below the specification (objective) and require incremental improvement. The latter method, DMADV, is used to design new processes or to improve a process that requires substantial improvement. Six Sigma was made central to the business strategy and operations at General Electric in 1995.[63]

The use of Six Sigma in health care is growing. Fanari and colleagues from Prairie Heart Institute in Springfield, Illinois, have described the impacts of Six Sigma quality improvement in their TAVR program. Sources of waste were identified, and the primary goal was to decrease cost and improvement reimbursement. Target improvements and results included improved documentation, billing, and coding of comorbid conditions to the TAVR diagnosis-related group (average gain in reimbursement US$340.8K over 6 months); decreased penalties for post–acute care transfer (decreased from 18% to 10% of cases); decreased pacemaker utilization (unchanged); and decreased intensive care unit utilization (decreased from 100% to 33% over 6 months). The estimated total cost savings per case was US$4.2K per TAVR.[64] As programs strive for efficiency, Six Sigma may be applied to various initiatives to improve processes and outcomes.

Gap Analysis

A gap analysis aims to describe the current state and the desired state, the differences between the 2 states and their root causes, and options for bridging the gaps as well as the barriers and facilitators. This methodology is useful for various program optimizations. For example, a gap analysis may be used for a specific initiative, such as a risk stratification protocol to determine the anesthesia mode for TAVR. Assessment of the current state may include data such as total number of TAVR cases; TAVR cases performed with general anesthesia versus monitored anesthesia care; and patient demographics, outcomes (procedural complications, adverse events), and process metrics (procedure duration, admitting unit, intensive care unit length of stay, total length of stay) observed by mode of anesthesia. The desired state may define the objectives and desired outcomes/measures as compared with national and/or local benchmarks. A gap analysis may also be used for large-scale program assessment of key performance pillars, eg, safety, quality, people, growth, value, and innovation. Some of the tools used for gap analysis include the PDSA cycle and SBAR.

Plan-Do-Study-Act Cycle

The PDSA cycle is a simple tool for process and quality improvement from the Agency for Healthcare Research and Quality.[57] After a team has set a goal, assigned responsibilities, and defined the measures to ascertain the impact of a change, the PDSA cycle allows for a change to be tested. Step 1 is to plan the test or observation, including data collection. Step 2 is to Do, or execute, the change on a small scale. Step 3, Study, is the analysis of data and the study of the results. Finally, step 4 is to Act, or make refinements to the action based on what was learned. Referred to as a modified scientific method, the PDSA cycle allows for a team to plan, try, observe, and improve changes in practice.[57] This tool may be used to review and implement small-scale practice changes in TAVR programs, such as an initiative to use a specific checklist to the nurse call to patients at 24 and 72 hours after hospital discharge or to conduct a patient satisfaction survey with a specific checklist during the discharge phone call.

Situation, Background, Assessment, Recommendation

Originally used in the military and adopted by hospital teams as a communication tool, the SBAR is now also used in health care as a framework for business cases and proposals.[57] Situation refers to a concise statement of the problem. Background provides brief, relevant information to describe the situation. Assessment is the analysis and evaluation of the situation. Recommendation is a description of the requested action(s). The SBAR may be used to communicate gaps and needs. Take the previous example of encounter volume from Table 11.3, in which 10,000 encounters were required for 200 TAVR procedures. Although this is not comprehensive, a sample SBAR is offered.

1. Situation

   We are on pace to double our TAVR volumes this year, but to treat 200 patients with TAVR, 10,000 encounters are required.
2. Background
   a. For patient safety, clinical excellence, and compliance with CMS and the TVT Registry, specific numbers of direct and indirect encounters (Table 11.3) are required. Currently we are able to schedule about 50% of these encounters and our wait time from referral to TAVR has grown from 4 to 8 weeks.

   b. The primary rate-limiting steps to evaluating and treating patients referred to the program include:
  - i. Limited access for scheduling history and physical and follow-up clinic appointments with the physicians (extended from a 2- to 6-week wait for next available new patient appointment times).
  - ii. A nurse practitioner spending 60% of his/her FTE scheduling appointments instead of performing clinical responsibilities.
3. Assessment
  Our new patient clinic appointments with physicians are taking 6 weeks to schedule owing to growing volumes of appointments for history and physicals and follow-up visits. Our nurse practitioner is not empowered to work at the top of his license. These delays may result in the following:
  - a. Clinical decline (death and disability) and attrition (transfer or referral to other centers) of patients.
  - b. Decreased role engagement and satisfaction with retention/turnover concerns of the nurse practitioner.
4. Recommendations
  To treat 200 patients with TAVR this year:
  - a. Urgently allocate up to 0.6-1.0 FTE of scheduler time (may be a nurse based on site-specific definition and scope of role) to enable the nurse practitioner to conduct history and physicals and follow-up visits. This will offload these billable visits to the nurse practitioner, capture revenue, and enable new patients to be seen by physicians more quickly.
  - b. Evaluate encounter volumes, throughput, and skill-task alignment before and after the allocation of nurse or scheduler time monthly and quarterly.
  - c. Comprehensively quantify the number of appointments and additional infrastructure requirements to meet the needs for 200 TAVRs.
  - d. Engage stakeholders in this analysis in 2 meetings: initial in 2 weeks and follow-up in 4 weeks.
  - e. Consider designated hire to plan for growth, informed by findings a to d.

Conclusions

Establishment of a TAVR program entails the application of evidence, guidelines, and quality and regulatory requirements to the hospital mission, vision, infrastructure, and processes. The many complex Inputs, Processes, Outputs, and Outcomes, when taken together, provide a framework for the dynamic iteration of TAVR program development and optimization. The alignment of medical device industry, professional societies, governmental agencies, and payers has accelerated the translation of evidence into clinical practice and the adoption of novel therapies. The focus has shifted from the TAVR procedure to the patient-centered, disease-based program, which uses clinical pathways to deliver the right care to the right patient at the right time. As the second decade of TAVR comes to a close, options for catheter-based treatment have expanded to all valvular and structural heart disease. Future advances leverage the foundation set in place by TAVR programs and the leadership provided by the multidisciplinary Heart Team, including the VPC.

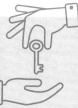

KEY TAKEAWAYS AND BEST PRACTICES

▶ Program development must begin with the end in mind, which includes an understanding of the historical, current, and future landscape of VHD and its treatment options.

▶ Consider a dynamic conceptual framework that incorporates Inputs, Processes, Outputs, and Outcomes using the 5 Ws (why, who, what where, when) and 3 Hs (how, how many, how well).

▶ Various methodologies (Triple Aim, Toyota Lean Production System, Six Sigma) and gap analysis tools (PDSA and SBAR) may be used for performance improvement and program optimization.

▶ The VPC is well suited to play a key role in program optimization and enhancement of program value.

References

1. Lauck S, Achtem L, Boone RH, et al. Implementation of processes of care to support transcatheter aortic valve replacement programs. *Eur J Cardiovasc Nurs.* 2011;12(1):33-38.
2. Hawkey MC, Lauck SB, Perpetua EM, et al. Transcatheter aortic valve replacement program development: recommendations for best practice. *Catheter Cardiovasc Interv.* 2014;84(6):859-867.
3. Kappetein AP, Head SJ, Généreux P, et al. Updated standardized endpoint definitions for transcatheter aortic valve implantation: the Valve Academic Research Consortium-2 Consensus Document. *J Am Coll Cardiol.* 2012;60(15):1438-1454.
4. Baumgartner H, Falk V, Bax JJ, et al. 2017 ESC/EACTS guidelines for the management of valvular heart disease. *Eur Heart J.* 2017;38(36):2739-2791.
5. Nishimura RA, Otto CM, Bonow RO, et al. 2014 AHA/ACC guideline for the management of patients with valvular heart disease: a report of the American College of Cardiology/American Heart Association Task Force on Practice Guidelines. *J Am Coll Cardiol.* 2014;63(22):e57-e185.
6. Vahanian A, Alfieri O, Al-Attar N, et al. Transcatheter valve implantation for patients with aortic stenosis: a position statement from the European Association of Cardio-Thoracic Surgery (EACTS) and the European Society of Cardiology (ESC), in collaboration with the European Association of Percutaneous Cardiovascular Interventions (EAPCI). *Eur Heart J.* 2008;29(11):1463-1470.
7. Mylotte D, Osnabrugge RLJ, Martucci G, Lange R, Kappetein AP, Piazza N. Adoption of transcatheter aortic valve implantation. *Interv Cardiol Rev.* 2013;9(1):37-40.
8. Mylotte D, Osnabrugge RLJ, Windecker S, et al. Transcatheter aortic valve replacement in Europe: adoption trends and factors influencing device utilization. *J Am Coll Cardiol.* 2013;62(3):210-219.
9. Tommaso CL, Bolman Iii RM, Feldman T, et al. Multisociety (AATS, ACCF, SCAI, and STS) expert consensus statement: operator and institutional requirements for transcatheter valve repair and replacement, part 1: transcatheter aortic valve replacement. *J Am Coll Cardiol.* 2012;59(22):2028-2042.
10. Centers for Medicare and Medicaid Services. *National Coverage Determination for Transcatheter Aortic Valve Replacement.* 2012. https://www.cms.gov/medicare-coverage-database/details/ncd-details. aspx?NCDId=355&ncdver=1&NCAId=257&ver=4&NcaName=Transcatheter+Aortic+Valve+Replacement+(TAVR)&bc=ACAAAAAACAAAAA%3D%3D&. Accessed 31 March 2017.
11. Walters D, Webster M, Pasupati S, et al. *The Cardiac Society of Australia and New Zealand Position Statement for the Operator and Institutional Requirements for a Transcatheter Aortic Valve Implantation (TAVI) Program.* 2014.

12. Webb J, Rodés-Cabau J, Fremes S, et al. Transcatheter aortic valve implantation: a Canadian Cardiovascular Society position statement. *Can J Cardiol.* 2012;28(5):520-528.

13. Eggebrecht H, Bestehorn M, Haude M, et al. Outcomes of transfemoral transcatheter aortic valve implantation at hospitals with and without on-site cardiac surgery department: insights from the prospective German aortic valve replacement quality assurance registry (AQUA) in 17919 patients. *Eur Heart J.* 2016;37(28):2240-2248.

14. Bonow RO, Brown AS, Gillam LD, et al. ACC/AATS/AHA/ASE/EACTS/HVS/SCA/SCAI/ SCCT/SCMR/STS 2017 appropriate use criteria for the treatment of patients with severe aortic stenosis. A report of the American College of Cardiology appropriate use criteria task force, American Association for Thoracic Surgery, American Heart Association, American Society of Echocardiography, European Association for Cardio-Thoracic Surgery, Heart Valve Society, Society of Cardiovascular Anesthesiologists, Society for Cardiovascular Angiography and Interventions, Society of Cardiovascular Computed Tomography, Society for Cardiovascular Magnetic Resonance, and Society of Thoracic Surgeons. *J Am Coll Cardiol.* 2017;70(20):2566-2598.

15. STS/ACC Transcatheter Valve Therapies Registry. *Data Collection and Requirements.* 2017. https://www.ncdr.com/webncdr/tvt/publicpage/data-collection.

16. Huded CP, Youmans QR, Puthumana JJ, et al. Lack of association between extracranial carotid and vertebral artery disease and stroke after transcatheter aortic valve replacement. *Can J Cardiol.* 2016;32(12):1419-1424.

17. Condado JF, Jensen HA, Maini A, et al. Should We Perform Carotid Doppler Screening Before Surgical or Transcatheter Aortic Valve Replacement? *Ann Thorac Surg.* 103(3):787-794.

18. *Society of Thoracic Surgeons/American College of Cardiology Transcatheter Valve Therapies Registry Database.* January 2018.

19. Canadian Cardiovascular Society TAVI Quality Working Group. *National Quality Report: Transcatheter Aortic Valve Implantation.* October 2016.

20. Ludman PF, van Domburg RT. The scientific value of TAVI surveys: insights and perspectives from European centres and European patients. *EuroIntervention.* 2016;12(7):823-826.

21. Kodali S. Updates from the U.S. TAVR Commercial Release of the Edwards Sapien Valve. Paper Presented at: Transcatheter Valve Therapies 2013. Vancouver, BC.

22. American Heart Association. Heart disease and stroke statistics 2010 update: a report from the American Heart Association. *Circulation.* 2010;121:e46-e215.

23. Nkomo VT, Gardin JM, Skelton TN, Gottdiener JS, Scott CG, Enriquez-Sarano M. Burden of valvular heart diseases: a population-based study. *Lancet.* 2006;368:1005-1011.

24. Iung B, Baron G, Butchart EG, et al. A prospective survey of patients with valvular heart disease in Europe: The Euro Heart Survey on Valvular Heart Disease. *Eur Heart J.* 2003;24(13):1231-1243.

25. He W, Goodkind D, Kowal P. *An Aging World: 2015.* 2016.

26. Mylotte D, Lefevre T, Søndergaard L, et al. Transcatheter aortic valve replacement in bicuspid aortic valve disease. *J Am Coll Cardiol.* 2014;64(22):2330-2339.

27. U.S. Census Bureau. *U.S. and World Population Clock 2014.* 2018. https://www.census.gov/popclock/.

28. Miller DC. Proliferation of approved TAVR centers in the United States: rational dispersion run amok. *Cardiac Interv Today.* 2017;11(3):29-33.

29. Nishimura R, O'Gara P, Bavaria J, et al. Multisociety expert consensus systems of care document 2017 AATS/ACC/ASE/SCAI/STS expert consensus systems of care document a proposal to optimize care for patients with valvular heart disease: a joint report of the American Association for Thoracic Surgery, American College of Cardiology, American Society of Echocardiography, Society for Cardiovascular Angiography and Interventions, and Society of Thoracic Surgeons (unpublished, open for public comment 2017). 2017.

30. Durko AP, Osnabrugge RL, Van Mieghem NM, et al. Annual number of candidates for transcatheter aortic valve implantation per country: current estimates and future projections. *Eur Heart J.* 2018:2635-2642.

31. Stub D, Lauck S, Lee M, et al. Regional systems of care to optimize outcomes in patients undergoing transcatheter aortic valve replacement. *JACC Cardiovasc Interv.* 2015;8(15):1944-1951.
32. Grover FL, Vemulapalli S, Carroll JD, et al. 2016 annual report of The Society of Thoracic Surgeons/American College of Cardiology Transcatheter Valve Therapy Registry. *J Am Coll Cardiol.* 2017;69(10):1215-1230.
33. O'Brien SM, Cohen DJ, Rumsfeld JS, et al. Variation in hospital risk–adjusted mortality rates following transcatheter aortic valve replacement in the United States. A report from the Society of Thoracic Surgeons/American College of Cardiology Transcatheter Valve Therapy Registry. *Circ Cardiovasc Qual Outcomes.* 2016;9(5):560-565.
34. Birkmeyer JD, Stukel TA, Siewers AE, Goodney PP, Wennberg DE, Lucas FL. Surgeon volume and operative mortality in the United States. *New Engl J Med.* 2003;349(22):2117-2127.
35. Fanaroff AC, Zakroysky P, Dai D, et al. Outcomes of PCI in relation to procedural characteristics and operator volumes in the United States. *J Am Coll Cardiol.* 2017;69(24):2913-2924.
36. Besthorn K, Eggebrecht H, Fleck E, Bestehorn M, Mehta RH, Kuck K-H. Volume-outcome relationship with transfemoral transcatheter aortic valve implantation (TAVI): insights from the compulsory German Quality Assurance Registry on Aortic Valve Replacement (AQUA). *EuroIntervention.* 2017;13(8):914-920.
37. Brennan JM, Holmes DR, Sherwood MW, et al. The association of transcatheter aortic valve replacement availability and hospital aortic valve replacement volume and mortality in the United States. *Ann Thorac Surg.* 2014;98(6):2016-2022.
38. Carroll JD, Vemulapalli S, Dai D, et al. Procedural experience for transcatheter aortic valve replacement and relation to outcomes: The STS/ACC TVT registry. *J Am Coll Cardiol.* 2017;70(1):29-41.
39. Wassef AWA, Alnasser S, Rodes-Cabau J, et al. Institutional experience and outcomes of transcatheter aortic valve replacement: results from an international multicentre registry. *Int J Cardiol.* 2017;245:222-227.
40. Bavaria JE, Tommaso CL, Brindis RG, et al. 2018 AATS/ACC/SCAI/STS expert consensus systems of care document: operator and institutional recommendations and requirements for transcatheter aortic valve replacement. A Joint Report of the American Association for Thoracic Surgery, the American College of Cardiology, the Society for Cardiovascular Angiography and Interventions, and the Society of Thoracic Surgeons. *J Am Coll Cardiol.* 2018.
41. Otto CM, Kumbhani DJ, Alexander KP, et al. 2017 ACC expert consensus decision pathway for transcatheter aortic valve replacement in the management of adults with aortic stenosis. A Report of the American College of Cardiology Task Force on Clinical Expert Consensus Documents. *J Am Coll Cardiol.* 2017.
42. Lauck SB, Wood DA, Baumbusch J, et al. Vancouver transcatheter aortic valve replacement clinical pathway. Minimalist approach, standardized care, and discharge criteria to reduce length of stay. *Circ Cardiovasc Qual Outcomes.* 2016;9(3):312-321.
43. Kamioka N, Wells J, Keegan P, et al. Predictors and clinical outcomes of next-day discharge after minimalist transfemoral transcatheter aortic valve replacement. *JACC Cardiovasc Interv.* 2018;11(2):107-115.
44. Lauck SB, Kwon J-Y, Wood DA, et al. Avoidance of urinary catheterization to minimize in-hospital complications after transcatheter aortic valve implantation: an observational study. *Eur J Cardiovasc Nurs.* 2017;17(1):66-74.
45. Centers for Medicare and Medicaid Services. *MEDCAC Meeting 7/25/2018-TAVR.* 2018. https://www.cms.gov/medicare-coverage-database/details/medcac-meeting-details.aspx?MEDCACId=75. Accessed 1 July 2018.
46. Julian DA. The utilization of the logic model as a system level planning and evaluation device. *Eval Program Plann.* 1997;20(3):251-257.

47. Asgar AW, Lauck S, Ko D, et al. The transcatheter aortic valve implantation (TAVI) quality report: a call to arms for improving quality in Canada. *Can J Cardiol.* 2018;34(3):330-332.

48. Doerr J. *Measure What Matters: OKRs the Simple Idea that Drives 10x Growth.* London, UK: Penguin Books; 2018.

49. National Institutes of Health. *Evaluation of Transcatheter Aortic Valve Replacement Compared to Surveillance for Patients With Asymptomatic Severe Aortic Stenosis (EARLY TAVR).* 2018. https://clinicaltrials.gov/ct2/show/NCT03042104. Accessed 18 January 2018.

50. National Institutes of Health. *Transcatheter Aortic Valve Replacement to Unload the Left Ventricle in Patients With Advanced Heart Failure (TAVR UNLOAD).* 2018. https://clinicaltrials.gov/ct2/show/NCT02661451. Accessed 18 January 2018.

51. Advisory Board Company. *Enhancing TAVR Program Value.* 2017.

52. Institute for Operations Research and the Management Sciences. *Operations Research.* 2018. https://www.informs.org/Explore/Operations-Research-Analytics. Accessed 18 February 2018.

53. Perpetua EM, Clark SE, Guibone K, Keegan PA, Speight MK. *Surveying the Landscape of Heart Team Coordination: The Role of the Advanced Practice Nurse. American College of Cardiology Scientific Sessions 2017, March 17, 2017.* Washington, DC; 2017.

54. Kenney C. *Transforming Health Care: Virginia Mason Medical Center's Pursuit of the Perfect Patient Experience.* New York, NY: Taylor & Francis Books; 2010.

55. Bloom B, Engelhart M, Furst E, Hill W, Krathwohl D. *Taxonomy of Educational Objectives; Handbook I: The Cognitive Domain.* New York: David McKay Co Inc; 1956.

56. Agency for Healthcare Research and Quality. *Plan-Do-Study-Act.* 2008. https://innovations.ahrq.gov/qualitytools/plan-do-study-act-pdsa-cycle.

57. Helmreich R, Merritt A. *Culture at Work in Aviation and Medicine: National, Organizational and Professional Influences.* Aldershot, Great Britain: Ashgate; 2001.

58. Institute for Healthcare Improvement. *Triple Aim Concept Design.* 2012.

59. Sorajja P. Mitral Valve Center of Excellence. Paper Presented at: American College of Cardiology Scientific Sessions 2017. Washington, DC.

60. Linley PA, Harrington S. Strengths coaching: A potential-guided approach to coaching psychology. *Int Coaching Psychol Rev.* 2006;1(1):37-46.

61. Monden Y. *Toyota Production System: An Integrated Approach to Just-in-Time.* Norcross, GA: Industrial Engineering and Management Press; 1993.

62. Mason Virginia. *Fast Facts: Virginia Mason Production System.* 2008. https://www.virginiamason.org/workfiles/pdfdocs/press/vmps_fastfacts.pdf.

63. Harry M, Schroeder R. *Six Sigma.* Random House, Inc; 2000.

64. Fanari Z, Zinselmeier T, Nandish S, Goswami N, Mishkel G. TCT-238 applying lean processes to TAVR work flow to reduce waste and improve cost saving of TAVR program. *J Am Coll Cardiol* 2017;70(18 suppl):B99.

CHAPTER 12

Measuring Success of Transcatheter Aortic Valve Replacement Programs

Sandra B. Lauck, PhD, RN | *Jopie Polderman, BSN, RN* |
Joan Michaels, MSN, CPHQ, AACC

OBJECTIVES

▶ Discuss quality indicators and evaluation frameworks
▶ Highlight opportunities to use quality reports to drive practice change and quality improvement

Introduction

Careful case selection, adherence to current indications, optimal outcomes, and longitudinal follow-up are essential components of transcatheter aortic valve replacement (TAVR) program development. The perfect storm of highly disruptive and evolving technology, the rapid pace of scientific evidence, the potential vulnerabilities of the mostly frail and elderly patient population, and the cost burden of treatment compound to keep TAVR programs under the intense scrutiny of policy makers, funders, clinicians, patients, and other stakeholders. Rigorous program evaluation is pivotal to quality assurance, stewardship of health resources, and support for new indications for treatment.

The requirements of a comprehensive TAVR program evaluation framework differ for various stakeholders. Although all parties share a common interest in quality of care, focus spans case selection and adherence to indications, clinical outcomes, access to care, and health service utilization. In addition, there is increasing interest in strengthening the use of quality indicators to improve accountability and transparency, drive changes in practice, and establish benchmarks of quality. To this end, this chapter proposes a TAVR evaluation framework that addresses diverse indicators. The overarching goal is to support a comprehensive and inclusive approach to measure success and to use program evaluation data to drive quality improvement.

Measuring Case Selection, Risk Evaluation, and Adherence to Indications

Indications for TAVR differ across regions and jurisdictions.[1-5] TAVR programs report patient characteristics, indicators of risk, estimated likelihood to derive benefit from treatment, and adherence to indications based on evidence and the policies set by regulators and funders. There is clinical consensus that case selection warrants the careful consideration of multiple variables and findings; we currently lack an appropriate risk score that captures the complexity of the condition of patients undergoing TAVR and can reliably drive case selection.[6] At this time, there is not a single number or variable that indicates appropriate case selection and adherence to indications. This leaves TAVR programs with the need to capture multiple patient characteristics to describe the population while we await robust risk-adjustment predictor models to inform treatment decision along the continuum of indications. The most salient patient characteristics relate to demographics, burden of cardiac disease and symptoms, comorbidities, and frailty and function.

Patient Demographics

In addition to reporting age and sex, the administrative documentation of marital status and place of residence can provide demographic indicators of social support and geographical distance to the TAVR site. Together, these variables can inform discharge planning and safe transition home and provide a limited measure of social characteristics. Additional information about social support, economic resources, and education can augment programs' awareness of socioeconomic challenges to promote equity of care. The recording of race is well established in the United States, whereas it is not systematically reported in other regions.

Cardiac History

Markers of severity and progression of aortic stenosis are essential to document case selection. Aortic valve area, highest mean gradient pressure, peak velocity, and the grading of valve regurgitation are standard measures obtained by echocardiography or angiography. Valve morphology (ie, tricuspid or bicuspid) can further help describe patients' profile.

The burden of cardiac disease and symptoms is captured to ascertain the severity of overall cardiac risk and degree of patients' symptoms and experience of aortic stenosis. The grading of New York Heart Association functional class and Canadian Cardiovascular Society (CCS) angina are helpful indicators of symptom status. Caution and awareness of inconsistent interrater reliability is warranted in the assessment of these indicators. The recording of left ventricular ejection fraction provides an objective measure to augment the assessment of cardiac function and heart failure.

Patients' history of coronary artery disease is expanded with the recording of previous coronary revascularization (percutaneous coronary intervention or coronary artery bypass graft) and the documentation of current coronary anatomy. Recording prior aortic valve procedures is particularly salient; it includes surgical aortic valve replacement (indicator of planned valve-in-valve procedure), aortic balloon valvuloplasty, and previous TAVR (indicator of planned TAV-in-TAV procedure). The documentation of procedure dates/years provides additional clinical context and indicators of acuity.

Heart rhythm considerations include the documentation of previous permanent pacemaker and/or implantable cardioverter-defibrillator with pacing function. This variable enables the evaluation of new pacemaker rates with the consideration of the denominator of patients "eligible" for a new device. In addition, preexisting atrial fibrillation is documented because of its association with outcomes.[7-9] For procedure planning purposes, the Heart Team may further conduct and document risks of impaired atrioventricular conduction delay to support device selection and anticipate patients' postprocedure pathway.

Comorbidities

Patients undergoing TAVR are routinely burdened with additional comorbidities. To ascertain risk and anticipate patients' postprocedure journey of care, renal function (estimated glomerular filtration rate, creatinine, and history of dialysis), pulmonary function (smoking history, pulmonary function tests, home oxygen, history of chronic lung disease), and neurological function (prior stroke and/or transient ischemic attack) are important variables to describe complexity. A history of porcelain aorta, peripheral arterial disease, and hypertension, treated and untreated, are pertinent to risk stratification. A record of height, weight, and body mass index, as well as preprocedure hemoglobin and serum albumin, provides important indications of clinical status.

Frailty

Frailty is a common comorbidity experienced by patients undergoing TAVR. It is also an important indication for recommending a transcatheter approach owing to excessive risk for a surgical approach. Yet, frailty is not appropriately captured in surgical risk scores or measured in a standard way in clinical practice across TAVR programs. The selection of rigorous, reliable, and clinically useful indicators can help programs highlight this unique risk factor of the TAVR population. Approaches to the measurement of frailty are discussed in a separate chapter.

Risk Scores

The measurement of procedural risk aims to provide an indicator of predicted risk of operative mortality for surgical aortic valve replacement that can inform TAVR case selection and adherence to current indications. The most pertinent risk scores include the Society of Thoracic Surgeons (STS) Predicted Risk of Mortality, the European System for Cardiac Operative Risk Evaluation (EuroSCORE), and the American College of Cardiology (ACC)/STS TAVR In-Hospital Mortality Risk Calculator. Both STS and EuroSCORE define surgical operative mortality as death within 30 days from the operation or later if the patient is still hospitalized.[10] Table 12.1 provides a summary of the variables used for risk adjustment in the 3 models discussed.

The Society of Thoracic Surgeons Predicted Risk of Mortality

The STS National Cardiac Database was created in 1989 to support national quality improvement and has become the largest clinical database, best of its kind.[11] The online calculator is available at http://riskcalc.sts.org/stswebriskcalc/#/. There is a hover function available that provides the definition of each variable.

TABLE 12.1. Variables Considered in Risk Score Models

	STS	EuroSCORE II	ACC/STS TAVR In-Hospital
Risk Estimate	SAVR	SAVR	TAVR
Outcomes estimates	Risk of mortality Morbidity or mortality Long length of stay Short length of stay Permanent stroke Prolonged ventilation Deep sternal wound infection Renal failure Reoperation		In-hospital mortality
Demographics	Age Sex Race	Age Sex	Age Sex Race
Cardiac function	Ejection fraction NYHA class Heart failure <2 weeks Cardiac symptoms Coronary artery disease Prior myocardial infarction Atrial fibrillation Valve disease	Ejection fraction NYHA class CCS class Prior myocardial infarction	NYHA class
Renal function	Creatinine Dialysis	Creatinine	Creatinine Dialysis
Other risk factors	Height and weight Chronic lung disease Cerebrovascular disease Peripheral arterial disease Diabetes mellitus Hypertension Immunocompromise	Chronic lung disease Peripheral arterial disease Diabetes mellitus Poor mobility Pulmonary hypertension	Chronic lung disease
Previous cardiac procedures	Prior Percutaneous coronary intervention Prior Coronary artery bypass Prior valve surgery	Prior cardiac surgery	
Clinical status	Procedure urgency status Resuscitation Cardiogenic shock Intra-aortic balloon pump Inotropes Active endocarditis	Procedure urgency status Active endocarditis	Procedure urgency status Cardiac arrest Cardiogenic shock Inotropes Mechanical assist device
Procedure considerations		Procedure type (weight of the intervention)	Access site

ACC, American College of Cardiology; CCS, Canadian Cardiovascular Society; EuroSCORE, European System for Cardiac Operative Risk Evaluation; NYHA, New York Heart Association; SAVR, surgical aortic valve replacement; STS, Society of Thoracic Surgeons; TAVR, transcatheter aortic valve replacement.

The risk model used in the evaluation of patients undergoing TAVR is the "AV replacement" (aortic valve) procedure, whereas "AV replacement + CAB" (aortic valve replacement + coronary artery bypass) is selected when coronary revascularization is considered, regardless of whether percutaneous coronary intervention will be performed. The model considers a wide variety of end points and generates risk scores for mortality, morbidity, long/short length of stay, permanent stroke, prolonged ventilation, deep sternal wound infection, renal failure, and reoperation. The STS predicted risk of mortality does not fully account for comorbidities pertinent to the population undergoing TAVR, such as severe respiratory disease, porcelain aorta, and frailty, and may underestimate the true surgical risk of patients. The risk scores for 30-day mortality are stratified as low (<4%), intermediate (4%-8%), and high (>8%).

The European System for Cardiac Operative Risk Evaluation

The clinical aim of the EuroSCORE is to provide a scoring system predicting early mortality in cardiac surgical patients in Europe on the basis of objective risk factors. Information was initially collected on 97 risk factors in nearly 20,000 consecutive patients in 128 hospitals in 8 European countries. In the model development, the outcome (survival or death) was related to the selected preoperative risk factors. The most important, reliable, and objective risk factors, weighted from 1 to 4, were then used to prepare a scoring system. The EuroSCORE was updated in 2011 and renamed EuroSCORE II.[12] The online calculator is available at http://www.euroscore.org/calc.html. Standardized variable definitions are available on the calculator page.

The EuroSCORE II provides 2 methods for calculating predicted outcome: the additive model and the logistic model. The additive score has been reported to overpredict risk, whereas the logistic model has been reported to have a more reliable risk-predictor ability, especially in higher-risk groups. The risk scores for 30-day mortality are stratified as low (0-2 points), medium (3-5 points), and high (>5 points); the models do not predict possible morbidity and do not take into consideration intraoperative variables.

The Transcatheter Aortic Valve Replacement In-Hospital Mortality Risk Calculator

The US ACC/STS Transcatheter Valve Therapy (TVT) novel risk estimate was developed from the data of nearly 14,000 consecutive patients treated in US sites between 2011 and 2014 and further validated in a subsequent cohort over nearly 7000 patients treated in 2014.[13] The model is recommended to be used for local quality improvement, monitoring for appropriateness of case selection, and guidance in the overall conversation about the TAVR procedure but not as a recommendation for or against any medical procedure. The online calculator is available at http://tools.acc.org/tavrrisk/#!/content/evaluate/.

The calculator takes into account a set of variables to predict patient risk. It generates a risk-adjusted estimate of in-hospital mortality (not 30-day as for STS and EuroSCORE) and a comparison with a current national average. In the future, the TAVR Risk Calculator will be strengthened with ongoing prospective data collection, inclusion of new variables, and modeling of 30-day mortality.

Measuring Clinical Outcomes

Valve Academic Research Consortium Clinical End Points

The evaluation of TAVR outcomes center on the standardized reporting of the Valve Academic Research Consortium (VARC-2).[14] VARC aims to combine expertise and reach a consensus agreement on the selection of appropriate clinical end points and standardized definitions of single and composite end points. VARC-2 definitions aim to expand the understanding of patient risk stratification and case selection and augment the validity of the EuroSCORE and STS Predicted Risk of Mortality score.[15] Valve program clinicians should become familiar with VARC-2 definitions to support data quality and appropriate reporting. The following is a review of the 8 VARC-2 clinical end points.[14,16]

Mortality

Procedural mortality includes all-cause mortality within 30 days or during the index procedure hospitalization if the postoperative length of stay is longer than 30 days. In addition, VARC-2 recommends the collection of immediate procedure mortality to capture intraprocedural events that result in death ≤72 hours following the procedure. If possible, the cause of death should be captured to discern all-cause, cardiovascular, and noncardiovascular mortality.

Myocardial Infarction

The collection of biomarkers of myocardial injury before the procedure, within 12 to 24 hours after the procedure, at 24 hours, and at discharge is recommended to capture myocardial injury. Acute ischemic events occurring >72 hours are considered spontaneous myocardial infarctions (not related to TAVR).

Stroke

There are significant challenges associated with the accurate assessment, documentation, and reporting of stroke. With the close scrutiny of this potentially devastating periprocedure complication, there is increasing attention to improving data capture and quality. The definition is aligned with the US Food and Drug Administration to assess the clinically relevant consequences of vascular brain injury for determining the safety and efficacy of treatment. To meet VARC-2 criteria, stroke must occur as an acute episode of focal or global neurological dysfunction caused by the brain, spinal cord, or retinal vascular injury as a result of hemorrhage or infarction. Unlike in a transient ischemic attack, tissue damage on neuroimaging studies or new sensory-motor deficit lasting >24 hours is present in stroke. The classification of stroke has evolved from "major" and "minor" to "disabling" and "nondisabling"; the severity is often best assessed by a medical specialist using the modified Rankin scale. Standard reporting includes all strokes, disabling and nondisabling strokes.

Bleeding Complications

The ascertainment of bleeding complications rests on the assessment of the impact on critical organ(s), hemodynamic changes, hemoglobin, and use of blood products. Bleeding complications are categorized as (1) life threatening or disabling, (2) major, and (3) minor. Careful attention to the VARC-2 definition is essential to identify the multiple variables and ensure appropriate reporting. The criteria include the following:

- Life-threatening or disabling bleeding: Fatal bleeding **or** bleeding in a critical organ (eg, intra-cranial) **or** bleeding causing severe hemodynamic decompensation **or** overt bleeding causing a decrease in hemoglobin ≥5 g/dL **or** requiring ≥4 units of red blood cells or whole blood.
- Major bleeding: Overt bleeding causing a decrease in hemoglobin ≥3 g/dL **or** requiring 2-3 units of red blood cells or whole blood **or** causing hospitalization **or** permanent injury requiring surgery.
- Minor bleeding: Any bleeding worthy of clinical mention (eg, access site hematoma) that does not qualify as another category of bleeding.

Acute Kidney Injury

VARC-2 has adopted the acute kidney injury system to classify the severity of renal dysfunction. The timing of diagnosis spans from the day of the procedure to 7 days. Acute kidney injury is classified in 3 stages:

- Stage 1: A 1.5- to 2-fold increase in baseline serum creatinine **or** increase of ≥0.3 mg/dL **or** urine output <0.5 mL/kg/h for >6 but <12 hours.
- Stage 2: A 2- to 3-fold increase in baseline serum creatinine **or** urine output <0.5 mL/kg/h for >12 but <24 hours.
- Stage 3: Greater than 3-fold increase in baseline serum creatinine **or** an increase of ≥4.0 mg/dL with an acute increase of at least 0.5 mg/dL **or** urine output <0.3 mL/kg/h for ≥24 hours **or** anuria for >12 hours.

Vascular Access Site Complications

VARC-2 recommends that information about access and closure techniques be carefully documented and defines both major and minor complications and percutaneous closure device failure. The 3 categories should be consulted in detail. The following highlight some of the indicators without providing a full set of the more complex definitions:

- Major complication: Any aortic dissection, aortic or annulus rupture, or left ventricle perforation **or** access-related vascular injury leading to death or other critical complication **or** distal embolization from a vascular source requiring surgery/amputation/irreversible organ damage **or** unplanned endovascular or surgical intervention associated with death or other critical complication **or** any new documented lower extremity ischemia.
- Minor complication: Access-related vascular injury *not* leading to death or other critical complication **or** distal embolization treated with embolectomy/thrombectomy *not* resulting in amputation/irreversible end-organ damage **or** unplanned endovascular stenting/surgical intervention not meeting the criteria for major complication **or** vascular repair.
- Percutaneous closure device failure: Failure to achieve hemostasis leading to alternative treatment (other than manual compression or adjunctive endovascular ballooning).

Preplanned surgical access or a planned endovascular approach (eg, "preclosure") are part of the procedure and are only documented as complications if an untoward event (eg, bleeding, limb ischemia) occurs. If the complication includes both access site and bleeding, both outcomes are recorded as separate adverse events.

Conduction Disturbances and Arrhythmias

The frequency of TAVR-related new and/or worsened conduction disturbances (eg, atrioventricular block, right or left bundle branch block, atrial fibrillation/flutter) and the incidence and indication for permanent pacemaker implantation are included as VARC-2 complications.

Other Transcatheter Aortic Valve Replacement–Related Complications

VARC-2 recommends documenting other complications including conversion to open heart surgery, unplanned use of cardiopulmonary bypass, coronary obstruction, cardiac tamponade, endocarditis, valve thrombosis/malpositioning/embolization, and the use of more than one TAVR device.

Valvular Function

Echocardiography is used to measure hemodynamic parameters, and transcatheter valve stenosis and regurgitation to document valve function.

Composite End Points

Device success, early safety (30 day), clinical efficacy (>30 day), and time-related valve safety are the VARC-2 families of composite end points. Detailed definitions should be consulted in the source documents to support data quality.

Valve Academic Research Consortium Clinical End Points: Quality of Life

The measurement of quality of life (QOL) is included as a VARC-2 indicator. The Kansas City Cardiomyopathy Questionnaire and the Minnesota Living with Heart Failure questionnaire are validated instruments that produce outcomes on a continuous, responsive, and sensitive scale. Generic health status can be captured using the Medical Outcomes Study Short Form 36, the Short Form 12, or the EuroQOL 5 Domains. The disease-specific measurements provide improved sensitivity, responsiveness, and clinical interpretability and are augmented by the findings of the generic QOL measures of additional domains.

There is a significant challenge associated with the management of missing QOL data because measurements cannot be obtained retrospectively and the assumption that data are missing at random cannot be made.[17] The interpretation of findings cannot be jeopardized by the attrition of the sickest patients who are unable to complete the measurements. Statistical adjustment techniques for missing data could cause QOL to falsely appear to improve over time. The valve program clinician can play an essential role in pursuing the completion of QOL data to strengthen the inclusion of patients' perspectives in the evaluation framework. This enables the reporting of the powerful composite end point that includes both quantity of life (mortality) and QOL.[18]

Measuring Access to Care

An evaluation framework for the measurement of access to care is helpful to report wait list activities, wait times, and overall program capacity to serve patients' needs. This is salient to TAVR program evaluation because wait time benchmarks and expectations differ across regions and models of health care funding.

Transcatheter Aortic Valve Replacement Clinic Activities

The measurement of TAVR clinic activities is an important indicator of access to care. Ideally, program volume reports should consider the following cohorts to fully describe wait list activities every month or fiscal period:

- Number of new referrals received;
- Number of patients under assessment;
- Distribution of treatment decision: (1) accepted for TAVR, (2) not accepted for TAVR (eg, futility of treatment), and (3) other;
- Number of patients actively waiting for the procedure.

These indicators augment the measurement of other clinic activities (eg, diagnostic tests, consultations) and can help provide a snapshot of change over time as programs grow.

Transcatheter Aortic Valve Replacement Wait Times

The CCS adopted the measurement of wait times as a quality indicator to capture patients' trajectory of care from the day of referral to the day of procedure.[19] The CCS highlights that the accurate and timely capture and reporting of wait times is essential to improve clinical wait list management, programmatic planning, and funding allocation. The availability of accurate and standardized measurement of wait times enables cross-regional comparisons and promotes equity of access to care. To this end, the following definitions are recommended to standardize data capture:

- Date of referral: The intent is to capture the date when a referral is made from a physician who knows the patient's clinical status (eg, cardiologist, internist, primary care provider) and believes the patient may benefit from TAVR.
- Date of acceptance: The intent is to capture the date when the Heart Team has the necessary information required to recommend TAVR and has agreed to perform the procedure. It is assumed that the patient confirms shortly after that he/she is ready, willing, and able to undergo the procedure and can be placed on the wait list.
- Placed "on hold": The intent is to subtract the time when a patient's clinical status or personal needs prevents the completion of the assessment or procedure. Patients who request a delay for personal reasons (travel, family events) or need other medical treatments (eg, other elective procedure, new hospitalization that prevents TAVR, clinical deterioration related to a health problem) before they can again be considered actively waiting for the TAVR procedures are placed on hold. Time spent on hold (eg, unavailable for care) can jeopardize accurate wait time reporting. The time placed "on hold" is subtracted from the time under assessment (between date of referral and date of acceptance) or from the time on the wait list (between the date of acceptance and date of procedure). Patients must be ready, willing, and able to proceed with the procedure to be considered as actively waiting for TAVR.
- Date of procedure: The intent is to capture the date when TAVR was performed. The date of admission can be different that the day of procedure. Figure 12.1 summarizes the time points of wait list activities required for appropriate reporting.

Wait List Management Strategies

In programs that experience wait list pressures, multidisciplinary discussions inclusive of administration can facilitate the implementation of wait list strategies to support access to care.

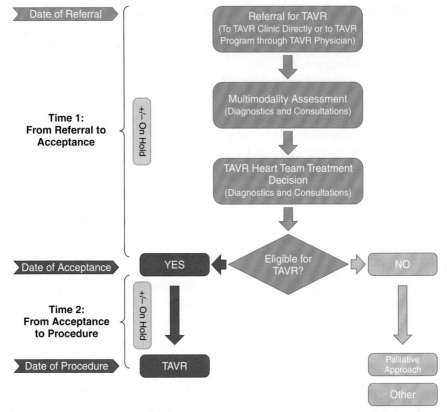

FIGURE 12.1. Time points for accurate reporting of wait time activities. (Used with permission from the Canadian Cardiovascular Society.)

The following illustrate potential interventions that can optimize patient safety and health service resources to manage wait list activities:

- Monitoring of patients' status on the waitlist: A telephone assessment of activities (eg, walking frequency and length, activities of daily living), symptoms (shortness of breath, chest pain, syncope/presyncope, and fatigue), and social support available can provide helpful information to the valve program clinician and the medical team to ascertain status on the wait list and determine patients' procedural priority.
- Appropriate queuing: The valve program clinician plays an essential role in prioritizing patients while ensuring equity of access. The complexity of procedure scheduling may not afford the flexibility and nimbleness required to meet the needs of urgent in-patients and the rapidly evolving clinical status of some out-patients. Thus, appropriate triage is an important competency and activity of the valve program clinician.

- Regular wait list activity report: The following variables are useful indicators of wait list activities to communicate regularly to stakeholders to support program planning:
  - Count of patients added to the wait list (ie, accepted and ready, willing, and able);
  - Count of patients on the wait list;
  - Count of procedures completed resulting in patients removed from the wait list (elective out-patients and urgent in-patients).
- Reporting of adverse events on the wait list: The regular reporting of changes in medical care needs (eg, emergency department visit, hospital readmission, unscheduled physician visit) and mortality while under assessment and on the wait list provides important clinical and administrative information to optimize programs.

Measuring the Transformation of Care

The increased interest in streamlining the moving parts of TAVR programs creates an opportunity to apply an evaluation framework to measure practice and operational change over time to augment the measurement of clinical outcomes. This combined approach enables programs to report on the quality of care and cost-effectiveness of modified processes. Measurements should be captured along patients' journey of care from procedure to safe transition home and throughout the process of change in operations and practices.

Transformation of Periprocedure Care

The transition to a minimalist strategy includes changes in practice and operations related to procedure location, staffing models, mode of anesthesia, use of invasive lines, and procedure times.[20] A comprehensive evaluation framework includes the following:

- Procedure location: Diversity of procedure location enables programs to be more versatile and less resource intensive while adapting to contemporary TAVR. The measurement of the total volume of procedures performed with ratio of use of surgical (ie, hybrid operating room) and cardiac (ie, cardiac catheterization laboratory) procedure rooms can help report changes in periprocedure operations.
- Staffing model: Streamlined models of staffing are an important component of minimalist TAVR. The documentation of the number and disciplines of periprocedure nurses and allied health professionals can support the reconfiguration of services and help recalibrate the human resource requirements.
- Model of anesthesia: For programs adopting a default strategy of local anesthesia or monitored anesthesia care, the documentation of change over time in anesthetic approach (ie, ratio of general anesthesia and local/monitored anesthesia care) provides a helpful illustration of change management. In addition, the measurement of planned and final anesthesia provides a documentation of crossover of modality and conversion to a higher degree of anesthesia.
- Use of invasive lines: The avoidance of invasive lines is associated with improved outcomes and shorter length of stay. The adoption of this change in practice can be captured by documenting the change in use of central venous catheter, removal of temporary pacemaker at the end of procedure, and avoidance of urinary catheterization.

- Procedure times: The cumulative impact of changes in anesthesia and avoidance of invasive lines is associated with shorter procedure times. The capture of points of (1) time of entry in procedure room, (2) time of first attempt at vascular access, (3) time of successful vascular closure, and (4) time of exit from room are required to measure implantation and total procedure times.

Transformation of Postprocedure Care

The primary goals of postprocedure TAVR care focus on the rapid return to baseline status, the avoidance of procedure-related complications and geriatric deconditioning, and patients' successful transition home. The implementation of a standardized postprocedure protocol has been shown to augment the benefits of a minimalist periprocedure approach and facilitate next-day discharge.[20] The measurement of the effectiveness of the multiple moving parts of a streamlined protocol (eg, reduced bedrest time, early hydration and nutrition, removal of invasive lines, avoidance of temporary pacemaker, facilitated elimination) can be captured in the measurement of time to first mobilization.

The critical care requirements of patients undergoing TAVR are evolving. There is increasing evidence that the accelerated transfer to the cardiac telemetry ward, and the avoidance of recovery in a critical care unit, is a safe strategy for select patients.[21] The measurement of postprocedure critical care hours enables the tracking of nursing care resource intensity.

Lastly, total hospital length of stay and disposition at discharge are increasingly recognized as TAVR program quality indicators. Shorter length of stay and discharge home are the end products of a bundle of changes that encompass case selection, a minimalist approach, and rapid reconditioning postprocedure care.[22] Monitoring changes in the length of stay and proportion of patients successfully discharged home without increased care requirements stresses the overarching goal of minimizing disruptions to patients' health status while promoting safety and optimal outcomes.

Measuring Cost-Effectiveness

The measurement of cost-effectiveness of TAVR is a priority for decision makers and a strategy for programs to complement outcome evaluation and improve the stewardship of health resources.

Value in Health Care

There is a consensus agreement that the society ought to increase the value of health services as a guiding principle in the assessment of innovation, decisions about funding, and implementation of health care reform.[23] The concept of value can be defined in widely varying ways informed by diverse perspectives. From a health economics standpoint, value can be conceptualized as the ratio of incremental benefits to incremental costs.[23] This definition captures the notion of "bang for the buck" or "best buy," the allocation of resources with an expectation of a net gain for individuals and a return on society's investment.[24]

Interest in the cost-effectiveness of TAVR remains high as funders, policy makers, clinicians, patients and their families, and society at large rightfully ask for evidence that this rapidly evolving treatment provides sufficient value to justify costs.[25] Stakeholders seek to adapt to the evolving clinical context to build consensus on how to best integrate this therapy in health services and funding models. Cost-effectiveness assessment takes into consideration costs, clinical effectiveness, and society's values and judgments.[26]

The costs of TAVR are, in theory, easy to define. One of the challenges is that regions and health systems differ in their capacity to capture high-quality costing data and ascertain true costs. In addition, the acquisition costs of devices can vary significantly across jurisdictions and be opaque owing to differing systems of pricing and contracts.[27]

Quantifying effectiveness is more challenging; it is driven first and foremost by clinical effectiveness—an innovative treatment such as TAVR has to be effective in and of itself before it can be cost-effective for different groups of patients.[25] Improvement in survival and morbidity and QOL are the essential components to demonstrate clinical effectiveness. These assessments must be cautiously interpreted in the greater context of disease progression and alternative treatments, including the costs of surgical valve replacement or "doing nothing"—continuing medical management, and considering a transition to a palliative approach.[28,29]

Finally, values and judgements informed by scientific and social perspectives play an important role in determining cost-effectiveness. The appraisal of the scientific evidence aims to determine the reliability and the generalizability of findings to "real-world" clinical care and the appropriate capture of changes in QOL, an essential component of cost-effectiveness analyses. This scrutiny is essential because all clinical trials have limitations and deficiencies and none are perfect.[27]

Thus, the fundamental notion of cost-effectiveness analysis is simple: how much does TAVR improve clinical outcomes compared with the next best alternative for a given patient (ie, surgical valve replacement or medical management), and how much does treatment cost compared with that alternative?[25] This principle is conventionally captured by the measurement of quality-adjusted life-years divided by the difference in costs, which yields the incremental cost-effectiveness ratio. A working knowledge of these concepts is helpful for valve program clinicians to fully participate in measuring success.

Quality-Adjusted Life-Year

A quality-adjusted life-year is commonly referred to as a QALY, a unit that simultaneously measures quality and quantity of life. It is a means to attribute a QOL value to a year of life. This unit reflects the idea that people are often willing to trade off some quantity of life if they can substantially reduce their symptom burden and improve their QOL and that a year of life in high-quality health should "count for" more than a year of life in poor quality health.[24] QALYs integrate benefits, harms, and burdens into a single number that can then be compared with the cost of treatment.[30,31]

Calculating a Quality-Adjusted Life-Year

The 2 dimensions that must be captured to calculate a QALY are (1) years of life (ie, mortality) and (2) QOL, captured as a utility value (for example, with the EuroQoL scale). A utility can have a value between 1 (representing perfect health) and 0 (representing death). One QALY equates to 1 year of perfect health.

The number of QALYs is the product of years of life multiplied by the utility value (number of QALYs = years of life × utility value). The following examples illustrate how to interpret the number of QALYs:

- If a person lives in **perfect health** for **1 year**, that person will have **1 QALY** (1 year of life × 1 utility value = 1 QALY)
- If a person lives in **perfect health** for **6 months**, that person will have **0.5 QALY** (1/2 year of life × 1.0 utility value = 0.5 QALY)
- If a person lives for **1 year** but in **a situation with imperfect health with a 0.3 utility value**, that person will have 0.3 QALY (1 year of life × 0.3 utility value = 0.3 QALY)

Cost-Effectiveness Plane: Quadrants

The comparison of QALY with cost can be depicted in a cost-effectiveness plane with 4 quadrants that show the incremental relationship between cost of treatment and QALY gained compared with the next best alternative (Figure 12.2). The categories of cost-effectiveness can be summarized as follows[26]:

- Quadrant A: High cost and low effectiveness—The intervention is more expensive and less effective. This treatment option should be rejected by society.
- Quadrant B: Low cost and low effectiveness—The intervention is less expensive but less effective. This option is unusual and rarely discussed.
- Quadrant C: Low cost and high effectiveness—The intervention is less expensive and more effective. This option is relatively uncommon; it should be readily adopted.
- Quadrant D: High cost and high effectiveness—The intervention is more expensive but more effective. This option can pose significant dilemmas for decision makers to ascertain how a health care system can afford the additional cost given the incremental benefits to individuals and society.

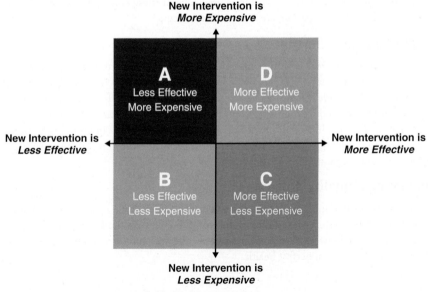

FIGURE 12.2. Cost-effectiveness plane.

Cost-Effectiveness Plane: Incremental Cost-Effectiveness Ratio

The incremental cost-effectiveness ratio (ICER) illustrates the relationship between QALY and cost and summarizes the difference in cost between 2 possible interventions, divided by the difference in their effect. Data are conventionally presented as a total cost incurred per QALY added.

There is no absolute or internationally recognized ICER given the substantial differences within and between health care systems in the accepted standards of care and the relevant comparators. The threshold between cost-effective and cost-ineffective interventions is influenced by social consideration and value judgements, irrespective of scientific evidence, because it is a measure of what society is willing to pay, considers affordable, and appraises as a good or reasonable investment. In economically wealthy countries, a cost of $50,000 per QALY gained is readily accepted, whereas treatments with a cost of more than $100,000 per QALY are generally considered too expensive. There is more debate when the ICER is between these 2 thresholds.[25] Figure 12.3 illustrates the delineation of an acceptable ICER based on the assessment of cost-effectiveness.

Quality Reports

The dissemination of quality reports is a powerful vehicle to promote continuous quality improvement through rigorous and transparent evaluation, comparison with benchmarks, and monitoring of change over time. The mandatory participation in regional/national registries and the adoption of standardized indicators have enabled the regular reporting of quality of care across jurisdictions and championed the importance of using quality data to drive quality of care. The following reports illustrate how data are reported in select health authorities to feed information back to stakeholders, establish national benchmarks, and promote a culture of accountability.

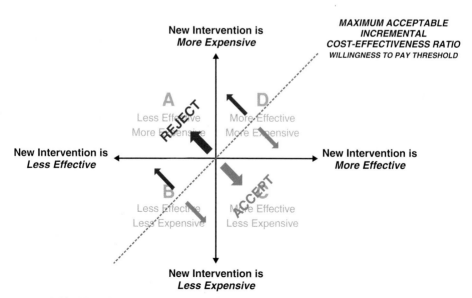

FIGURE 12.3. Threshold for acceptable incremental cost-effectiveness ratio.

The American College of Cardiology/Society of Thoracic Surgeons Transcatheter Valve Therapy Registry Report

The STS/ACC TVT Registry was launched in 2011 and is designed to support a national surveillance system to assess the characteristics, treatments, and outcomes of patients receiving transcutaneous valve therapies. Participation in the national registry is mandatory to meet the reimbursement requirements of the Centers for Medicare & Medicaid Services. To date, over 100,000 cases have been centrally reported. Patient-level data are submitted by participating hospitals to the TVT Registry. The purposes of the TVT Registry include:

- Collecting pertinent and standardized data elements from participating hospitals, health care providers, and others that measure and assess the quality of care for patients receiving TVT;
- Providing confidential periodic reports to participating hospitals, health care providers, and others, to evaluate and improve the quality of care in these areas; and
- Permitting and fostering appropriate research based on the data collected by means of the TVT Registry. A unique aspect of the TVT Registry is that it also requires 30-day and 1-year follow-up data. Patients are followed up for 5 years through the Centers for Medicare & Medicaid Services linked data.

Data are submitted in the Web-based STS/ACC TVT Registry data collection tool. Data quality is augmented by the data quality report process, which provides surveillance for errors and completeness. Individual information is summarized in an automated report that is shared with the implanting site. Participating sites receive a quarterly outcomes report with benchmarking data that enables comparisons across centers.

The Canadian Cardiovascular Society Transcatheter Aortic Valve Replacement Quality Report

In 2016, the CCS published the first iteration of national quality indicators in collaboration with a working group with representatives from all Canadian centers.[19] The goal was to develop an evaluation framework to provide evidence-based findings to catalyze local, regional, and national quality improvement; to support patients' access to appropriate, high-quality care; and to foster a national strategy to optimize patient outcomes and health service utilization. The project aimed to overcome the challenges associated with the absence of a national registry and the historical difficulties in pooling patient-level data across Canadian jurisdictions by linking provincial jurisdictions. The first Canadian TAVR Quality Report was released in 2016 and provided a proof of concept of the feasibility of the project and important information to begin a national benchmarking exercise.

The selection of the CCS TAVR quality indicators was driven by the Donabedian conceptual framework that is widely adopted to examine health services and evaluate quality of health care using structural, process, and outcome indicators.[32] The criteria used by the CCS TAVR Working Group to conduct the selection of indicators included (1) the perceived importance of the variable, (2) the feasibility of measurement, and (3) the likelihood of obtaining quality data across jurisdictions. The current CCS TAVR Quality Indicators include the following:

- Structural indicators: documentation of Heart Team treatment decision; TAVR wait times; length of stay.
- Process indicators: evaluation of procedural risk; evaluation of QOL.
- Outcome indicators: 30-day and 1-year mortality; in-hospital stroke; new permanent pacemaker; transfusion of blood products; all-cause 30-day and 1-year hospital readmission.

The level of reporting has evolved from an initial agreement to compare indicators across 4 geographical regions to the adoption of site-level reporting.[33] The intent is to foster a commitment to accountability and transparency and stress the importance of collective engagement to address the complexity of TAVR quality assurance. To this end, the CCS TAVR Working Group has published a "TAVR Toolkit" to support improved data quality and to provide stakeholders with practice-ready strategies to use data reporting as a mechanism to embed quality improvement (available at https://www.ccs.ca/en/).

European Registries

In a 2016 systematic review of European registries, 7 national TAVR registries were identified.[34] These include the following:

- Belgian National Registry[35]
- French Aortic National CoreValve and Edwards (FRANCE 2) Registry[36,37]
- German Aortic Valve Registry (GARY)[38,39]
- Italian transcatheter aortic valve implantation (TAVI) registries[40,41]
- Spanish TAVI Registry[42]
- Swiss TAVI Registry[43]
- United Kingdom TAVI Registry[44]

The adoption of standardized quality indicators across international regions is an essential component of monitoring of quality of care.

Conclusion

The measurement of success for patients undergoing TAVR and TAVR programs is an essential component of quality care and stewardship of resources. The primary objective of a comprehensive evaluation framework is to drive best practices and quality improvement. The high level of scrutiny applied to TAVR is likely to remain unchanged as indications, technology, and procedural approaches evolve and as stakeholders grapple with ensuring appropriate access to care and optimal outcomes.

KEY TAKEAWAYS AND BEST PRACTICES

▶ The goals of measuring the success of TAVR programs include evaluating case selection, clinical outcomes, QOL, access to care, and quality improvement.

▶ Adherence to standardized definitions and the pursuit of data quality are essential to program evaluation and enable comparison across programs and regions.

▶ VARC-2 indicators are the most commonly reported clinical indicators. Valve program clinicians require a working knowledge of these important markers of quality.

References

1. Nishimura RA, Otto CM, Bonow RO, et al. 2014 AHA/ACC guideline for the management of patients with valvular heart disease: executive summary: a report of the American College of Cardiology/American Heart Association Task Force on Practice Guidelines. *J Am Coll Cardiol.* 2014;63(22):2438-2488.

2. Otto CM, Kumbhani DJ, Alexander KP, et al. 2017 ACC expert consensus decision pathway for transcatheter aortic valve replacement in the management of adults with aortic stenosis: a report of the American College of Cardiology Task Force on Clinical Expert Consensus Documents. *J Am Coll Cardiol.* 2016.

3. Bonow RO, Brown AS, Gillam LD, et al. ACC/AATS/AHA/ASE/EACTS/HVS/SCA/ SCAI/SCCT/SCMR/STS 2017 appropriate use criteria for the treatment of patients with severe aortic stenosis: a report of the American College of Cardiology Appropriate Use Criteria Task Force, American Association for Thoracic Surgery, American Heart Association, American Society of Echocardiography, European Association for Cardio-Thoracic Surgery, Heart Valve Society, Society of Cardiovascular Anesthesiologists, Society for Cardiovascular Angiography and Interventions, Society of Cardiovascular Computed Tomography, Society for Cardiovascular Magnetic Resonance, and Society of Thoracic Surgeons. *J Am Coll Cardiol.* 2017;70(20):2566-2598.

4. Nishimura RA, O'Gara PT, Bonow RO. Guidelines update on indications for transcatheter aortic valve replacement. *JAMA Cardiol.* 2017;2(9):1036-1037.

5. Vahanian A, Alfieri O, Andreotti F, et al. Guidelines on the management of valvular heart disease (version 2012): the Joint Task Force on the Management of Valvular Heart Disease of the European Society of Cardiology (ESC) and the European Association for Cardio-Thoracic Surgery (EACTS). *Eur J Cardio-Thorac Surg.* 2012;42(4):S1-S44.

6. Cerrato E, Nombela-Franco L, Nazif TM, et al. Evaluation of current practices in transcatheter aortic valve implantation: the WRITTEN (WoRldwIde TAVI ExperieNce) survey. *Int J Cardiol.* 2017;228:640-647.

7. Hengstenberg C, Chandrasekhar J, Sartori S, et al. Impact of pre-existing or new-onset atrial fibrillation on 30-day clinical outcomes following transcatheter aortic valve replacement: results from the BRAVO 3 randomized trial. *Catheter Cardiovasc Interv.* 2017;90(6):1027-1037.

8. Biviano AB, Nazif T, Dizon J, et al. Atrial fibrillation is associated with increased pacemaker implantation rates in the placement of AoRTic Transcatheter Valve (PARTNER) trial. *J Atrial Fibrillation.* 2017;10(1):1494.

9. Tarantini G, Mojoli M, Windecker S, et al. Prevalence and impact of atrial fibrillation in patients with severe aortic stenosis undergoing transcatheter aortic valve replacement: an analysis from the SOURCE XT Prospective Multicenter Registry. *JACC Cardiovasc Interv.* 2016;9(9):937-946.

10. Arangalage D, Cimadevilla C, Alkhoder S, et al. Agreement between the new EuroSCORE II, the Logistic EuroSCORE and the Society of Thoracic Surgeons score: implications for transcatheter aortic valve implantation. *Arch Cardiovasc Dis.* 2014;107(6-7):353-360.

11. Ferguson TB Jr. The Society of Thoracic Surgeons' National Cardiac Database: provider engagement in continuous quality improvement. *Am Heart Hosp J.* 2003;1(2):180-182.

12. Roques F, Michel P, Goldstone A, et al. The logistic euroscore. *Eur Heart J.* 2003;24(9):882-883.

13. Edwards FH, Cohen DJ, O'Brien SM, et al. Development and validation of a risk prediction model for in-hospital mortality after transcatheter aortic valve replacement. *JAMA Cardiol.* 2016;1(1):46-52.

14. Kappetein AP, Head SJ, Genereux P, et al. Updated standardized endpoint definitions for transcatheter aortic valve implantation: the Valve Academic Research Consortium-2 consensus document. *J Am Coll Cardiol.* 2012;60(15):1438-1454.

15. Zhang S, Kolominsky-Rabas PL. How TAVI registries report clinical outcomes—A systematic review of endpoints based on VARC-2 definitions. *PLoS One.* 2017;12(9):e0180815.

16. Kappetein AP, Head SJ, Genereux P, et al. Updated standardized endpoint definitions for transcatheter aortic valve implantation: the Valve Academic Research Consortium-2 consensus document. *EuroIntervention.* 2012;8(7):782-795.

17. Bell ML, Fairclough DL. Practical and statistical issues in missing data for longitudinal patient-reported outcomes. *Stat Methods Med Res.* 2014;23(5):440-459.

18. Arnold SV, Afilalo J, Spertus JA, et al. Prediction of poor outcome after transcatheter aortic valve replacement. *J Am Coll Cardiol.* 2016;68(17):1868-1877.

19. Asgar AW, Lauck S, Ko D, et al. Quality of care for transcatheter aortic valve implantation: development of canadian cardiovascular society quality indicators. *Can J Cardiol.* 2016;32(8):1038.e1-4.

20. Lauck SB, Wood DA, Baumbusch J, et al. Vancouver transcatheter aortic valve replacement clinical pathway: minimalist approach, standardized care, and discharge criteria to reduce length of stay. *Circ Cardiovasc Qual Outcomes.* 2016;9(3):312-321.

21. Kamioka N, Wells J, Keegan P, et al. Predictors and clinical outcomes of next-day discharge after minimalist transfemoral transcatheter aortic valve replacement. *JACC Cardiovasc Interv.* 2018;11(2):107-115.

22. Lauck SB, Wood DA, Achtem L, et al. Risk stratification and clinical pathways to optimize length of stay after transcatheter aortic valve replacement. *Can J Cardiol.* 2014;30(12):1583-1587.

23. Braithwaite RS, Rosen AB. Linking cost sharing to value: an unrivaled yet unrealized public health opportunity. *Ann Intern Med.* 2007;146(8):602-605.

24. Braithwaite RS, Mentor SM. Identifying favorable-value cardiovascular health services. *Am J Manag Care.* 2011;17(6):431-438.

25. Hlatky MA. Considering cost-effectiveness in cardiology clinical guidelines: progress and prospects. *Value Health.* 2016;19(5):516-519.

26. Rawlins MD. Cost, effectiveness, and value: how to judge? *JAMA.* 2016;316(14):1447-1448.

27. Rawlins MD. Evidence, values, and decision making. *Int J Technol Assess Health Care.* 2014;30(2):233-238.

28. Indraratna P, Ang SC, Gada H, et al. Systematic review of the cost-effectiveness of transcatheter aortic valve implantation. *J Thorac Cardiovasc Surg.* 2014;148(2):509-514.

29. Sud M, Tam DY, Wijeysundera HC. The economics of transcatheter valve interventions. *Can J Cardiol.* 2017;33(9):1091-1098.

30. Braithwaite RS, Omokaro C, Justice AC, et al. Can broader diffusion of value-based insurance design increase benefits from US health care without increasing costs? Evidence from a computer simulation model. *PLoS Med.* 2010;7(2):e1000234.

31. Neumann PJ, Rosen AB, Weinstein MC. Medicare and cost-effectiveness analysis. *New Engl J Med.* 2005;353(14):1516.

32. Ayanian JZ, Markel H. Donabedian's lasting framework for health care quality. *New Engl J Med.* 2016;375(3):205-207.

33. Asgar AW, Lauck S, Ko D, et al. The Transcatheter Aortic Valve Implantation (TAVI) quality report: a call to arms for improving quality in Canada. *Can J Cardiol.* 2018;34(3):330-332.

34. Krasopoulos G, Falconieri F, Benedetto U, et al. European real world trans-catheter aortic valve implantation: systematic review and meta-analysis of European national registries. *J Cardiothorac Surg.* 2016;11(1):159.

35. Bosmans JM, Kefer J, De Bruyne B, et al. Procedural, 30-day and one year outcome following CoreValve or Edwards transcatheter aortic valve implantation: results of the Belgian national registry. *Interact Cardiovasc Thorac Surg.* 2011;12(5):762-767.

36. Eltchaninoff H, Prat A, Gilard M, et al. Transcatheter aortic valve implantation: early results of the FRANCE (FRench Aortic National CoreValve and Edwards) registry. *Eur Heart J.* 2011;32(2):191-197.

37. Gilard M, Eltchaninoff H, Iung B, et al. Registry of transcatheter aortic-valve implantation in high-risk patients. *New Engl J Med.* 2012;366(18):1705-1715.

38. Beckmann A, Hamm C, Figulla H, et al. The German Aortic Valve Registry (GARY): a nationwide registry for patients undergoing invasive therapy for severe aortic valve stenosis. *Thorac Cardiovasc Surg.* 2012;60(05):319-325.

39. Zahn R, Gerckens U, Grube E, et al. Transcatheter aortic valve implantation: first results from a multi-centre real-world registry. *Eur Heart J.* 2010;32(2):198-204.

40. D'onofrio A, Salizzoni S, Agrifoglio M, et al. Medium term outcomes of transapical aortic valve implantation: results from the Italian Registry of Trans-Apical Aortic Valve Implantation. *Ann Thorac Surg.* 2013;96(3):830-836.

41. Buja P, Napodano M, Tamburino C, et al. Comparison of variables in men versus women undergoing transcatheter aortic valve implantation for severe aortic stenosis (from Italian Multicenter CoreValve registry). *Am J Cardiol.* 2013;111(1):88-93.

42. Sabaté M, Cánovas S, García E, et al. In-hospital and mid-term predictors of mortality after transcatheter aortic valve implantation: data from the TAVI National Registry 2010-2011. *Rev Esp Cardiol (Engl Ed).* 2013;66(12):949-958.

43. Wenaweser PM, Stortecky S, Heg DH, et al. Short-term clinical outcomes among patients undergoing transcatheter aortic valve implantation in Switzerland: the Swiss TAVI registry. *EuroIntervention.* 2014;10(8):982-989.

44. Blackman DJ, Baxter PD, Gale CP, et al. Do outcomes from transcatheter aortic valve implantation vary according to access route and valve type? The UK TAVI Registry. *J Interv Cardiol.* 2014;27(1):86-95.

CHAPTER 13

Transforming the Way We Care for Transcatheter Aortic Valve Replacement Patients

Sandra B. Lauck, PhD, RN | *Patricia A. Keegan, DNP, NP-C, AACC*

OBJECTIVES

▶ Discuss strategies to move change forward in TAVR programs
▶ Discuss opportunities to adopt strategies to promote safe and early discharge home, improve outcomes, and reduce health care costs

Background

The Need to Revisit Historical Practices

Advances in technology, case selection, anatomical screening and imaging, procedural approaches, and expertise create new opportunities to revisit historical practices. There has been a dramatic global increase in the number of procedures and a universal acceptance that patients of all risk profiles will be increasingly treated with a transcatheter option as evidence continues to emerge.[1,2] The unique needs of elderly patients undergoing transcatheter aortic valve replacement (TAVR) and the distinct risks associated with a minimally invasive catheter-based procedure are prompting clinicians to examine early practices informed by cardiac surgery to tailor care to patients' individual requirements.[3] It is imperative that TAVR programs evolve from the historical blueprint where TAVR was considered as *"One Off,"* a low-volume procedure requiring significant resources and planning for the potentially catastrophic *"What Ifs."* Historically, the operations and practices of TAVR programs were guided by "surgical thinking," including recommendations or requirements for the use of a hybrid operating room, the presence of cardiac surgery teams and perfusion services, and the use of established cardiac surgery postprocedure protocols developed for open heart surgery, an often maximally invasive procedure. In addition, interventional cardiology processes have not been fully adapted to meet patient and procedural needs. There is varying practice about the use of invasive monitoring devices, mode of anesthesia and echocardiographic monitoring, critical care nursing requirements, and optimal length of stay.

In the era of 30-day mortality rates as low as 1.1%,[4] TAVR programs require processes of care that reflect contemporary practices, operations, and outcomes and are adapted to patients and current technology. We can reflect back on the first-in-human implantation by Dr Cribier in a cardiac catheterization laboratory in Rouen, France, and remind ourselves that the earliest vision was to adopt minimalist strategies involving access and sedation. Evidence is rapidly emerging that the implementation of a clinical pathway tailored to the unique needs of patients and benchmarked to contemporary TAVR practices can help transform care, improve outcomes, streamline health resource utilization, and decrease costs to help fulfill this vision.[5,6] Valve program clinicians, in close partnership with the Heart Team, are leaders in the transformation of TAVR care.

A New Standard for Transcatheter Aortic Valve Replacement Programs?

Procedural success is insufficient to ensure that the unique group of primarily elderly patients with advanced valvular disease and other comorbidities have an optimal outcome following TAVR. Achieving low mortality and high patient satisfaction requires a concerted effort to identify opportunities for quality improvement along patients' continuum of care, from referral, admission, discharge home, and follow-up.

In the past decade of TAVR, programs have learned important lessons. From a program development perspective, these can be summarized as follows:

- *It is not all about the valve.* Careful attention to all components of care from admission to transition home is essential.
- Most patients undergoing TAVR are elderly. *We must mitigate the risks of complications caused by the geriatric giants* (new onset of confusion, falls, incontinence, impaired homeostasis, iatrogenic disorders). These can jeopardize the success of the valve replacement.
- Procedural and program *success is when the patient goes home* without in-hospital complications to benefit from improved quantity and quality of life.
- *A cardiac surgery pathway and "mindset" are inappropriate* for TAVR.
- TAVR programs require *TAVR-specific processes of care* to meet the unique needs of the patients and the procedure.

The purpose of this chapter is to explore the substantial challenges and opportunities associated with multidisciplinary change management in the already complex TAVR context and to offer strategies for teams to consider to transition practice and operations to match contemporary TAVR.

Transforming Transcatheter Aortic Valve Replacement: Challenges and Opportunities

Bigger than Transcatheter Aortic Valve Replacement: Promoting Change in Program Development

Organizations strive to improve care provided to enhance patient outcomes. At times, change is necessary for organizational growth, patient benefit, and staff engagement. Continuous quality improvement is a marker of high-performing health care organizations and an imperative for patient safety. Change can be difficult and even traumatic, and personnel may have apprehension when moving to a new system of care. Unfortunately, change is not easy. Challenges include institutional barriers, lack of motivation, limited access to technology, lack of knowledge, physician and patient factors, and limited time.[7]

When deciding to enact change, conducting a baseline assessment can help the organization identify potential and actual barriers to making the change. Baseline assessments can be conducted in various ways, including using a gap analysis or SWOT analysis (strengths, weaknesses, opportunities, threats). Barriers create gaps in recommended practices and can have a negative effect on the process.[8] This process is potentially fragile, fraught with expected and unexpected twists and turns, and requires thoughtful planning and the complex engagement of stakeholders. Failure to involve the right people or teams at the right time can elicit fear, lack of desire to make changes, and ultimately failure to complete the change. This can contribute to the "sabotage" of the vision, to delays and other complications, and to short- and long-term challenges.

Understanding Change Management

Having some understanding of the complexity of organizational change management can help valve program clinicians to work closely with teams to pioneer the review of practice and program operations and champion the contributions of nurses and allied health professionals to transform TAVR care. Lewin's change theory is commonly used in the health care arena to enact change.[9] This theory proposes that individuals and groups are influenced by restraining forces as well as driving forces and the tension between these forces maintains equilibrium.[10] Examples of organizational restraints include resources, organizational structures, and threshold for risk, whereas drivers include patient safety, quality improvement, shift to patient-centered processes, efficiencies, and cost containment. Lewin's model consists of 3 steps: unfreezing, changing, and refreezing.[11] During the unfreezing step, problem awareness is created. Once the problem is recognized and acknowledged, it is then possible to undo the current process.[10] During changing, otherwise known as moving, alternative action is sought out. Benefits of change and strategies are explored and efforts to negate barriers are identified. Lastly, during refreezing, the behavior change becomes habit and resists further change (Figure 13.1).[10,12]

Another helpful conceptualization is the Lean system approach for change (Lean change management). This model was developed by Toyota Motor Company to address manufacturing problems and improve efficiencies.[12] Many concepts are transferrable to supporting innovation in health care. In Lean, value is created by limiting waste, in terms of human resource utilization, process, time, or equipment. Areas addressed during the Lean process focus on overproduction, inventory, motion, transportation, overprocessing, defects, waiting, and

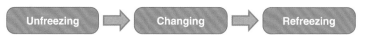

FIGURE 13.1. Lewin's theory of change. During the unfreezing step, problem awareness is created. Once the problem is recognized and acknowledged, it is then possible to undo the current process.[10] During changing, otherwise known as moving, alternative action is sought out. Benefits of change and strategies are explored while efforts to negate barriers are identified. Lastly, during refreezing, the behavior change becomes habit and resists further change.

underutilizing staff.[12] When using Lean in health care, the patient is the center of the initiative and the guiding priority throughout the process. The "5S" model is a helpful road map to enact Lean principles:

- Sort: Eliminate waste
- Set in order: Apply organizational method
- Shine: Clean work area
- Standardize: Standardize work practices
- Sustain: Commit to new standard while constantly seeking improvement[13]

There are a number of benefits to standardizing care across a health system to match innovation. Patient safety is advanced when guidelines to improve clinical care, reduce errors, and actions known to improve outcomes are put into place. Elimination of practices that lack evidence or are no longer considered the standard of care are enacted across the health care system.[14] This transformation can have a cumulative impact on both the restraints and drivers of change and on the process of going from unfreezing to refreezing to reset expectations and adapt to advances.

Identifying the Champions of Change

In addition to gaining awareness of opportunities for quality improvement, fostering a culture of champions is imperative to moving change forward. Unit champions can work with the implementation lead(s) to introduce new practices to the identified areas. These essential team members can assist in the process of moving new innovations or processes through the phases of initiation, development, and implementation.[15] Champions can work to address perceived barriers and are on the front line to assess resistance. Choosing the appropriate champions who can inform change management, be role models and inspire their peers, and tackle challenges as they arise are key in the success of evidence-based practice adoption.

Making Change

Any strategy aimed at increasing the integration of research-based knowledge into practice is called an implementation intervention.[16] These strategies refer to tactics aimed at the adoption of recommendations supported by evidence. The Cochrane Effective Practice and Organization of Care (EPOC) group has developed a taxonomy to classify interventions into 4 categories depending on the change desired: professional, financial, organizational, and regulatory.[17] EPOC investigators stress that interventions designed to identify barriers before implementation are more likely to succeed than those that fail to attend to this important step.[8,18] The following implementation strategies to change provider behavior have been proposed using the EPOC taxonomy:

- Distribution of educational materials
- Educational meetings
- Local consensus regarding clinical issues and management approach
- Outreach visits that can help provide feedback on performance
- Local opinion leaders
- Audit and feedback

As the field of transcatheter therapies continues to grow and challenges programs to meet patient need while achieving outstanding outcomes and providing careful stewardship of resources, improvements in the way we provide care will continue to be at the forefront of keeping pace with change. Partnering with members of the Heart Team, patients, families, and those who provide care at the bedside is imperative to overcoming barriers to the update of evidence-based care.

Opportunities to Transform Transcatheter Aortic Valve Replacement and Promote Early Discharge

Multiple centers have proposed strategies to transition to risk-stratified individualized procedure planning, the adoption of minimalist periprocedure strategies, and a postprocedure recovery protocol. The Emory Hospital team showed that the adoption of a minimalist strategy can be supported by careful case selection and procedure planning.[6] The Multicenter Multimodality, Multidisciplinary but Minimalist TAVR (3M TAVR) study demonstrated the safety and effectiveness of the Vancouver Clinical Pathway in facilitating next-day discharge after transfemoral TAVR by implementing a minimalist periprocedure approach, rapid recovery postprocedure protocol, and criteria-driven discharge in select patients.[19] This growing evidence is creating a sea of change in the acceptance of new benchmarks for optimal procedural approaches, accelerated reconditioning, length of stay, outcomes, and cost savings.

There are significant potential programmatic rewards to transforming TAVR care and promoting shorter length of stay as standard practice and as a quality indicator. Optimizing length of stay in the elderly TAVR population is associated with lower readmission rates, avoiding malnutrition, and reducing in-hospital infection rates.[20] Although change is challenging, the benefits of recalibrating clinical operations and standards of care offer programs a chance to make large steps toward patient safety and health resource stewardship.

Strategies to Transform Transcatheter Aortic Valve Replacement

Time for a Transcatheter Aortic Valve Replacement Clinical Pathway

Clinical pathways are clinical tools for the planning and evaluation of standardized care and treatment goals developed by care teams to support the implementation of evidence-based practices and consensus expert opinions.[21] These tools can be an effective strategy to improve outcomes, shorten length of stay, reduce costs and gaps in care, increase patient satisfaction and participation in their care, and enhance multidisciplinary communication.[22] The development of a TAVR clinical pathway supports technological advances focused on the development of procedural expertise, including anatomical and functional screening to generate the evidence needed to guide how we care for patients undergoing TAVR (Figure 13.2). Importantly, tailored TAVR care can help mitigate the risks of the cascade of in-hospital clinical events in the complex geriatric population, including infections, falls, delirium, and overall deconditioning,[23] and reduce the intensity of health services that have grown to support programs.

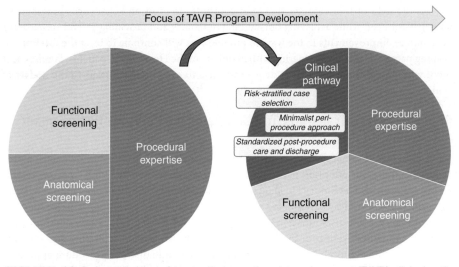

FIGURE 13.2. Incorporation of transcatheter aortic valve replacement (TAVR) clinical pathway in the focus of program development.

The goals of a TAVR clinical pathway are to:

- Reduce variation in care
- Minimize disruption and deconditioning
- Facilitate rapid return to baseline status
- Promote safe and rapid discharge home
- Streamline processes of care and reduce costs

The following are strategies for multidisciplinary teams to consider to meet these goals.

Not All Patients Undergoing Transcatheter Aortic Valve Replacement Are the Same: Risk-Stratified Case Selection

Multimodality assessment and case selection led by a multidisciplinary heart valve team are foundational components of current treatment decision.[24] The careful evaluation of vascular and cardiac anatomy, multimorbidities, disability, cognition, and frailty is essential to determine procedural success.[25] With widening indications and increasing variation of patients' presentation, there is growing heterogeneity of clinical risk profiles. The risks for periprocedure complications of patients undergoing TAVR (eg, vascular access anatomy) differ from their risks for discharge and transition home (eg, availability of social support) and warrant distinct strategies to evaluate and mitigate.[3] To this end, the Heart Team must add to the consideration of *"Can TAVR be done?"* and *"Should TAVR be done?"* the emerging questions of *"How should TAVR be done for this patient?"* and *"Is the patient suitable for early/next-day discharge?"* to identify opportunities to change practice while ensuring patient safety. Select anatomical, comorbid, and functional objective factors outlined in Table 13.1 can help determine patients' suitability for a default strategy of minimalist approach and early/next-day discharge. Figure 13.3 provides an example of documentation of Heart Team risk-stratified case selection and procedure planning.

TABLE 13.1. Clinical Factors to Guide TAVR Risk Stratification for a Strategy of Minimalist Approach and Next-Day Discharge

Periprocedure Factors	
Anatomical considerations	• Adequate aortoiliofemoral CT angiogram • Anticipated successful percutaneous vascular access and closure • Low risk of coronary obstruction • Absence of anticipated device sizing and/or implantation angle issues • Absence of airway barriers to emergency intubation • Appropriate transthoracic echocardiography imaging windows available
Other considerations	• Patient is able to lie flat for duration of procedure • Patient is able to follow periprocedure instructions • If body mass index >35: Heart Team confirmation that patient is suitable for a minimalist approach
Postprocedure and Discharge Factors	
Recovery considerations	• Patient is expected to return to baseline status • Absence of high-risk factors for needing a new permanent pacemaker (eg, preexisting right bundle branch block, prolong first-degree atrioventricular block)
Next-day discharge considerations	• Patient has social support for 48 h after discharge • Patient is able to follow postprocedure instructions • Activities of daily living score 6/6

CT, computed tomography; TAVR, transcatheter aortic valve replacement.

Moving Away from the Periprocedure Surgical Model

Procedure location is associated with established protocols, roles, responsibilities, and constraints. The decision to locate hybrid procedure rooms within the adjacency of the operating rooms or the cardiac catheterization laboratory may trigger a blueprint of services, human resources, and operations as these 2 clinical areas are conventionally managed by different programs. The consideration of space, imaging and monitoring equipment, and safety standards must be augmented by a review of contemporary requirements. Multiple regions and centers are increasing program capacity by using an adapted cardiac catheterization laboratory, streamlining the model of nursing and allied health professionals, and developing an emergency intervention plan to manage the increasingly rare occurrence of conversion to hemodynamic decompensation, heart surgery, or surgical vascular repair.

Transcatheter Aortic Valve Replacement in the Cardiac Catheterization Laboratory

The addition of periprocedural capacity in the cardiac catheterization laboratory requires the consensus agreement of the implanting physicians and/or surgeons, cardiac catheterization laboratory staff, anesthesia, and imaging services, in addition to concerted agreements with perfusion services and the operating room to support emergencies, in ways similar to the provision of services during percutaneous coronary revascularization and other interventional cardiology procedures. Staff education and simulation training are effective tools to foster team engagement, standardize practice, and emphasize patient safety.

THV Team Rounds – Aortic Porgram
Treatment Decision and Procedure Planning

Status: ☐ Elective ☐ In-Patient	Assessments Completed		
☐ Nursing Assessment	☐ Documented Surgical Opinion		
☐ Angiogram	☐ TEE	☐ CT Scan	☐ TTE

Treatment Recommendation

Assessments reviewed:
☐ Nursing Assessment   ☐ Angiogram   ☐ Echo   ☐ CT   ☐ Other:

Decision:

☐ Accepted for TAVI:	☐ TF	☐ TA	☐ Subclavian
☐ Not Accepted for TAVI:	☐ Re-Refer to Surgery		☐ Consider Re-Referral for TAVI
	☐ Palliative		☐ Responsibility for Dictation:

Risk Stratification

Anatomical/Peri-Procedure Risks: Suitable for Cath Lab		Functional/Post-Procedure Risks: Suitable for Next Day Discharge
☐ Adequate femoral artery size and anatomy		☐ Social support for next day discharge
☐ No anticipated vascular percutaneous access or closure issues		☐ No significant mobility issues
☐ No subannular calcification	☐ BMI < 30	☐ ADL 6/6
☐ eGFR > 30 ml/min	☐ Able to follow verbal commands	☐ Discharge plan
☐ Able to lie flat	☐ Other:	☐ Other:

Procedure Planning

Planned TF access size:	CT area: cm²	X-ray angle:

| Valve eligibility: | ☐ Eligible for all standard devices | |
| | ☐ Eligible for specific device(s) only: ☐ S3 ☐ EvolutR ☐ Portico ☐ J-Valve ☐ Other: | |

| TF approach: | ☐ Local anesthesia/conscious sedation | ☐ General anesthesia |
| | ☐ Cath lab | ☐ Hybrid OR |

| Pre-procedure requirements: | ☐ None | ☐ PCI: | ☐ Pre-TAVI *or* ☐ Single stage |
| | | ☐ BAV | ☐ Other: |

Surgical back-up: ☐ Standard consent for TAVI/emergency intervention   ☐ Not suitable for heart surgery:

Screen for research:

Urgency: ☐ Standard   ☐ Urgent (in next month)

Comments:

FIGURE 13.3. Example of documentation of risk-stratified case selection and procedure planning. ADL, activity of daily living; BAV, balloon aortic valvuloplasty; BMI, body mass index; CT, computed tomography; eGFR, estimated glomerular filtration rate; PCI, percutaneous coronary intervention; TA, transapical; TAVI, transcatheter aortic valve implantation; TEE, transesophageal echocardiography; TF, transfemoral; THV, transcatheter heart valve; TTE, transthoracic echocardiography. (Reprinted with permission by Centre for Heart Valve Innovation, St. Paul's Hospital, Vancouver Canada.)

Nursing and Allied Health Model of Staffing

There is no consensus on the optimal model of periprocedure staffing in contemporary TAVR. The expertise of operating nurses prioritizes the asepsis imperatives of valve implantation, assistance with anesthesia, and management of emergency surgery. Similarly, the expertise of the cardiac catheterization team with transcatheter techniques and invasive hemodynamic monitoring and their familiarity with balloon valvuloplasty and emergency percutaneous coronary intervention are well suited to the needs of patients undergoing TAVR. Similar to cardiology and cardiac surgery trainees who are gaining experience beyond the confines of their specialty, periprocedure TAVR nurses and allied health professionals are increasingly training across the specialty of the operating room and the cardiac catheterization laboratory. This transition to a "hybrid model of staffing" requires administrative and clinical leadership, investment in education and training, and the fostering of constructive partnerships between clinical areas that may be unaccustomed to close collaboration. The competencies of TAVR nursing are informed by the knowledge and expertise of operating room and cardiac catheterization laboratory nursing (Figure 13.4). The disciplinary home of the nurse may be less than important than the expert knowledge required to support TAVR periprocedure care.

Emergency Intervention Planning and Simulation Training

As indications broaden, the tolerable threshold for complications will continue to decrease. The treatment of lower-risk patients places increased scrutiny on adhering to the highest standards of care in the event of complications. The consensus agreement of multidisciplinary agreements for roles, responsibilities, and processes in the event of complications is essential to patient safety. Emergency intervention planning should outline the process for emergency vascular repair, emergency percutaneous coronary intervention, management of severe hemodynamic instability, intervention for pericardial tamponade, and conversion to cardiac surgery. Simulation training can help strengthen teamwork and competency, improve patient safety, and help move the team mindset to adapting to the increasingly lower rates of severe complications.

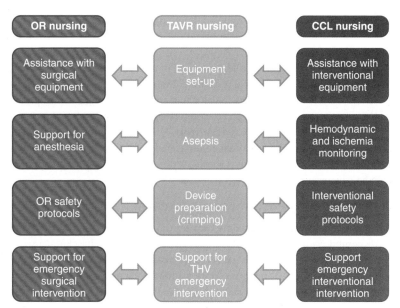

FIGURE 13.4. Opportunities to build model of transcatheter aortic valve replacement (TAVR) nursing. CCL, cardiac catheterization laboratory; OR, operating room.

Less May Be Better: Implementation of Minimalist Strategies

Changes to Anesthesia Strategies

There is increasing clinical interest and evidence supporting the use of local anesthesia, conscious sedation, or other strategies of monitored anesthesia care as a safe and viable option for patients undergoing TAVR. The European Society of Cardiology Transcatheter Valve Treatment Sentinel Registry reported a 20% increase in the adoption of local anesthesia from 37% in 2013 to 57% 1 year later without negative effects on patient outcomes.[26] The development of a minimalist approach in a cardiac catheterization laboratory at Emory University Hospital enabled 98% of patients selected for the pathway modality to avoid general anesthesia and contributed to the decrease of median length of stay from 5 to 3 days and a $9900 cost reduction while maintaining excellent outcomes.[6] In the Vancouver program, the pivotal support of anesthesiologists and their ongoing support for all TAVR procedures contributed to a rapid and successful transition in the mode of anesthesia for over 90% of patients.[5] Studies have reported that the use of conscious sedation is associated with similar or lower rates of in-hospital events and 30-day mortality than general anesthesia, decreased requirements for critical care and shorter hospital length of stay, and cost savings.[27,28] Although there is no consensus on the optimal mode of anesthesia,[29] there are opportunities for the multidisciplinary team to explore the selection of a cohort of patients for whom a minimalist anesthesia strategy may be suitable.

Avoidance of Invasive Monitoring Equipment

The requirements for the insertion of invasive monitoring devices should be reviewed by the multidisciplinary team to ensure that each device is warranted and used optimally. The routine placement of a central venous catheter may be avoided in cases in which peripheral access may be sufficient. The avoidance of neck site insertion pain and the unimpaired mobilization can facilitate patients' rapid reconditioning without compromising patient safety if this strategy is deemed acceptable by the implanting team. Similarly, the rapid removal of the temporary pacemaker is essential to promote rapid mobilization and reduce the risk of deconditioning.

Historically, the use of urinary catheterization for patients undergoing TAVR was an established practice in many centers.[25] The standard of care developed as a carryover practice from cardiac surgery in view of the long procedure times during the early TAVR years and the management of potential complications. TAVR clinicians are becoming increasingly aware that urinary catheterization is associated with in-hospital delirium and mortality, a decreased likelihood of discharge home in the elderly, and mortality.[30,31] The avoidance of urinary catheterization is a small but pivotal component of the multifaceted shift from historical to contemporary TAVR; this change in practice is simple, is feasible if there is multidisciplinary support, and can yield immediate benefits to improve quality of care.[32]

Rapid Reconditioning Postprocedure Protocol

The primary goals of TAVR postprocedure care are to (1) mitigate the risks of TAVR-related and geriatric complications and (2) facilitate patients' rapid return to baseline status and avoid complications related to the "geriatric giants" of in-hospital admission of the elderly.[33] Thus, the rapid reconditioning TAVR postprocedure protocol includes assessments that focus on monitoring the safe return to baseline status, nurse-led interventions to promote early mobilization and activities of daily living, and communicating with patients and families and health to collectively achieve the goal of next day discharge home.

Focus on Rapid Return to Baseline Status

Complications after TAVR have become infrequent.[4,6] Nevertheless, careful monitoring of potential vascular access complications, hemodynamic instability, new conduction delays, and signs of stroke is essential. In parallel and concurrently with this monitoring, rapid reconditioning requires the accelerated removal of invasive devices and the promotion of mobilization, hydration, and nutrition in preparation for discharge. The main components of the accelerated postprocedure protocol with a goal of next-day discharge are outlined in Table 13.2.

The protocol combines established standards of interventional cardiology and minimally invasive surgery recovery protocols. It outlines a period of intense monitoring during the first 4 hours to assess vital signs, cardiac rhythm, vascular hemostasis, neurological status, and signs of pain. The removal of central venous and/or radial arterial catheters in the first 4 hours and the avoidance of postprocedure urinary catheterization are pivotal to meet the goals of care.

Early mobilization and resumption of baseline self-care activity, elimination, hydration, and nutrition optimize patients' use of their physiological reserve in the early recovery period and increase their resilience and ability to recover quickly from the multiple disruptions caused by admission for TAVR.

Early mobilization is the central intervention to expedite rapid reconditioning. Following successful percutaneous closure of the TAVR femoral access site and the removal of the

TABLE 13.2. Vancouver TAVR Postprocedure Clinical Pathway

Interventions/ Component of Care	0-6 h	6-12 h	12-18 h	18-24 h	24-36 h
Goal of Care #1: Return to Baseline Hemodynamic and Neurological Status					
Vital signs	Q15 min × 4 Q1 h × 3	Q4 h			
Neuro vital signs and Cincinnati Stroke Scale assessment	Q15 min × 4 Q30 min × 2 Q1 h × 3	Q4 h			
#1 Goal status	☐ Met ☐ Unmet:	☐ Met ☐ Unmet:	☐ Met ☐ Unmet:	☐ Met ☐ Unmet:	☐ Met ☐ Unmet:
Goal of Care #2: Vascular Access Hemostasis					
Vascular access monitoring	Q15 min × 4 Q1 h × 3	Q4 h			
Diagnostic tests	CBC			CBC	
Pain assessment	Assess and treat access sites and/or back/postural pain discomfort as required. Avoid opioids and sedative hypnotics to minimize risk of delirium. Communicate abnormal findings early				
#2 Goal status	☐ Met ☐ Unmet:	☐ Met ☐ Unmet:	☐ Met ☐ Unmet:	☐ Met ☐ Unmet:	☐ Met ☐ Unmet:

(Continued)

TABLE 13.2. Vancouver TAVR Postprocedure Clinical Pathway (Continued)

Goal of Care #3: Absence of New Conduction Delay					
Cardiac rhythm monitoring	Continuous monitoring. Analyze PR interval and cardiac rhythm with each set of vital signs.				
Diagnostic tests	12-Lead ECG				
Communication	Inform physician of any new intraventricular conduction delay				
#3 Goal status	☐ Met ☐ Unmet:	☐ Met ☐ Unmet:	☐ Met ☐ Unmet:	☐ Met ☐ Unmet:	☐ Met ☐ Unmet:
Goal of Care #4: Removal of Invasive Monitoring Devices					
Peripheral/central vascular access	If Goal of Care #1 achieved, remove central venous and peripheral arterial catheters	Apply saline lock to peripheral intravenous access			Remove saline lock before discharge
#4 Goal status	☐ Met ☐ Unmet:	☐ Met ☐ Unmet:	☐ Met ☐ Unmet:	☐ Met ☐ Unmet:	☐ Met ☐ Unmet:
Goal of Care #5: Early Mobilization and Return to Baseline Elimination, Hydration, and Nutrition					
Mobilization and activity	Head of bed flat × 2 h, then ↑ 30° Bedrest × 4 h then stand at side of bed	Mobilize short distance Up in chair		Facilitate uninterrupted sleep Encourage self-care behavior	Mobilize for 5-10 min every 4-6 h
Elimination— Avoid urinary catheterization	Monitor eGFR × 1 Mobilize to commode and/or standing position when bedrest completed	Mobilize to toilet Anticipate low urine output in the early recovery period until return to baseline hydration status eGFR POD1			
Hydration and nutrition	NPO until hemostasis and confirmed clinical stability IV infusion 50-75 mL/h	If LVEF ≥50%: Encourage fluids If LVEF <50%: Encourage fluids within limit of any pre-procedure fluid restrictions Up in chair for meals Encourage nutritional intake and preferred foods			
#5 Goal status	☐ Met ☐ Unmet:	☐ Met ☐ Unmet:	☐ Met ☐ Unmet:	☐ Met ☐ Unmet:	☐ Met ☐ Unmet:

TABLE 13.2. Vancouver TAVR Postprocedure Clinical Pathway (Continued)

	Goal of Care #6: Readiness for Next Day Discharge			
Patient and family education	Teaching about maintaining vascular access hemostasis	Teaching about importance of return to baseline status (eg, motivation for mobilization) Begin discharge teaching	Complete discharge teaching	
Discharge planning		Confirm discharge plan with patient and family	Assess readiness for discharge	Confirm discharge criteria
#6 Goal status	☐ Met ☐ Unmet:	☐ Met ☐ Unmet:	☐ Met ☐ Unmet:	☐ Met ☐ Unmet:	☐ Met ☐ Unmet:

CBC, complete blood count; ECG, electrocardiogram; eGFR, estimated glomerular filtration rate; IV, intravenous; LVEG, left ventricular ejection fraction; NPO, nothing by mouth; POD, post operative day; Q, every; TAVR, transcatheter aortic valve replacement.

contralateral vascular sheaths, many centers report the adoption of bedrest time spanning 3 to 4 hours. A nurse-led progressive activity protocol is an effective strategy to begin mobilization. The early mobilization protocol is used as a means to resume normal patterns of activities of daily living. This reduces the need for postprocedure urinary catheterization by promoting normal elimination patterns and facilitates the resumption of nutritional and fluid intake to avoid dehydration and excessive muscle wasting in the elderly. Together, these interventions help patients transition to early self-care behavior in preparation for discharge.

Bypassing Critical Care or Early Transfer to the Cardiology Ward

The need for postprocedure critical care continues to evolve. The standardization of care coupled with the predictability of clinical course and outcomes allow for the development of "a program within the program" to avoid critical care for select lower-risk patients or the transition to a default strategy of transfer from the procedure room to the cardiology wards. Proposed criteria for accelerated transfer to the ward are listed in Table 13.3.

Collaboration and education with nurses across the postprocedure units is an essential requisite to modify the historical practice of extensive critical care nursing and support ward nurses in the implementation of the TAVR postprocedure protocol. A valve program clinician–led program of mentorship between the critical care nurses and the cardiology ward can support this transition. Additional support may be obtained from social workers, physical therapists, or other allied health professionals if needed, while nurses play the central role of coordinating care during the 24- to 36-hour admission.

Discharge Home

The transformation of TAVR care is a shift to early and safe discharge home following a successful implantation and with minimal disruptions to patients' health status; this shift is evolving as a benchmark of procedural success, quality of care, and cost-effectiveness. To this end, patients

TABLE 13.3. Criteria for Transitions of Care of Patients Undergoing TAVR

Criteria for Early Transfer to Cardiology Ward After TAVR
<ul><li>Minimum 2-h critical care monitoring</li><li>Hemodynamic stability and SBP < 180 mm Hg</li><li>Hemostasis of TAVR and non-TAVR vascular access sites</li><li>Absence of new conduction delay</li><li>Physician order that patient is suitable for early transfer</li></ul>
Criteria for Next-Day Discharge After TAVR
<ul><li>Multidisciplinary consensus of readiness for discharge and physician's order</li><li>Absence of persistent (>3 h) intraventricular conduction delays</li><li>Absence of laboratory contraindications (ie, clinically important change in hemoglobin and eGFR)</li><li>Return to baseline mobilization</li><li>Confirmed availability of family member for 24 h to remain with patient</li><li>Discharge teaching completed and confirmed follow-up plan</li></ul>

eGFR, estimated glomerular filtration rate; SBP, systolic blood pressure; TAVR, transcatheter aortic valve replacement.

and families are essential partners. Discharge planning must begin at the time of clinic visit to ascertain social support and discharge resources, set common expectations about length of stay, and develop a "Going Home after TAVR" plan. The failure to attend to this early planning can be associated with delayed discharge, miscommunication, and avoidable complications. Patient and family education resources that outline patients' expected journey of care and the target early discharge time and stress the importance of patient and family partnerships to contribute to optimal outcomes is an important component; these resources should be made available as soon as possible to enable careful planning and avoid unexpected challenges.

Close communication between the implanting physician(s) and the postprocedure nursing team is important to ensure that care does not deviate from the established protocol and that support is provided to attend to arising issues (eg, oozing from the vascular access site, new conduction delay, urinary retention) to maintain patients on the TAVR protocol. The agreement that implanting physician(s) remain the most responsible physician(s) until the time of discharge can promote continuity of care, minimize care disruptions, and guide patients' care to early discharge. Criteria for next-day discharge are outlined in Table 13.3.

Conclusions

The transformation of TAVR needs for champions, resources, and collective commitment to reconfiguring the Heart Team to mirror patients' journey of care (Figure 13.5). Valve program clinicians are natural leaders of this change and are well positioned to tackle the challenges inherent to quality improvement. The many moving parts of the recalibration of TAVR (Figure 13.6) is not about "all or nothing." Rather, an iterative approach grounded in quality improvement and the adoption of a "modular approach" to change can help set priorities that are aligned with local contexts and cultures of care and enact small changes over time.

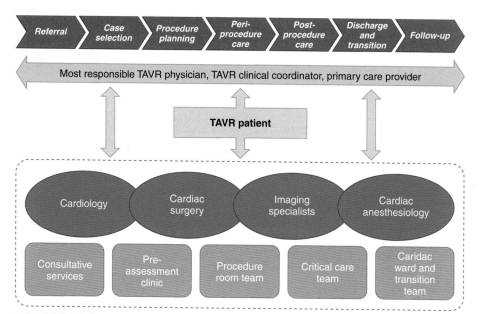

FIGURE 13.5. The big Heart Team of the transformation of transcatheter aortic valve replacement (TAVR).

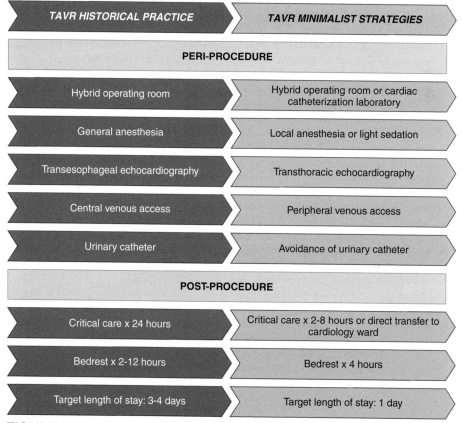

TAVR HISTORICAL PRACTICE	TAVR MINIMALIST STRATEGIES
PERI-PROCEDURE	
Hybrid operating room	Hybrid operating room or cardiac catheterization laboratory
General anesthesia	Local anesthesia or light sedation
Transesophageal echocardiography	Transthoracic echocardiography
Central venous access	Peripheral venous access
Urinary catheter	Avoidance of urinary catheter
POST-PROCEDURE	
Critical care x 24 hours	Critical care x 2-8 hours or direct transfer to cardiology ward
Bedrest x 2-12 hours	Bedrest x 4 hours
Target length of stay: 3-4 days	Target length of stay: 1 day

FIGURE 13.6. Summary of changes associated with the transformation of transcatheter aortic valve replacement (TAVR).

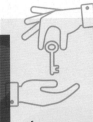

KEY TAKEAWAYS AND BEST PRACTICES

▶ TAVR programs have unique opportunities to revisit historical practices and recalibrate processes of care to match contemporary technology and patient needs.

▶ Change management strategies can help accelerate the uptake of new approaches.

▶ Risk-stratified case selection, minimalist periprocedure approach, rapid reconditioning postprocedure protocol, and criteria-driven discharge are effective interventions to decrease length of stay, improve outcomes, and lead to cost savings.

References

1. Waksman R, Pichard AD. Will TAVR become the default treatment for patients with severe aortic stenosis? *J Am Coll Cardiol.* 2015;66(2):122-124.

2. Webb JG, Lauck S. Transcatheter aortic valve replacement in transition. *JACC Cardiovasc Interv.* 2016;9(11):1159-1160.

3. Lauck SB, Wood DA, Achtem L, et al. Risk stratification and clinical pathways to optimize length of stay after transcatheter aortic valve replacement. *Can J Cardiol.* 2014;30 (12):1583-1587.

4. Thourani VH, Kodali S, Makkar RR, et al. Transcatheter aortic valve replacement versus surgical valve replacement in intermediate-risk patients: a propensity score analysis. *Lancet (London, England).* 2016;387(10034):2218-2225.

5. Lauck SB, Wood DA, Baumbusch J, et al. Vancouver transcatheter aortic valve replacement clinical pathway: minimalist approach, standardized care, and discharge criteria to reduce length of stay. *Circ Cardiovasc Qual Outcomes.* 2016;9(3):312-321.

6. Babaliaros V, Devireddy C, Lerakis S, et al. Comparison of transfemoral transcatheter aortic valve replacement performed in the catheterization laboratory (minimalist approach) versus hybrid operating room (standard approach): outcomes and cost analysis. *JACC Cardiovasc Interv.* 2014;7(8):898-904.

7. Tacia L, Biskupski K, Pheley A, Lehto RH. Identifying barriers to evidence-based practice adoption: a focus group study. *Clin Nurs Stud.* 2015;3(2):90.

8. Baker R, Camosso-Stefinovic J, Gillies C, et al. Tailored interventions to address determinants of practice. *Cochrane Database Syst Rev.* 2015;2015(4):CD005470.

9. Shirey MR. Lewin's theory of planned change as a strategic resource. *J Nurs Adm.* 2013;43(2):69-72.

10. Wojciechowski E, Pearsall T, Murphy P, French E. A case review: integrating Lewin's theory with Lean's system approach for change. *Online J Issues Nurs.* 2016;21(2):4.

11. Lewin K. Frontiers in group dynamics: concept, method and reality in social science; social equilibria and social change. *Hum Relat.* 1947;1(1):5-41.

12. Green P, Arnold SV, Cohen DJ, et al. Relation of frailty to outcomes after transcatheter aortic valve replacement (from the PARTNER trial). *Am J Cardiol.* 2015;116(2):264-269.

13. Kanamori S, Sow S, Castro MC, Matsuno R, Tsuru A, Jimba M. Implementation of 5S management method for lean healthcare at a health center in Senegal: a qualitative study of staff perception. *Glob Health Action.* 2015;8:27256.

14. Golden SH, Hager D, Gould LJ, Mathioudakis N, Pronovost PJ. A gap analysis needs assessment tool to drive a care delivery and research agenda for integration of care and sharing of best practices across a health system. *Jt Comm J Qual Patient Saf.* 2017;43(1):18-28.
15. Shaw EK, Howard J, West DR, et al. The role of the champion in primary care change efforts: from the State Networks of Colorado Ambulatory Practices and Partners (SNOCAP). *J Am Board Fam Med.* 2012;25(5):676-685.
16. Cahill LS, Carey LM, Lannin NA, Turville M, O'Connor D. Implementation interventions to promote the uptake of evidence-based practices in stroke rehabilitation. *Cochrane Database Syst Rev.* 2017.
17. Blanke P, Soon J, Dvir D, et al. Computed tomography assessment for transcatheter aortic valve in valve implantation: the vancouver approach to predict anatomical risk for coronary obstruction and other considerations. *J Cardiovasc Comput Tomogr.* 2016;10(6):491-499.
18. Sepehri A, Beggs T, Hassan A, et al. The impact of frailty on outcomes after cardiac surgery: a systematic review. *J Thorac Cardiovasc Surg.* 2014;148(6):3110-3117.
19. Wood DA LS, Cairns J, Humphries KH, et al. The Vancouver Multidisciplinary, Multimodality, but Minimalist Clinical Pathway Facilitates Safe Next Day Discharge Home at Low, Medium, and High Volume Transfemoral Transcatheter Aortic Valve Replacement Centres: The 3M TAVR Study. *JACC Cardiovascular Interventions.* 2018 [in press].
20. Arbel Y, Zivkovic N, Mehta D, et al. Factors associated with length of stay following trans-catheter aortic valve replacement - a multicenter study. *BMC Cardiovasc Disord.* 2017;17(1):137.
21. Barbieri A, Vanhaecht K, Van Herck P, et al. Effects of clinical pathways in the joint replacement: a meta-analysis. *BMC Med.* 2009;7:32.
22. Aziz EF, Javed F, Pulimi S, et al. Implementing a pathway for the management of acute coronary syndrome leads to improved compliance with guidelines and a decrease in angina symptoms. *J Healthcare Qual.* 2012;34(4):5-14.
23. Merten H, Johannesma PC, Lubberding S, et al. High risk of adverse events in hospitalised hip fracture patients of 65 years and older: results of a retrospective record review study. *BMJ Open.* 2015;5(9):e006663.
24. Holmes DR, Rich JB, Zoghbi WA, Mack MJ. The heart team of cardiovascular care. *J Am Coll Cardiol.* 2013;61(9):903-907.
25. Hawkey MC, Lauck SB, Perpetua EM, et al. Transcatheter aortic valve replacement program development: recommendations for best practice. *Catheter Cardiovasc Interv.* 2014;84(6):859-867.
26. Dall'Ara G, Eltchaninoff H, Moat N, et al. Local and general anaesthesia do not influence outcome of transfemoral aortic valve implantation. *Int J Cardiol.* 2014;177(2):448-454.
27. Hyman MC, Vemulapalli S, Szeto WY, et al. Conscious sedation versus general anesthesia for transcatheter aortic valve replacement: insights from the National Cardiovascular Data Registry Society of Thoracic Surgeons/American College of Cardiology Transcatheter Valve Therapy Registry. *Circulation.* 2017;136(22):2132-2140.
28. Toppen W, Johansen D, Sareh S, et al. Improved costs and outcomes with conscious sedation vs general anesthesia in TAVR patients: time to wake up? *PLoS One.* 2017;12(4):e0173777.
29. Villablanca PA, Mohananey D, Nikolic K, et al. Comparison of local versus general anesthesia in patients undergoing transcatheter aortic valve replacement: a meta-analysis. *Catheter Cardiovasc Interv.* 2017.
30. Wald HL, Ma A, Bratzler DW, Kramer AM. Indwelling urinary catheter use in the postoperative period: analysis of the national surgical infection prevention project data. *Arch Surg.* 2008;143(6):551-557.

31. Eide LS, Ranhoff AH, Fridlund B, et al. Comparison of frequency, risk factors, and time course of postoperative delirium in octogenarians after transcatheter aortic valve implantation versus surgical aortic valve replacement. *Am J Cardiol.* 2015;115(6):802-809.

32. Lauck SB, Kwon JY, Wood DA, et al. Avoidance of urinary catheterization to minimize in-hospital complications after transcatheter aortic valve implantation: an observational study. *Eur J Cardiovasc Nurs.* 2017:1474515117716590.

33. Olenek K, Skowronski T, Schmaltz D. Geriatric nursing assessment. *J gerontological Nurs.* 2003;29(8):5-9.

Index

Note: Page numbers followed by "f" indicate figures, "t" indicate tables and "b" indicate boxes.